DATE			

BAKER & TAYLOR BOOKS

NEUROSCIENCE PERSPECTIVES

Editor: Peter Jenner
Pharmacology Group
Biomedical Sciences Division
King's College London
Manresa Road
London SW3 6LX

Titles in this series:

Antipsychotic Drugs and their Side-Effects

edited by

Thomas R.E. Barnes

Department of Psychiatry,
Charing Cross and Westminster Medical School,
London, UK

ACADEMIC PRESS

Harcourt Brace & Company, Publishers
London San Diego New York
Boston Sydney Tokyo Toronto

ACADEMIC PRESS LIMITED
24/28 Oval Road,
London NW1 7DX

United States Edition published by
ACADEMIC PRESS INC.
San Diego, CA 92101

This book is printed on acid free paper

A catalogue record for this book
is available from the British Library

ISBN 0-12-079035-1

Typeset by GCS, Leighton Buzzard, Beds.
Printed and bound in Great Britain
by Hartnolls Limited, Bodmin, Cornwall

Contents

Contents

Contents

Contents

Contributors

Thomas R.E. Barnes Department of Psychiatry, Charing Cross and Westminster Medical School, St. Dunstan's Road, London W6 8RP,UK

David M. Coward Sandoz Pharma Ltd. Clinical Research & Development, CH-4002 Basle, Switzerland

Stephen H. Curry Drug Metabolism and Pharmacokinetics, Fisons Pharmaceuticals, 755 Jefferson Road, PO Box 1710, Rochester, NY 14603, USA

John M. Davis University of Illinois at Chicago, Illinois State Psychiatric Institute, 1153 North Lavergne Avenue, Chicago, IL 60651, USA

J. Guy Edwards Southampton University Medical School, Royal South Hants Hospital, Southampton SO9 4PE, UK

Jes Gerlach Research Institute of Biological Psychiatry, St. Hans Hospital, Department P, DK-4000 Roskilde, Denmark

Paul Harrison Department of Psychiatry, University of Oxford, Warneford Hospital, Oxford OX3 7JX, UK

Steven R. Hirsch Department of Psychiatry, Charing Cross and Westminster Medical School, St. Dunstan's Road, London W6 8RP, UK

Susan D. Iversen Merck Sharp and Dohme Research Laboratories, Neuroscience Research Centre, Terlings Park, Harlow, Essex CM20 2QR, UK

Philip G. Janicak University of Illinois at Chicago, Illinois State Psychiatric Institute, 1153 North Lavergne Avenue, Chicago, IL 60651, USA

D.A.W. Johnson University Hospital of South Manchester, Manchester M20 8LR, UK

John M. Kane Department of Psychiatry, Long Island Jewish Medical Center, 75–59 263rd Street, Glen Oaks, NY 11004, USA

Brian E. Leonard Department of Pharmacology, University College, Galway, Republic of Ireland

Peter F. Liddle Department of Psychology, Royal Postgraduate Medical School, Hammersmith Hospital, Du Cane Road, London W12 0HS, UK

Robin G. McCreadie Department of Clinical Research, Crichton Royal Hospital, Dumfries DG1 4TG, UK

Nadia M.J. Rupniak Merck Sharp and Dohme Research Laboratories, Neuroscience Research Centre, Terlings Park, Harlow, Essex CM20 2QR, UK

Rajiv P. Sharma University of Illinois at Chicago, Illinois State Psychiatric Institute, 1153 North Lavergne Avenue, Chicago, IL 60651, USA

Abhin Singla University of Illinois at Chicago, Illinois State Psychiatric Institute, 1153 North Lavergne Avenue, Chicago, IL 60651, USA

John L. Waddington Department of Clinical Pharmacology, Royal College of Surgeons in Ireland, 123 St. Stephen's Green, Dublin 2, Republic of Ireland

Series Preface

The neurosciences are one of the most diverse and rapidly changing areas in the biological sphere. The need to understand the workings of the nervous system pervades a vast array of different research areas. By definition research in the neurosciences encompasses anatomy, pathology, biochemistry, physiology, pharmacology, molecular biology, genetics and therapeutics. Ultimately we are striving to determine how the human brain functions under normal circumstances and perhaps more importantly how function changes in organic disease and in altered states of mind. The key to many of these illnesses will unlock one of the major therapeutic challenges remaining in this era.

The difficulty lies in the vastness of the subject matter. However I try, I find it almost impossible to keep abreast of the changes occurring in my immediate sphere of interest, let alone those exciting advances being made in other areas. The array of journals dealing with neurosciences is enormous and the flow of reprints needed to keep me updated is daunting. Inevitably piles of papers accumulate on my desk and in my briefcase. Many lie there unread until sufficient time has passed for their content to be overtaken by yet more of the ever rising tide of publications.

There are various approaches that one can take to deal with this problem. There is the blinkered approach in which you pretend that literature outside your area does not exist. There is the ignore it totally option. Indeed, one colleague of mine has ceased to read the literature in the belief that, if there is a publication of critical importance to his research, someone will tell him about it. I am not that brave and instead I arrived at what I thought was the ideal solution. I started to read critical reviews of areas of current interest. But I soon came unstuck as I realized that, for many subjects of importance to the neurosciences, such authoritative works did not exist.

Instead of simply moaning that the literature was incomplete, I conceived the idea of *Neuroscience Perspectives*. For purely selfish reasons I wanted to have available a series of individual edited monographs dealing in depth with issues of current interest to those working in the neuroscience area. Already a number of volumes have been published which have been well received and the series is thriving with books on a range of topics in preparation or in production. Each volume is designed to bring a multidisciplinary approach to the subject matter by pursuing the topic from the laboratory to the clinic. The editors of the individual volumes are producing balanced critiques of each topic to provide the reader with an up-to-date, clear and comprehensive view of the state of the art.

As with all ventures of this kind, I am simply the individual who initiates a chain of events leading to the production of the series. In reality, it is key individuals at Academic Press who are really responsible for the success of *Neuroscience Perspectives*.

In particular, Dr Carey Chapman and Leona Daw have the unenviable task of recruiting editors and authors and keeping the ship on an even keel.

Finally, I hope that *Neuroscience Perspectives* will continue to be enjoyed by my colleagues in the neurosciences. Already the series is being read, understood and enjoyed by a wide audience and it is fast becoming a reference series in the field.

Peter Jenner

Neuroscience Editorial Advisory Board

Preface

Over the past 40 years, conventional neuroleptic agents have proved to be the most consistently effective compounds for psychotic illness, particularly schizophrenia. However, there has been an increasing awareness of the limitations of such treatment: only partial amelioration of psychotic symptoms in a large proportion of patients and a relative lack of effect on both the negative symptoms and the chronic course of the illness. The therapeutic efficacy has been at the cost of a wide range of adverse effects, including motor side-effects such as parkinsonism, akathisia, dystonia and tardive dyskinesia. Judicious use of antipsychotic drugs may help to avoid side-effects, as evidence from clinical studies suggests that moderate doses are adequate for an antipsychotic effect in the majority of patients, with a greater risk of motor side-effects at higher doses. This notion is supported by studies of *in vivo* neuroreceptor occupancy during antipsychotic treatment. Nevertheless, the recent discovery and characterization of multiple dopamine receptors raises the possibility of selective drugs with an inherently better side-effect potential. Also, clozapine, a drug with an atypical pharmacological profile and a low incidence of motor side-effects, was found to be effective for both positive and negative symptoms in patients who had proved unresponsive to conventional antipsychotics. Although the explanation for the atypicality of clozapine remains uncertain, these findings led to the investigation of antipsychotic potential for compounds which, like clozapine, had both dopamine and 5-HT_2 receptor blocking activity, but not clozapine's relatively high incidence of agranulocytosis. These novel antipsychotic drugs may be classified as combination receptor blockers, and several have shown promise in clinical trials. Other novel antipsychotic agents recently introduced or under investigation may be broadly classified as selective dopamine blockers at the D_2 or D_1 receptor, partial dopamine agonists, and non-dopamine drugs, including 5-HT receptor blockers, sigma receptor antagonists and NMDA receptor agonists.

This volume brings together reviews of the pharmacology of the conventional and atypical neuroleptics, their clinical use and adverse effects. All the authors are acknowledged experts in their field and active researchers. I would like to thank them all for their hard work and the time they committed to their chapters. I am especially indebted to those who, for various reasons, had to complete their contributions in less time than is usual. I am also grateful to Professor Peter Jenner for inviting me to edit this timely book and to Dr Carey Chapman of Academic Press for her regular prompting. I hope that the book will prove useful to neurobiologists and psychopharmacologists as well as psychiatrists and other clinicians who prescribe these drugs.

Thomas Barnes

PART I
BASIC SCIENCE

THE PHARMACOLOGY OF THE PHENOTHIAZINES, BUTYROPHENONES, THIOXANTHINES AND DIPHENYLBUTYLPIPERIDINES

Brian E. Leonard

Department of Pharmacology, University College, Galway, Republic of Ireland

Table of Contents

1.1 Introduction

Schizophrenia is a group of illnesses of unknown origin that occurs in approximately 1% of the adult population in most countries in which surveys have been conducted.

ANTIPSYCHOTIC DRUGS AND THEIR SIDE-EFFECTS
ISBN 0-12-079035-1

The economic and social costs of schizophrenia are considerable, as approximately 40% of all hospitalized psychiatric patients in most industrialized countries suffer from schizophrenia and related disorders. At least 25 major family studies have been published in the last three decades; all have consistently shown a risk for the disease in the relatives of schizophrenics that is substantially greater than that expected in the general population. While most of these studies have been criticized on methodological grounds, it is generally accepted that schizophrenia does have a genetic basis (Kendler, 1987).

Schizophrenia usually begins during adolescence or young adulthood and is characterized by a spectrum of symptoms that typically include disordered thought, social withdrawal, hallucinations (both aural and visual), delusions and bizarre behaviour. So far, there is no known cure and the disease is chronic and generally progressive. Nevertheless, the introduction of the phenothiazine neuroleptic chlorpromazine by Delay and Deniker in France in 1952 initiated the era of pharmacotherapy in psychiatric medicine and has led to the marketing of dozens of clinically diverse antipsychotic drugs that have played a major role in limiting the disintegration of the personality of the schizophrenic patient.

Although the discovery that chlorpromazine and related phenothiazine neuroleptics were effective in the treatment of schizophrenia was serendipitous, investigators soon attempted to define the mechanism of action of this group of drugs that had begun to revolutionize psychiatric treatment. It was hoped that the elucidation of the mechanism of action of such neuroleptics would not only enable more selective and potent drugs to be discovered, but also give some insight into the pathology of schizophrenia.

A major advance came with the discovery by Carlsson & Lindqvist (1963) that chlorpromazine, haloperidol and other related neuroleptics not only antagonized the stimulant action of L-dopa in animals but also enhanced the accumulation of the main metabolites of dopamine and noradrenaline in rat brain. These findings led to the suggestion that the neuroleptics must be blocking the postsynaptic receptors for dopamine, and to some extent noradrenaline, thereby leading to a stimulation of the presynaptic nerve terminal through a feedback mechanism. The seminal paper by Carlsson & Lindqvist (1963) helped to lay the basis of the dopamine hypothesis of schizophrenia and the mode of action of neuroleptic drugs. Later studies in Canada and the USA showed that there was a good correlation between the average clinical dose of neuroleptic administered and the affinity of the drug for postsynaptic dopamine receptors (Seeman *et al.*, 1976; Creese & Hess, 1986; Creese *et al.*, 1976). The dopamine hypothesis of schizophrenia, which has been reviewed by Carlsson (1988) amongst others, has reasonably good support from pharmacological studies but the supporting evidence from post mortem material (Crow *et al.*, 1982), and from studies on schizophrenic patients by means of imaging techniques such as positron emission tomography, are more controversial (Wong *et al.*, 1986; Farde *et al.*, 1987). Whatever the final outcome, however, the dopamine hypothesis has had a major impact on drug development. Even though dopamine may not be the only neurotransmitter involved in the illness, the hypothesis is leading to an investigation of the interconnection between dopamine and other transmitters which may be more directly involved in the pathology of the illness.

1.2   Effects of neuroleptics on dopaminergic and other neurotransmitter systems

Because of the discovery that all neuroleptics in clinical use are dopamine receptor antagonists, and that an abnormality in the dopaminergic system might underlie the pathology of the condition, the action of neuroleptics on the dopaminergic system has been extensively studied over the past two decades. Four major anatomical divisions of the dopaminergic system have been described:

(1) The nigrostriatal system, in which fibres originate from the A9 region of the pars compacta and project rostrally to become widely distributed in the caudate nucleus and the putamen.

(2) The mesolimbic system, where the dopaminergic projections originate in the ventral tegmental area, the A10 region, and then spread to the amygdala, pyriform cortex, lateral septal nuclei and the nucleus accumbens.

(3) The mesocortical system. In this system the dopaminergic fibres also arise from the A10 region (the ventral tegmental area) and project to the frontal cortex and septo-hippocampal regions.

(4) The tubero-infundibular system, which originates in the arcuate nucleus of the hypothalamus and projects to the median eminence.

Following its release, dopamine produces its physiological effects by activating postsynaptic receptors which have been classified as D_1 or D_2 (Kebabian & Calne, 1979). The D_1 receptors are linked to adenylate cyclase which, when activated, produces cyclic adenosine monophosphate (cAMP) as a secondary messenger (Kebabian *et al.*, 1972). The D_2 receptors are not linked to adenylate cyclase and may owe their physiological effects to their ability to inhibit adenylate cyclase activity (Stoof & Kebabian, 1981). The D_2 receptors are probably the most important postsynaptic receptors mediating behavioural and extrapyramidal activity; most effective neuroleptics block the D_2 receptors while bromocriptine activates them.

Agonist stimulation of D_1 receptors results in cAMP synthesis which is followed by phosphorylation of intracellular proteins including dopamine and adenosine monophosphate-regulated phosphoprotein (termed DARPP-32) (Walaas & Greengard, 1984). The receptor-binding affinity of a dopamine agonist is dependent on the degree of association of the receptor and the guanine nucleotide-binding regulatory protein, which is regulated by guanosine triphosphate (GTP) and calcium or magnesium ions (Rodbell, 1980). Thus, the D_1 receptor may exist in a high or low agonist affinity state depending on the balance between GTP (favours low affinity) and the divalent cations (favours high affinity) (Jacobs & Cuatrecasas, 1976). The high-affinity D_1 receptor state was at one time classified as a D_3 receptor (Seeman, 1980).

In the mammalian brain, the D_1 receptors are located postsynaptically in the striatum, nucleus accumbens, olfactory tubercle, substantia nigra, etc., but their precise physiological function in the brain is currently unclear. The partial D_1 receptor agonist SKF 38393 stimulates grooming and stereotypic motor behaviour in rodents, effects that are blocked by the D_1 antagonist SCH 23390; this antagonist also blocks the behaviours initiated by the selective D_2 receptor agonist quinpirole (LY 171555). This suggests that there is a functional interaction between the D_1 and D_2 receptors (Fleminger et al., 1983; Breese & Creese, 1986). The relative selectivities of some agonists for D_1 receptors have been placed in the following order by Creese (1987): SKF 38393 $>$ fenoldopam $>$ $>$ apomorphine $=$ dopamine $=$ ADTN $>$ N-propylnorapomorphine $>$ bromocriptine $>$ pergolide $>$ quinpirole, while the antagonists order is: SCH 23390 $>$ $>$ α-fluphenthixol $=$ fluphenazine $=$ (+)butaclamol $=$ chlorpromazine $>$ haloperidol $>$ pimozide $>$ spiroperidol $>$ domperidone $>$ (-)sulpiride. Agonist stimulation of the D_2 receptors leads to a decrease in cAMP formation, the receptor adenylate cyclase interaction being mediated by a guanine nucleotide-binding regulatory protein (Munemura et al., 1980). The binding affinity of agonist to the D_2 receptor is regulated by GTP and mono- and divalent cations (Sibley et al., 1982); the high agonist affinity state of the D_2 receptor (Sibley et al., 1982) being formerly termed the D_4 receptor. Some D_2 receptors may be coupled to calcium channels or phosphoinositol turnover and not indirectly to adenylate cyclase (Memo et al., 1985).

Unlike the D_1 receptor, the function of the D_2 receptor in the brain is at least partially understood. The anterior lobe mammotrophs of the pituitary control lactation via prolactin release; dopamine acting on the D_2 receptor acts as the prolactin release inhibitory factor (McDonald et al., 1984). In the intermediate lobe, dopamine inhibits release of α-melanocyte-stimulating hormone. In the striatum, D_2 receptors inhibit acetylcholine release, while on the dopaminergic nerve terminals, the D_2 receptors function as autoreceptors and inhibit the release of the amine. D_2 receptors occur on the dopaminergic neurons in the substantia nigra where they inhibit the firing of the neurons. Lastly, in the chemoreceptor trigger zone, stimulation of the D_2 receptors elicits emesis. The selective agonist for D_2 receptors is quinpirole (LY 171555) while the selective antagonist is spiroperidol (spiperone).

Increased motor activity and stereotyped behaviour arise as a result of activation of central D_2 receptors in rodents, while in man psychosis, stereotyped behaviour and thought disorders arise (Raisman et al., 1985; Creese, 1987). Conversely, neuroleptic drugs with selective D_2 antagonist properties (for example, the benzamides such as sulpiride) are antipsychotic and can lead to parkinsonism in man or catalepsy in rodents, although the propensity of the benzamide neuroleptics to cause these effects is much less than the phenothiazine neuroleptics that have mixed D_1 and D_2 receptor antagonist properties. By contrast, the butyrophenone neuroleptics, such as haloperidol, are approximately 100 times more potent as D_2 receptor antagonists than as D_1 antagonists (Seeman, 1980). The results of such studies suggest that the major classes of neuroleptics in therapeutic use owe their activity to their ability to block D_2 and/or D_1 receptors, particularly in the mesocortical and mesolimbic regions of the brain. Side-effects, such as parkinsonism and increased prolactin release would seem to be associated with the antagonistic effects of these drugs on D_2 and/or D_1 receptors in the nigrostriatal and tubero-infundibular systems.

While the precise importance of D_1 and D_2 receptors in the clinical effects of neuroleptics is still uncertain, there is experimental evidence from studies in primates that oral dyskinesia (which may be equivalent to tardive dyskinesia in man) is related to an imbalance in D_1 and D_2 receptor function, the dyskinesia arising from a relative overactivity of D_1 receptors (Peacock *et al.*, 1990). Thus the elucidation of the precise function of these receptor subtypes may be important not only in determining the mode of action of neuroleptics but also in understanding their side-effects.

In the last three years, the use of molecular biological techniques to identify and clarify dopamine receptors has led to the discovery of five dopamine receptor genes. As a consequence of this development the hypothesis linking the mode of action of antipsychotic drugs to the specific antagonism of D_2 receptors has had to be modified. Five types of dopamine receptors have now been cloned; the D_3 receptor has been identified in rat and human brains; and D_4 and D_5 receptors have been identified in the human brain (Schwartz *et al.*, 1993). The functional activity of these dopamine receptor subtypes has also been elucidated. D_1 and D_2 receptors appear to be positively coupled to adenyl cyclase by means of the G_s protein coupling unit, whereas the D_2, D_3 and D_4 receptors are linked to their secondary messenger systems via the G_1 protein subunit. While the precise details of the link between the D_3, D_4 and D_5 receptors and the subsequent intracellular changes are still being determined, it now appears that dopamine may affect target cells through changes in three major secondary messenger systems, namely cyclic AMP, phospholipase A_2 and phospholipase C. Thus the nature of the physiological response to dopamine depends not only on the receptor subtype involved, but also on the nature of the G protein and secondary effector systems located in the nerve cell.

In addition to the identification of five different types of dopamine receptors, the detection of mRNAs for the receptor subtypes in the brain have enabled the distribution of the receptors to be determined. Thus the D_1 and D_2 receptors are the most abundantly expressed in all the main dopaminergic areas of the mammalian brain. In contrast, the D_3 receptors are mainly restricted to those brain regions receiving dopamine inputs from the A_{10} cell region (anterior nucleus accumbens, bed nucleus of the stria terminals and other limbic areas, and in parts of the cerebellum). Thus the localization of the D_3 receptors to the limbic regions of the brain implies that this dopamine receptor subtype is functionally abnormal in schizophrenia, a situation which is modified by the antipsychotic action of neuroleptics. There is also evidence that D_3 receptors can act as autoreceptors in the substantia nigra and ventral tegmental area.

The precise distribution of the D_4 and D_5 receptors is less clear at present, but it would appear that the D_4 receptors are more abundant in limbic areas than in striatal areas, whereas the D_5 receptors are restricted mainly to the lateral mammillary nuclei, anterior pretectal nuclei and some hippocampus layers.

The discovery of the different subtypes of dopamine receptor has enabled the potencies of several 'standard' and atypical neuroleptics to be compared (Schwartz *et al.*, 1993). Haloperidol acts as an antagonist in the different types of dopamine receptors in the order $D_2 > D_3 > D_4 > D_1 > D_5$, whereas the benzamide neuroleptic sulpiride inhibits these receptors in the order $D_2 > D_3 > D_4 > > > D_1 > > D_5$. Clozapine, the atypical neuroleptic which has received extensive interest in recent years because of its proven benefit in the treatment of schizophrenia patients who fail to respond adequately to conventional neuroleptic treatment (Meltzer, 1991), has a unique inhibitory profile on dopamine receptors. Clozapine's order of potency is $D_4 > D_2 > > D_1 > D_5 > > D_3$. Conversely, the 'selective' D_1 dopamine antagonist SCH-23390 is found to be equally potent in inhibiting both D_1 and D_5 receptors, but has no significant inhibitory action on D_2, D_3 and D_4 receptors.

This is a very rapidly advancing field and the precise relevance of selectivity of action of neuroleptics on these subtypes of dopamine receptors is still subject to debate. It is not without interest however, that, apart from clozapine and SCH-23390, most typical and atypical neuroleptics are almost equipotent in inhibiting D_2 and D_3 receptors. Clearly neuroleptics that specifically target the limbic and in particular the mesocortical regions of the brain are less likely to cause extrapyramidal side-effects and therefore have therapeutic benefits over the nonselective neuroleptics that are currently widely used.

1.3 Heterogeneity of dopaminergic neurons in the mesocortical system

While the neurons projecting to the mesocortical regions appear to have somatodendritic and autoreceptors like any other dopaminergic neurons in the mammalian brain, there is evidence that the dopaminergic cells projecting to the prefrontal and cingulate cortices have fewer autoreceptors (Bannon *et al.*, 1983). The absence of such modulatory receptors may contribute to the unique properties of the mesocortical dopaminergic system. Thus, these neurons have a higher firing rate (Chiodo *et al.*, 1984), a higher dopamine turnover rate (Bannon & Roth, 1983) and a diminished responsiveness to dopaminergic agonists and antagonists relative to other dopamine-rich areas of the brain (Bannon & Roth, 1983). These differences between the mesocortical and other dopaminergic areas of the brain may explain the lack of tolerance development following chronic neuroleptic administration (Roth, 1984), and also a resistance to the development of depolarization-induced inactivation following the chronic administration of neuroleptics (Chiodo & Bunney, 1983). This may account for findings that dopaminergic neurons projecting to the prefrontal and cingulate cortices of rodents appear to be resistant to the development of the biochemical tolerance that follows the chronic administration of antipsychotic drugs at clinically relevant doses (Bannon et al., 1982; Scatton, 1977). Furthermore, the dopamine receptors in the pyriform cortex of the rat brain have been shown to be particularly sensitive to both typical and atypical neuroleptics (Van Ree et al., 1989). Such resistance to change is in marked contrast to the nigrostriatal, mesolimbic and mesopyriform dopaminergic neurons, which readily develop tolerance in response to chronic neuroleptic administration in both rodents and primates (Roth et al., 1980). It is also of interest to note that the mesocortical dopaminergic neurons, unlike the other dopaminergic systems in the brain, show particular sensitivity to the effect of tyrosine on dopamine synthesis (Tam & Roth, 1987). It has been hypothesized that the high rate of neuronal firing of these neurons is attributable to a lack of negative feedback on the nerve terminals due to the relative deficiency of autoreceptors (Chiodo et al., 1984). Perhaps the finding that the mesocortical dopaminergic neurons lack effective auto-receptor regulation could account for the relatively unsuccessful use of selective dopamine autoreceptor agonists for the treatment of schizophrenia, although there would appear to be some use for such agents in the treatment of subtypes of the illness (Corsini et al., 1981; Tamminga et al., 1983; Del Zompo et al., 1986). By contrast, it could be anticipated that selective dopamine autoreceptor agonists could be of clinical value in the treatment of such movement disorders as Huntington's disease and tardive dyskinesia, in which non-mesocortical dopaminergic neurons may play a causal role (Häggström et al., 1983).

The potential beneficial effect of the dopamine autoreceptor agonist, trans-dihydrolisuride, in the treatment of parkinsonism has already been shown to be of some benefit to patients (Corsini et al., 1985). It is possible that the novel partial dopamine receptor agonist (+)N-0437 (2-(N-propyl)-N-2-thienylethylamino 5 hydro-xytetralin), which has been shown to be selectively active in a number of behavioural tests, may help to elucidate the usefulness of dopamine agonists in the treatment of schizophrenia (Timmerman et al., 1990).

The relationship between pre- and postsynaptic receptors, and a summary of the suspected sites of action of the different classes of drugs that modulate the functioning of the dopaminergic system in the striatum, are shown in Figure 1.

While there is extensive experimental evidence showing that all clinically effective neuroleptic drugs block dopamine receptors, and a general agreement that blockade of the D_2 receptors in mesocortical regions is particularly important for antipsychotic activity, only with the advent of positron emission tomography (PET) has it been possible to determine the relative importance of these receptor subtypes in

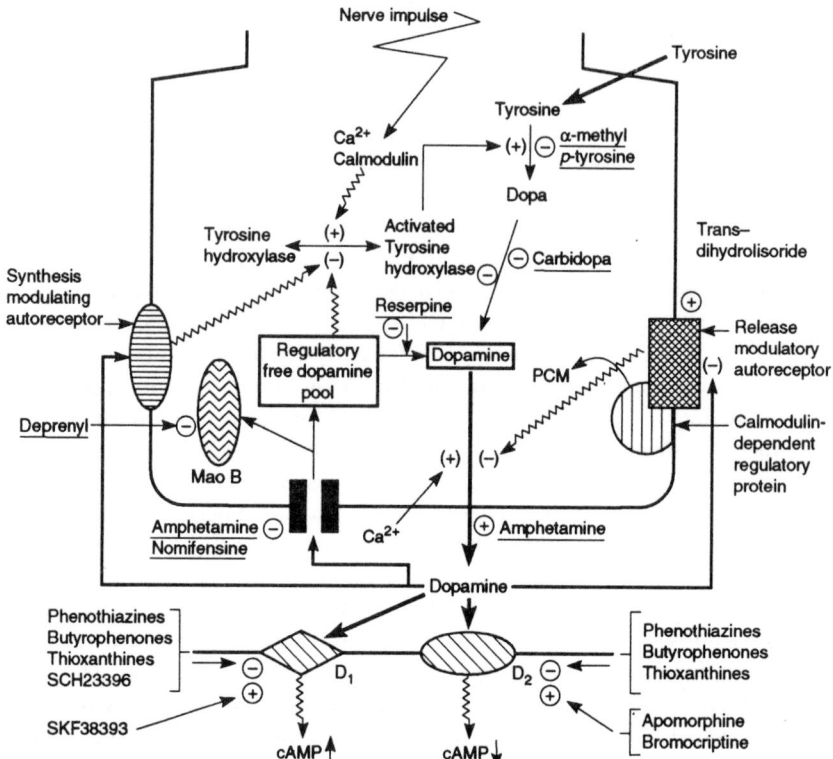

Figure 1 Schematic diagram of the possible sites of action of drugs that modify dopaminergic function in striatal and other non-mesocortical regions of the mammalian brain. PCM, Protein-*o*-methyl transferase which catalyses the transfer of methyl groups from S-adenosyl methionine to calmodulin-dependent regulatory protein. This may regulate C^{2+}-calmodulin-dependent transmitter synthesis and release (Billingsley *et al.*, 1985). For consideration of the role of synthesis and release modulating dopamine autoreceptors in the striatum, see Roth *et al.* (1987). Sites of action of drugs are underlined.

schizophrenia patients on neuroleptic therapy. Thus Farde *et al.* (1989) calculated the occupancy of D_2 receptors in cortical regions of the brains of schizophrenics treated with phenothiazines (chlorpromazine, trifluoperazine or perphenazine), a thioxanthine (flupenthixol), butyrophenones (haloperidol, melperone), a diphenylbutyl-piperazine (pimozide) or the atypical neuroleptics (sulpiride, raclopride or clozapine). The results of this study showed that with this structurally disparate group of drugs, 65–89% of D_2 receptors were occupied. Wiesel *et al.* (1989) have also shown that over 70% of D_2 receptors are occupied in the brains of schizophrenics following effective treatment with melperone. By contrast, no D_1 receptors were occupied by sulpiride or perphenazine, while 42% of the receptors were occupied by clozapine. From such a study it may be speculated that the D_2 receptor antagonist may be essential for the therapeutic effect of neuroleptics!

1.4 Interaction of neuroleptics with non-dopaminergic receptors

Despite the evidence from post-mortem brains studies that the density of D_2 receptors is increased in the nucleus accumbens and striatum of schizophrenic patients (Seeman *et al.*, 1987), it is uncertain whether such changes are a reflection of the underlying pathology of the disease or due to prolonged treatment with neuroleptics (Reynolds *et al.*, 1983). Nevertheless there is some indirect evidence to suggest that dopamine receptors are abnormal in schizophrenia. Abnormal involuntary movements have frequently been reported to occur in schizophrenics who have never been treated with neuroleptic drugs (Meltzer, 1976; Blowers *et al.*, 1982). There is also experimental evidence to suggest an abnormality of serotoninergic function in schizophrenia (reviewed by Stahl & Wets, 1987), and direct evidence from the analysis of post-mortem brains indicates that the density of 5-HT_2 receptors in the frontal cortex is lower in schizophrenics (Mita *et al.*, 1986). The finding that the 5-HT_2 receptor sensitivity is decreased in schizophrenic brains is difficult to interpret in the light of the studies on the effects of the atypical neuroleptic clozapine on the functional activity of D_2 and 5-HT_2 receptors in schizophrenic patients; clozapine would appear to reduce the functional activity of both receptor types as assessed by the action of apomorphine and the selective 5-HT_2 agonist MK212 on plasma prolactin and growth hormone responses (Meltzer, 1989).

In addition to their effects on serotonin receptors, neuroleptics have also been shown to increase the concentration of enkephalins in the striatum (Hong *et al.*, 1978; Chou *et al.*, 1984), while dopamine agonists facilitate the inhibitory effects of the endogenous opioids on dopamine-sensitive cells in the prefrontal cortex (Palmer & Hoffer, 1980). Thus the opioid system may play a role in the action of neuroleptics. Giardino *et al.* (1990) have shown that chronic administration of haloperidol and sulpiride to rats increases the binding of [^{3}H]naloxone to the medial and lateral/basal cortical areas; in the striatum both drugs increased the binding of the opioid antagonist. The precise mechanism whereby the endogenous opioids modulate dopaminergic activity in the cortex and striatum is uncertain, but there is experimental evidence to suggest that opioids inhibit the release of dopamine from dopaminergic terminals arising from the substantia nigra and ventral tegmental area (Heijna *et al.*, 1990) and that these effects involve the action of the opioids on presynaptic kappa receptors. Clearly, this is an area that needs further consideration with respect to the mode of action of antipsychotic drugs.

Kim *et al.* (1983) showed that the concentration of glutamate in the cerebrospinal fluid (CSF) of untreated schizophrenics is lower than normal but returns to control values following effective treatment with neuroleptics. More recently, it has been found that such dissociation anaesthetics as ketamine and phencyclidine have potent psychotomimetic effects that resemble many of the features seen in acute schizophrenia (Snyder, 1980) and that such effects may be attributed to the anaesthetics blocking the ion channel that is controlled by the action of glutamate and related excitatory amino acids on the N-methyl-D-aspartate receptor (Olney et al., 1986). In their seminal review of the interactions between glutaminergic and monoaminergic systems in the basal ganglia, Carlsson & Carlsson (1990) showed that even in the almost complete absence of brain dopamine, a pronounced behavioural activation is produced in mice following suppression of glutaminergic neurotransmission. They suggest that a diminished glutaminergic function may be an important pathophysiological component of schizophrenia. Phencyclidine, and related dissociation anaesthetics that cause psychotomimetic symptoms in man, appears to bind to a class of PCP/sigma receptors, and several atypical neuroleptics (such as rimcazole, BMY 14802 and HR375) appear to owe their antipsychotic activity to their antagonistic action on these receptors; haloperidol also has a high affinity for these receptors (Junien & Leonard, 1989). Thus, despite the value of the dopamine hypothesis of schizophrenia in unifying the pharmacological actions of neuroleptics with the biological features of the illness, the future assessment of their mode of action may also involve a critical role for the excitatory amino acid neurotransmitters.

1.5 Action of neuroleptics on different types of neurotransmitter receptor

In recent years traditional neuroleptics, as exemplified by chlorpromazine, have been structurally modified to produce drugs with greater affinity for dopamine receptors while retaining some of their activity on other receptor systems (for example, on α_1-adrenoceptors, 5-HT$_2$ receptors and histamine H$_1$ receptors). In the non-phenothiazine series, a high degree of specificity for the D$_2$ receptors has been achieved with sulpiride and pimozide, with haloperidol showing antagonistic effects on the 5-HT$_2$ and α_1-adrenoceptors in addition to its selectivity for D$_2$ receptors. The cis (Z) isomers of the thioxanthines are potent neuroleptics that, in addition to their selectivity for D$_2$ receptors also show antagonistic effects on D$_1$, 5-HT$_2$ and α_1-adrenoceptors; cis (Z)-flupenthixol has a greater effect on D$_1$ receptors than cis (Z)-clopenthixol. In the phenothiazines series of neuroleptics, thioridazine has a lower antimuscarinic potency than chlorpromazine but appears to be equally active as an antagonist of 5-HT$_2$ and D$_2$ receptors; like chlorpromazine, however, it is a potent α_1-adrenoceptor antagonist. By contrast, perphenazine, a potent phenothiazine neuroleptic, is only slightly less selective in blocking D$_2$ receptors than haloperidol but, unlike the latter, has a greater antagonistic effect on histamine receptors. The atypical neuroleptics, exemplified by clozapine and fluperlapine, have relatively little effect on either D_1 or D_2 receptors but a major antagonistic action on 5-HT_2 receptors. It should be noted, however, that Murray & Waddington (1990) have shown that clozapine has some preferential, although unselective, action *in vivo* as D_1 receptor antagonist (see also Chapter 2). Both these drugs are fairly potent antihistamines and α_1-adrenoceptor antagonists; fluperlapine also has quite potent antimuscarinic properties. The extreme selectivity for neurotransmitter receptors is shown by SCH 23390, which is highly selective as a D_1 receptor antagonist with only a slight antagonistic effect on 5-HT_2 receptors.

As the clinical effects of the specific D_1 antagonist SCH 23390 are presently unknown, it is difficult to draw any firm conclusion regarding the relative importance of the D_1/D_2 receptor interaction and the antipsychotic effect of these drugs. It is clear that all neuroleptics in current use are D_2 receptor antagonists and while the selective D_2 antagonist sulpiride appears to have low antipsychotic potency, other benzamides (such as remoxipride and raclopride) are at least 100 times more potent than sulpiride in animal behavioural tests, which might indicate their greater antipsychotic potency. For the typical neuroleptics in wide clinical use (for example, chlorpromazine, thioridazine, haloperidol, pimozide, flupenthixol and clopenthixol), there would appear to be a correlation between their D_2 antagonistic potency and their clinical potency; presumably the ability of these drugs to block 5-HT_2 receptors to varying extents is also evidence that the serotoninergic system is involved in their clinical activity in some way.

The actions of neuroleptics on histamine, muscarinic and α_1-adrenergic receptors explain the side-effects of these drugs, such as sedation, anticholinergic and hypotensive effects, which are generally considered to be undesirable side-effects. The spectrum of activity of the commonly used neuroleptics and the atypical neuroleptics on various classes of neurotransmitter receptor has been considered by Tamminga & Gerlach (1987).

1.6 Structure–activity relationships and pharmacokinetic aspects

For a neuroleptic to act on a neurotransmitter receptor, the molecular conformation is of fundamental importance. However, the specific conformation in which the molecule is bound to the receptor *in vivo* is largely unknown since most molecules possess a fairly flexible structure capable of assuming different conformations which are in equilibrium. Schmutz & Picard (1980) have described the detailed structural features of a series of tricyclic neuroleptics that have been shown to have antipsychotic activity. The butyrophenone and diphenylbutylpiperidine series of neuroleptics are tertiary amines; in the former series the 4-fluorobenzyl moiety, and in the latter the bis-(4-fluorophenyl)-methyl moieties, are linked by a straight unbranched propylene chain to the nitrogen of a 4-substituted piperidine or a 4-substituted piperazine ring. The structures of a series of tricyclic neuroleptics (exemplified by the phenothiazine and thioxanthine series) and the butyrophenones and diphenylbutylpiperidines are illustrated in Figures 2 and 3.

Janssen & van Bever (1980) have summarized the essential structure–activity relationships of the major series of neuroleptics as follows:

(1) All butyrophenones and diphenylbutylpiperidines generally have fully extended side-chains.
(2) The clinically more potent compounds possess a planar aromatic ring attached to the 4 position of the piperidine or piperazine ring and capable of orienting itself perpendicularly to the plane of the ring.
(3) Most clinically potent compounds possess an H-bond donating moiety attached to the 4 position of the piperidine or piperazine ring towards the side of the lone pair of the basic nitrogen atom.

The neuroleptics in current clinical use are highly lipophilic and surface active. Thus non-specific binding to non-neuronal constituents is of fundamental importance to their pharmacokinetics. Furthermore, the high surface activity of these compounds is directly related to their local anaesthetic effects, changes in the fragility of the erythrocyte membrane (Seeman, 1966), and their inhibitory effect on neutrophil phagocytosis which may occur in patients following prolonged treatment with high therapeutic doses of these drugs (Elferink, 1979). However, whereas the specific affinity of neuroleptics for neurotransmitter receptors occurs in the nanomolar range, the non-specific effects on membranes generally occur only in millimolar concentrations.

Non-specific binding of drugs to plasma proteins is an important factor that affects the distribution and elimination of a drug as well as the duration and intensity of its pharmacological response (see Koch-Wesel & Sellers, 1976 and Wilkinson & Shand, 1975, for discussion). Thus variations in the plasma concentrations and affinity for plasma protein-binding sites can make a significant contribution to the inter-individual variability of drug plasma levels. The variation in plasma binding of neuroleptics may partly explain the lack of correlation between the total and free plasma concentration and the consequent effects of the drug on the brain. Most neuroleptics are highly bound to plasma proteins. The phenothiazines chlorpro-mazine and promethazine, for example, are more than 90% protein bound (Quinn & Calvert, 1976) and similar high degrees of protein binding have been reported for thioridazine (Nyberg et al., 1978), perphenazine and fluphenazine (Brinkschulte & Breyer-Pfaff, 1979). The main sites for neuroleptic binding to plasma proteins are found on the α_1-acid glycoprotein, lipoproteins and albumin, plasma globulins being of minor importance (Verbeck et al., 1983).

Clinical treatment frequently necessitates the administration of more than one drug.

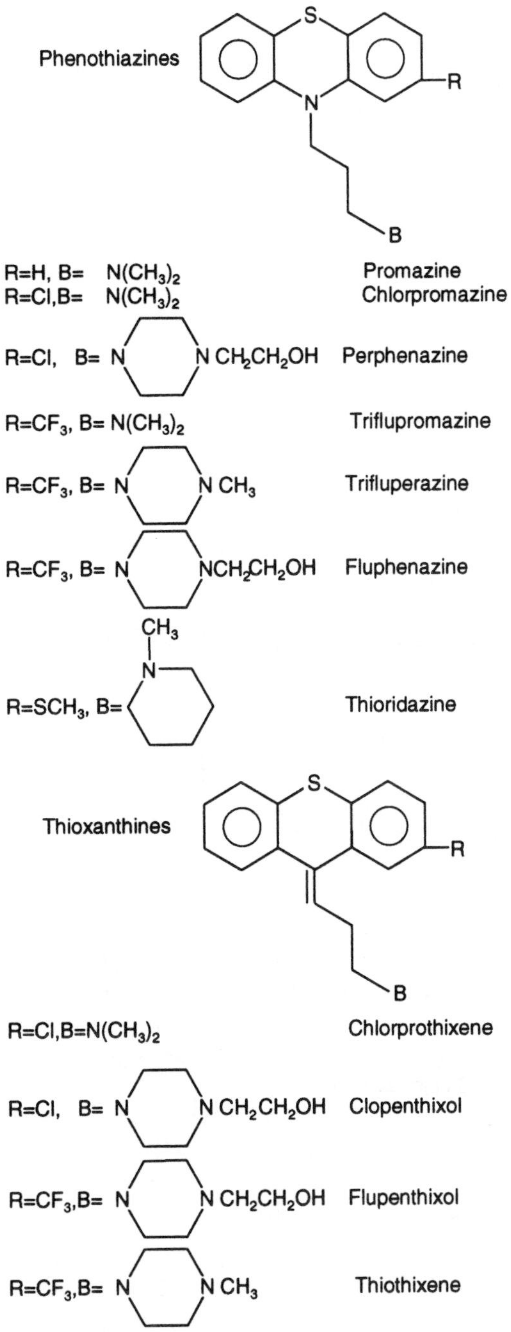

Figure 2 Phenothiazine and thioxanthine series of neuroleptics.

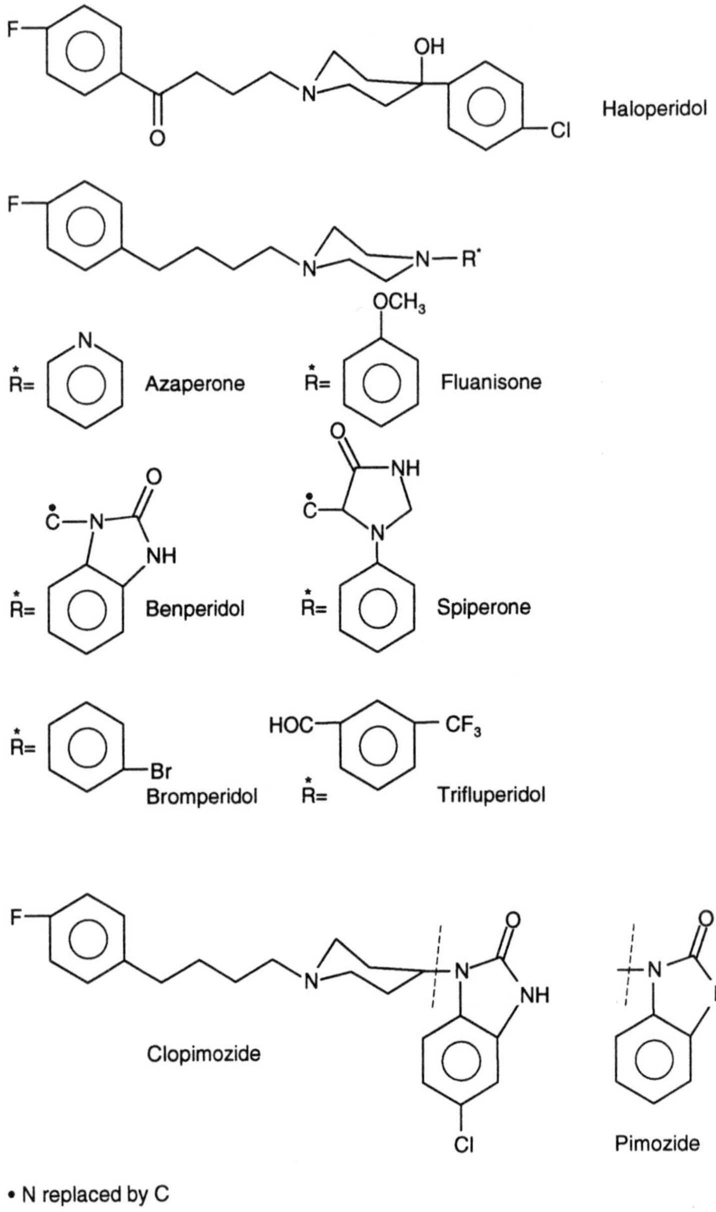

Figure 3 Butyrophenone and diphenylbutylpiperidine series of neuroleptics.

If these drugs compete for similar plasma protein-binding sites, the drug with the lower binding affinity will be displaced, leading to an increase in the free drug concentration.

A practical example of this in the treatment of psychiatric patients occurs with the concurrent administration of tricyclic antidepressants to patients given neuroleptics, both types of drug competing for common binding sites. This interaction may be of clinical importance (Sharples, 1975).

The widespread role of calmodulin in mediating calcium-dependent activities throughout the nervous system raises the possibility that neuroleptics may produce some of their pharmacological effects by altering cellular function via their inhibitory effects on calmodulin. The phenothiazines are amongst the most potent calmodulin antagonists found (Weiss & Levine, 1978). However, it seems improbable that their pharmacological effects can be attributed to their calmodulin inhibitory properties as a large number of lipophilic compounds that have diverse pharmacological properties (for example, α-adrenoceptor antagonists and neuropeptides) also interact with calmodulin (Roufogalis et al., 1983). Norman and co-workers (1979) have shown that the ability of drugs to inhibit calmodulin is closely related to their lipophilicity. However, it is well established that the partition coefficients of the neuroleptics are not correlated with their antipsychotic potency. Thus it would appear that the earlier assumptions that the binding of neuroleptics to calmodulin should be considered to be specific and possibly of relevance to their pharmacological actions cannot be sustained.

1.7 Behavioural and pharmacological properties of the neuroleptics

It is well established that all the major neuroleptics used clinically have a qualitatively similar effect in animals (Janssen et al., 1965). These effects may be summarized as follows:

(1) High doses of neuroleptics cause catalepsy in most animal species, the catalepsy being manifest as an akinetic state of immobility which may persist for several hours depending on the half-life of the drug.
(2) Spontaneous locomotion is inhibited.
(3) Apomorphine-induced locomotor hyperactivity, stereotypy, gnawing and climbing behaviour in rodents are inhibited. In addition, major neuroleptics inhibit vomiting in dogs.
(4) The effect of apomorphine on rodent behaviour is dose-dependent. Thus low doses (<0.1 mg/kg) reduce spontaneous locomotor activity whereas higher doses (>0.15 mg/kg) induce hypermobility and stereotypy. The effects of low doses of apomorphine are attributed to a selective stimulation of dopamine autoreceptors

which is responsible for inhibition of climbing behaviour, gnawing and penile erections. 'Classical' neuroleptics block these behavioural effects and also inhibit the hypermotility and stereotypy induced when apomorphine activates the postsynaptic dopamine receptors.

In an attempt to develop an animal model for the detection of neuroleptic activity based on selective enhancement of central dopaminergic activity, Kenny and co-workers examined the effects of chronic apomorphine administration on the behaviour of the male Wistar rat (Kenny & Leonard, 1980a, b; Kenny et al., 1980). High, chronic doses of apomorphine (0.75 mg/kg twice daily) induced either sniffing–burrowing or a fighting stereotypy. Concurrent chlorpromazine treatment at non-sedative doses increased the latency and reduced the duration of both types of stereotyped behaviours, whereas thioridazine only reduced those parameters in the group showing 'fighting' stereotypy (Kenny & Leonard, 1980b). Such findings suggest that thioridazine is more selective in its action on central dopamine receptors than a 'standard' alkylamine phenothiazine and points to the potential value of such an animal model for the detection of atypical neuroleptics.

(5) Conditional avoidance responses in rodents are inhibited by major neuroleptics.

It is of interest that the atypical neuroleptics exemplified by clozapine, the benzamide neuroleptics (such as sulpiride) and novel neuroleptics like zotepine do not have the same profile as the 'classical' neuroleptics such as the phenothiazines and butyrophenones. For example, whereas clozapine inhibits spontaneous locomotor activity and apomorphine-induced hyperactivity and climbing behaviour, it does not reverse apomorphine- or amphetamine-induced stereotypy or apomorphine-induced vomiting in the dog.

A summary of the pharmacological properties of the phenothiazines, thioxanthines, butyrophenones and diphenylbutylpiperidines is given in Tables 1 and 2.

As has already been discussed, there is considerable experimental evidence to show that D_1 and D_2 and dopamine autoreceptors are functionally closely interrelated, which makes the task of separating the precise behavioural roles of these receptors difficult to evaluate in man, or even in animals. There has been considerable attention paid to the differentiation of the mesolimbic, mesocortical and the nigrostriatal dopaminergic systems in an attempt to unravel the reasons for the reduced extrapyramidal side-effects shown by the atypical neuroleptics when compared to the 'classical' neuroleptics. Unfortunately, the specific functional aspects of the mesocortical and mesolimbic systems, which in man probably subserve the emotional affective state, cannot be easily studied in animals. Furthermore, there is experimental evidence to show that the mesolimbic system can modulate the activity of the nigrostriatal system (Tassin et al., 1978), thereby making it difficult to study the functions of this system in relative isolation. An additional problem that arises when attempting to define the precise action of neuroleptics on the function of the various subclasses of dopamine receptors arises from the observation that the septo-hippocampal formation appears to be involved in the organization and control of

Table 1 Pharmacological properties of some tricyclic neuroleptics in various pharmacological and biochemical tests.

	Catalepsy (μmol/kg)	Amphetamine antagonism (μmol/kg)	Apomorphine antagonism (μmol/kg)	[^{3}H]Haloperidol binding (K_i, nM)	[^{3}H]QNB binding ED$_{50}$ (μM)	Adenylate cyclase inhibition (K_i, nM)
Phenothiazines						
Promazine	143	99.7	>250	72	0.65	2800
Chlorpromazine	6.47	1.69	18.3	10.2	1.00	48
Perphenazine	0.84	0.14	0.67	—	11.0	—
Triflupromazine	4.37	0.75	4.63	2.1	1.0	—
Trifluoperazine	1.25	0.17	1.14	2.1	13.0	19
Fluphenazine	0.33	0.08	0.26	0.88	12.0	4.3
Thioridazine	34.4	22.4	>390	15.0	0.15	130
Thioxanthines						
Chlorprothixene	34.8	4.26	4.11	4.4	—	37
Clopenthixol (*cis*, α)	1.0	1.5	—	3.1	—	16
Flupenthixol (*cis*, α)	0.32	0.17	0.66	0.98	—	1.0
Thiothixene (*cis*, α)	5.86	0.46	0.25	1.5	—	—

ED$_{50}$, median effective dose

Data summarized from Janssen & van Bever (1975), Janssen *et al.* (1965), Burt *et al.* (1976), Iversen *et al.* (1976) and Snyder *et al.* (1974).

Table 2 Pharmacological properties of some butyrophenones and diphenylbutylpiperazines.

	Amphetamine antagonism in rat, ED_{50} (mg/kg)	Catalepsy in rat, ED_{50} (mg/kg)	Apomorphine antagonism in dog, ED_{50} (mg/kg)
Haloperidol	0.038	0.18	0.018
Azaperone	2.50	8.00	0.98
Benperidol	0.012	0.18	0.0005
Droperidol	0.023	0.38	0.0010
Fluanisone	0.20	2.00	0.070
Spiperone	0.020	0.036	0.00024
Trifluperidol	0.025	0.13	0.053
Clopimozide	0.085	0.50	—
Pimozide	0.10	0.18	0.011

Data summarized from Janssen & van Bever (1980).

other neurotransmitter systems that complicate attempts to associate specific behavioural effects of the neuroleptics with specific neurotransmitter changes (Bischoff et al., 1979). While the actions of neuroleptics on muscarinic, α_1-adrenergic and histaminergic receptors in the brain probably underly such adverse effects as dry mouth, postural hypotension and sedation which are particularly prominent with some of the low-potency phenothiazines, it is also established that many of the 'classical' neuroleptics affect GABA, glutamate and neuropeptide activity in the brain which might have some bearing on their behavioural profile. The interactions between the neuroleptics and the $5\text{-}HT_2$ receptors and glutamate receptors have already been mentioned.

In animal studies, tolerance to the pharmacological effects of the neuroleptics has been reported to occur following chronic neuroleptic treatment. It is well established that an increase in the number of postsynaptic dopamine receptors (possibly D_1) occurs following subacute neuroleptic treatment (Burt et al., 1977). Following chronic treatment, the inhibition of apomorphine-induced stereotyped behaviour by neuroleptics is reduced, the tolerance affecting the nigrostriatal system more rapidly than the mesocortical and mesolimbic systems. Such observations help to explain the fact that tolerance to the antipsychotic effects of the neuroleptics is less pronounced than the neurological effects of the drugs (Hippius, 1973). The chronic effects of neuroleptics on the incidence of such neurological features as vacuous chewing movements in rodents has been used to assess the potential of a neuroleptic to cause tardive dyskinesia. This may be exemplified by the study of Gunne & Johansson (1989), who administered haloperidol and melperone to rats for a period of 12 months; only haloperidol produced vacuous chewing movements following chronic treatment, thereby suggesting that the novel neuroleptic melperone has a lower propensity to cause tardive dyskinesia, and possibly parkinsonism, than haloperidol. These findings are supported by the clinical data showing that the incidence of extrapyramidal side-effects is low after melperone but not after the administration of a 'standard' neuroleptic such as thiothixene (Bjerkenstedt, 1989).

1.8 Clinical pharmacology of the neuroleptics

Despite the wide differences in the potency of the neuroleptics in current use, and their differences in specificity regarding their effects on various neurotransmitter systems in the mammalian brain, there is little evidence to suggest that their overall efficacy in treating the symptoms of schizophrenia, mania and other psychoses differ markedly (Hollister *et al.*, 1974).

Thus the 'classical' neuroleptics appear to be effective in attenuating the positive symptoms of schizophrenia (hallucinations and delusions), without affecting appreciably the negative symptoms of the illness (Lecrubier & Douillet, 1982), although a critical analysis of the actions of neuroleptics on the positive and negative symptoms by Goldberg (1985) suggests that both the positive and negative symptoms, which may coexist in the patient simultaneously or at different times during the course of the illness, may be favourably influenced by those drugs. Whether these effects on the positive and negative symptoms may be explained in terms of changes in the functional activity of different subtypes of dopamine and other neurotransmitter receptors (cf. MacKay, 1980) is presently uncertain.

Clearly dopamine receptor adaptation occurs in response to chronic neuroleptic treatment and this may be important in understanding both the efficacy and side-effects of the drugs. Thus, while the blockade of dopamine receptor functions is quite rapid, the time of onset of the clinical response takes several days (Nedopil *et al.*, 1983). Further, while the extrapyramidal side-effects show a sequence of changes beginning with dyskinesia which may give rise to akathisia and parkinsonian-like movements after several weeks or months of treatment, tardive dyskinesia, should it occur, may take months or even years to be manifest. While attempts have been made to explain the complexity of these adverse neurological effects in terms of changes in dopamine receptor sensitivity arising as a consequence of prolonged dopamine receptor blockade in the basal ganglia, knowledge that the commonly used neuroleptics also interact with multiple neurotransmitter systems in that region of the brain make such an explanation implausible. Nevertheless, there is clear evidence from clinical studies on schizophrenic patients being treated with neuroleptics that changes in central dopaminergic function are related to the clinical response to treatment. Thus Pickar *et al.* (1984) have shown that free plasma homovanillic acid concentration, the main metabolite of dopamine, correlates significantly with the antipsychotic effect of the phenothiazines. Undoubtedly the increased use of positron emission tomographic techniques to study neurotransmitter receptors in schizophrenic patients during neuroleptic treatment will provide invaluable evidence regarding the precise sites of action of these drugs in the brain.

The serum concentrations of 'classical' neuroleptics, together with their metabolites, vary considerably in patients even when the dose of drug administered has been standardized. Such inter-individual variation may account for the differences in the therapeutic effects and side-effects. High inter-individual variations in the steady-state plasma levels have been reported for pimozide, fluphenazine, flupenthixol and haloperidol (Nedopil et al., 1983), some of these differences being attributed to differences in absorption and metabolism between patients.

Various factors may account for the variability in response to neuroleptics. These include differences in the diagnostic criteria, concurrent drug administration (such as tricyclic antidepressants) which may affect the absorption and metabolism of the neuroleptics, different times of blood sampling and variations due to the different types of assay method used (Meltzer et al., 1983). In some cases, the failure to obtain consistent relationships between the plasma neuroleptic concentration and the clinical response may be explained by the contribution of active metabolites to the therapeutic effects. Thus chlorpromazine, thioridazine, levomepromazine and loxapine have active metabolites which reach peak plasma concentrations within the same range as those of the parent compounds (Forsman et al., 1977). As these metabolites have often pharmacodynamic and pharmacokinetic activities which differ from those of the parent compound (Forsman et al., 1977), it is essential to determine the plasma concentrations of both the parent compound and its metabolites in order to establish whether or not a relationship exists between the plasma concentration and the therapeutic outcome.

Even in the case of drugs like haloperidol which do not have active metabolites, an unequivocal relationship could not be found between the clinical effects and the plasma concentrations (McCreadie et al., 1984). Awad (1989) has reviewed the influence of demographic features, clinical characteristics, blood concentrations, potency for blocking dopamine receptors and early clinical response as factors determining the outcome of neuroleptic treatment and prediction of clinical response.

1.9   Hormonal changes resulting from neuroleptic treatment

Acute dopamine receptor blockade by neuroleptics has long been known to induce a dose-dependent increase in prolactin as a consequence of the decreased activity of the inhibitory D_2 receptors that govern the release of the hormone from the anterior pituitary (Meltzer et al., 1983). However dose–response studies show that the dose of a neuroleptic required to raise the plasma prolactin concentration is lower than that necessary to have an optimal therapeutic effect (Langer et al., 1980). Furthermore, the time of onset of the rise in prolactin is short (hours), whereas the antipsychotic effect of a neuroleptic takes many days or even weeks. There is also evidence that raised serum prolactin levels persist throughout drug treatment, which suggests that tolerance of the tubero-infundibular dopaminergic system to the action of neuroleptics does not occur (Gruen *et al.*, 1978), but not all investigators agree with such a view. Thus Naber & Mueller-Spahn (1984) reported that male schizophrenics who had been treated with neuroleptics for periods of 3–22 years had prolactin levels that were within the normal range. There is little evidence to suggest that a relationship exists between the symptoms of schizophrenia, or response to drug therapy, and changes in plasma prolactin concentrations.

The secretion of growth hormone is under the control of the dopaminergic, noradrenergic and possibly other neurotransmitter systems and the acute apomorphine growth hormone challenge test has been used to assess the D_2 dopaminergic receptor function in untreated schizophrenics and in patients during neuroleptic treatment. Apomorphine-stimulated growth hormone secretion is reported to be higher in untreated schizophrenics and blunted following both acute and chronic neuroleptic treatment (Mueller-Spahn *et al.*, 1984), returning to control values within a few weeks of drug withdrawal.

Sexual dysfunction in schizophrenic patients on long-term neuroleptic therapy is well established (see Chapter 15) and may result from changes in luteinizing and follicle-stimulating hormone release and the consequent decrease in oestrogen and testosterone release; menstrual cycle disruption is a common feature of neuroleptic treatment which may be complicated by hyperprolactinaemia (Brambilla *et al.*, 1975). However, it seems unlikely that the change in gonadotrophin secretion is a unique feature of schizophrenia, as patients with depression (Siris *et al.*, 1980) and anorexia nervosa (Carter *et al.*, 1982) also show such abnormalities. Furthermore, detailed studies of the luteinizing hormone and follicle-stimulating hormone levels in a group of male and female patients on very long-term neuroleptic therapy could not confirm an abnormality in sex hormone dysfunction due to drug treatment (Naber & Mueller-Spahn, 1984). Thus it must be concluded that unequivocal evidence showing that prolonged neuroleptic treatment results in sexual dysfunction due to a defect in gonadotrophin release awaits confirmation.

1.10 Conclusion

The use of the 'classical' neuroleptics, as exemplified by the phenothiazines, thioxanthines, butyrophenones and diphenylbutylpiperidines, have been a landmark in the pharmacotherapy of schizophrenia and psychotic disorders. The efficacy of such drugs in the alleviation of the symptoms of schizophrenia is universally accepted. However, it is also evident that they have a spectrum of adverse effects that frequently renders their long-term use problematic. Such side-effects as akathisia, parkinsonism, tardive dyskinesia and the all too frequent changes in peripheral autonomic activity are largely predictable from the structure of the molecules and the basic animal pharmacology data. Such adverse effects, and the difficulty encountered in reducing their frequency and severity by concurrent medication, has stimulated the development of such 'atypical' neuroleptics as the benzamides and clozapine which, hopefully, will combine efficacy with a reduction in the side-effects. The pharmacological and clinical properties of some of these compounds will form the basis of other chapters in this monograph.

References

Awad, A.G. (1989) *Can. J. Psychiat.* **34**, 711–720.

Bannon, M.J. & Roth, R.H. (1983) *Pharmacol. Rev.* **35**, 53–68.

Bannon, M.J., Reinhard, J.F., Bunney, E.B. & Roth, R.H. (1982) *Nature* **296**, 444–446.

Bannon, M.J., Wolf, M.E. & Roth, R.H. (1983) *Eur. J. Pharmacol.* **91**, 119–125.

Billingsley, M.L., Kincaid, R.L. & Lovenburg, W. (1985) *Proc. Natl. Acad. Sci., USA* **82**, 5612–5616.

Bischoff, S., Scatton, B. & Korf, J. (1979) *Brain Res.* **165**, 161–165.

Bjerkenstedt, L. (1989) *Acta Psychiat. Scand.* **80** (Suppl. 352), 35–39.

Blowers, A.J., Borison, R.L. & Blowers, C.M. (1982) *Br. J. Psychgiat.* **39**, 363–364.

Brambilla, F., Guerrine, A. & Guastalla, A. (1975) *Psychopharmacologia* **44**, 17–22.

Breese, G.R. & Creese, I. (1986) In *Neurobiology of Central D1 Dopamine Recetors*, New York, Plenum Press.

Brinkschulte, M. & Breyer-Pfaff, U. (1979) *Arch. Pharmacol* **30**, 1–7.

Burt, D.R., Creese, I. & Snyder, S.H. (1976) *Molec. Pharmacol.* **12**, 800–812.

Burt, D.R., Creese, I. & Snyder, S.H. (1977) *Science* **196**, 326–328.

Carlsson, A. (1988) *Neuropsychopharmacology* **1**, 179–186.

Carlsson, A. & Lindqvist, M. (1963) *Acta Pharmacol.* **20**, 140–144.

Carlsson, M. & Carlsson, A. (1990) *Trends Neurosci.* **13**, 272–276.

Carter, D.A., McGarrick, G.M. & Norton, K.R.W. (1982) *Psychoneuroendocrinology* **7**, 201–207.

Chiodo, L.A. & Bunney, B.S. (1983) *Neuropharmacology* **22**, 1087–1093.

Chiodo, L.A., Bannon, M.J., Grace, A.A. *et al.* (1984) *Neuroscience* **12**, 1–16.

Chou, J., Tang, J., Yang, H.Y.T. & Costa, E. (1984) *J. Pharmacol. Exp. Ther.* **229**, 170–174.

Corsini, G.U., Pitzalis, G.F., Bernardi, F. *et al.* (1981) *Neuropharmacology* **20**, 1309–1313.

Corsini, G.U., Bonuccelli, U., Rainer, E. & Del Zomps, M. (1985) *J. Neural Transm.* **64**, 105–111.

Creese, I. (1987) In *Psychopharmacology: The Third Generation of Progress* (ed. Melzer, H.Y.), pp. 257–264, New York, Raven Press.

Creese, I. & Hess, E.J. (1986) *Clin. Neuropharmacol.* **9** (suppl. 4), 14–16.

Creese, I., Burt, D.R. & Snyder, S.H. (1976) *Science* **192**, 481–487.

Crow, T.J., Cross, A.J., Johnstone, E.C. *et al.* (1982) *J. Clin. Psychopharmacol.* **2**, 336–340.

Del Zompo, M., Bocchetta, A., Piccardi, M.P. & Corsini, G.U. (1986) *Prog. Brain Res.* **65**, 41–48.

Elferink, J.G.R. (1979) *Biochem. Pharmacol.* **28**, 965–968.

Farde, L., Wiesel, F.A., Hall, H. *et al.* (1987) *Arch. Gen. Psychiat.* **44**, 671–672.

Farde, L., Wiesel, F.A., Nordstrom, A.-L. & Sedvall, G. (1989) *Psychopharmacology* **99**, S28–S31.

Fleminger, S., van de Waterbeend, H., Rupiniak, N.M. & Reavill, C. (1983) *J. Pharm. Pharmacol.* **35**, 363–368.

Forsman, A., Fosch, G. & Larson, M. (1977) *Curr. Ther. Res.* **21**, 606–661.

Giardino, L., Calza, L., Piazza, P.V. *et al.* (1990) *J. Psychopharmacol.* **4**, 7–12.

Goldberg, S.C. (1985) *Schizophrenia Bull.* **11**, 453–456.

Gruen, P.H., Sachar, E.J. & Langer, G. (1978) *Arch. Gen. Psychiat.* **35**, 108–116.

Gunne, L.M. & Johansson, P. (1989) *Acta Psychiat. Scand.* **80** (Suppl. 352), 48–50.

Häggström, J.-E., Gunne, L.M, Carlsson, A. & Wikström, H. (1983) *J. Neural Transm.* **58**, 135–142.

Heijna, M.H., Padt, M., Hogenboom, F. *et al.* (1990) *Eur. J. Pharmacol.* **181**, 267–278.

Hippius, H. (1973) In *Lexikon der Psychiatrie* (ed. Mueller, C.), Berlin, Springer-Verlag.

Hollister, L.E., Overall, J.E. & Kimbell, I. (1974) *Arch. Gen. Psychiat.* **30**, 94–99.

Hong, S.J., Yang, Y.T., Fratta, W. & Costa, E. (1978) *J. Pharmacol. Exp. Ther.* **205**, 141–147.

Iversen, I.L., Rogawski, M.A. & Miller, R.J. (1976) *Molec. Pharmacol.* **12**, 251–262.

Jacobs, S. & Cuatrecasas, P. (1976) *Biochim. Biophys. Acta* **433**, 482–495.

Janssen, P.A.J. & van Bever, W.F.M. (1975) In *Current Developments in Psychopharmacology* (eds Essman, W.B. & Valzelli, L.), Vol. 2, pp. 167–184, New York, Spectrum

Janssen, P.A.J. & van Bever, W.F.M. (1980) In *Psychotropic Agents. Pt. 1. Antipsychotics and Antidepressants* (eds Hoffmeister, F. & Stille, G.), pp. 27–34, Berlin, Springer-Verlag.

Janssen, P.A.J., Niemegeers, C.J.E. & Schellekens, K.H.L. (1965) *Arznemitt. Forsch.* **15**, 104–117.

Junien, J.-L. & Leonard, B.E. (1989) *Clin. Neuropharmacol.* **12**, 353–374.

Kebabian, J.W. & Calne, D.B. (1979) *Nature* **277**, 93–96.

Kebabian, J.W., Petzold, G.L. & Greengard, P. (1972) *Proc. Natl. Acad. Sci., USA* **79**, 2145–2149.

Kendler, K.S. (1987) In *Psychopharmacology: The Third Generation of Progress* (ed. Melzer, H.Y.), pp. 705–713, New York, Raven Press.

Kenny, M. & Leonard, B.E. (1980a) *Prog. Neuro-Psychopharmacol.* **4**, 161–170.

Kenny, M. & Leonard, B.E. (1980b) *J. Neurosci. Res.* **5**, 291–298.

Kenny, M., Lynch, M. & Leonard, B.E. (1980) *J. Neurosci. Res.* **5**, 35–42.

Kim, J.S. *et al.* (1983) *Eur. Neurol.* **22**, 367.

Koch-Wesel, J. & Sellers, E.M. (1976) *New Engl. J. Med.* **294**, 526–531.

Langer, G., Buehringer, W., Schoenbeck, G. *et al.* (1980) In *Psychoendocrine Dysfunction* (eds Shah, N.S. & Donald, A.H.), pp. 599–612, New York, Plenum Publishing.

Lecrubier, Y. & Douillet, A. (1982) In *Special Aspects of Psychopharmacology*, pp. 375–382.

MacKay, A.V.P. (1980) *Br. J. Psychiat.* **137**, 379–386.

McCreadie, R.G., MacKie, M. & Wiles, D.H. (1984). *Br. J. Psychiat.* **144**, 625–629.

McDonald, W.M., Sibley, D.R., Kilpatrick, B.F. & Caron, M.C. (1984) *Molec. Cell. Endocrinol.* **36**, 201–209.

Meltzer, H.Y. (1976) *Schizophrenia Bull.* **2**, 106–135.

Meltzer, H.Y. (1989) *Psychopharmacology* **99**, S18–S27.

Meltzer, H.Y. (1991) *Schizophrenia Bull.* **17**, 263–287.

Meltzer, H.Y., Kane, J.M. & Kolakowska, T. (1983) In *Neuroleptics: Neurochemical, Behavioural and Clinical Perspectives* (eds Enna, S.J. & Coyle, I.I.), pp. 255–279.

Memo, M., Carboni, E., Trabucchi, M. *et al.* (1985) *Brain Res.* **347**, 253–257.

Mita, T., Hanada, S., Nishino, N. & Juno, T. (1986) *Biol. Psychiat.* **21**, 1407–1414.

Mueller-Spahn, F., Ackenheil, M., Albus, M. *et al.* (1984) *Psychopharmacology* **84**, 436–440.

Munemura, M., Eskay, R.L. & Kebabian, J.W. (1980) *Endocrinology* **106**, 1795–1803.

Murray, A.M. & Waddington, J.L. (1990) *Eur. J. Pharmacol* **186**, 79–86.

Naber, D. & Mueller-Spahn, F. (1984) In *Psychoendocrine Dysfunction* (eds Shah, N.S. & Donald, A.H.), New York, Plenum Publishing.

Nedopil, N., Pflieger, R. & Ruether, E. (1983) *Pharmacopsychiatry* **16**, 201–205.

Norman, J.A., Drummond, A.H. & Moser, P. (1979) *Molec. Pharmacol.* **16**, 1089–1094.

Nyberg, G., Akelson, R. & Martensson, E. (1978) *J. Clin. Pharmacol.* **14**, 341–350.

B.E. Leonard

Olney, J.W., Price, M.T., Fuller, T.A. *et al.* (1986) *Neurosci. Lett.* **68**, 29–35.
Palmer, A.R. & Hoffer, B.J. (1980) *J. Pharmacol. Exp. Ther.* **213**, 205–215.
Peacock, L., Lublin, H. & Gerlach, J. (1990) *Eur. J. Pharmacol.* **186**, 49–59.
Pickar, D., Labarea, R., Linnoila, M. *et al.* (1984) *Science* **225**, 954–956.
Quinn, J. & Calvert, R. (1976) *J. Pharm. Pharmacol.* **28**, 59.
Raisman, R., Cash, R., Ruberg, M. *et al.* (1985) *Eur. J. Pharmacol.* **113**, 476–468.
Reynolds, G.P. Rossor, M.N. & Iversen, L.L. (1983) *J. Neural Transm.* (Suppl. 1) **18**, 273–277.
Rodbell, M. (1980) *Nature* **284**, 17–22.
Roth, R.H. (1984) *Ann. N.Y. Acad. Sci.* **430**, 27–53.
Roth, R.H., Vacapoulos, N.G., Bustos, G. & Redmond, D.E. (1980) *Adv. Biochem. Psychopharmacol.* **24**, 513–520.
Roth, R.H., Wolf, M.E. & Deutch, A.Y. (1987) In *Psychopharmacology: The Third Generation of Progress* (ed. Meltzer, H.Y.), pp. 81–94, New York, Raven Press.
Roufogalis, B.D., Minocherhomjee, A.M. & Al-Jobore, A. (1983) *Can. J. Biochem. Cell. Biol.* **61**, 927–933.
Scatton, B. (1977) *Eur. J. Pharmacol.* **46**, 363–369.
Schmutz, J. & Picard, C.W. (1980) In *Psychotropic Agents, Part 1, Antipsychotics and Antidepressants* (eds Hoffmeister, F. & Stille, G.), pp. 1–26, Berlin, Springer-Verlag.
Schwartz, J.-C. Giros, B., Martres, M.-P. and Sokoloff, P. (1993) In *New Generation of Antipsychotic Drugs: Novel Mechanisms of Action* (eds. Brunello, N. Mendelwitz, J. and Racagni, G.) vol. 4, pp. 1–4. Basel, Karger.
Seeman, P. (1966) *Int. Rev. Neurobiol.* **9**, 145–221.
Seeman, P. (1980) *Pharmacol. Rev.* **32**, 229–313.
Seeman, P., Lee, T., Chou-Wng, M. & Wong, K. (1976) *Nature* **26**, 177–179.
Seeman, P., Bzowcz, N.H., Guan, H.C. *et al.* (1987) *Neuropharmacology* **1**, 5–15.
Sharples, D. (1975) *J. Pharm. Pharmacol.* **27**, 379–382.
Sibley, D.R., de Lean, A. & Creise, I. (1982) *J. Biol. Chem.* **257**, 6351–6361.
Siris, S.G., Siris, D.P., van Kammen, D.P. *et al.* (1980) *Am. J. Psychiat.* **137**, 211–214.
Snyder, S.H. (1980) *Nature* **285**, 355–356.
Snyder, S.H., Greenberg, D. & Yamamura, H.I. (1974) *Arch. Gen. Psychiat.* **31**, 58–61.
Stahl, S.M. & Wets, K. (1987) In *Handbook of Schizophrenia 2. Neurochemical and Neuropharmacology of Schizophrenia* (eds Henn, F.A. & de Lisi, L.E.), pp. 257–296.
Stoof, J.C. & Kebabian, J.W. (1981) *Nature* **294**, 366–368.
Tam, S.-Y. & Roth, R.H. (1987) *Biochem. Pharmac.* **34**, 1595–1598.
Tamminga, C.A. & Gerlach, J. (1987) In *Psychopharmacology: The Third Generation of Progress* (ed. Meltzer, H.Y.), pp. 1129–1140, New York, Raven Press.
Tamminga, C.A., Golts, M.D. & Miller, M.R. (1983) *Acta Pharmac. Suecica* (Suppl. 2), 153–158.
Tassin, J.P., Stinus, L., Simon, M. *et al.* (1978) *Brain Res.* **141**, 267–273.
Timmerman, W., Tepper, P.G., Bohus, B.G.J. & Horn, A.J. (1990) *Eur. J. Pharmacol.* **181**, 253–260.
Van Ree, J.M., Elands, J., Kiraly, I. & Wolterink, G. (1989) *Eur. J. Pharmacol.* **166**, 441–452.
Verbeck, R.K., Cardinal, J.A., Hill, A.G. & Midha, K.K. (1983) *Biochem. Pharmacol.* **32**, 2565–2570.
Walaas, S.I. & Greengard, P. (1984) *J. Neurosci.* **4**, 84–98.
Weiss, B. & Levine, R.M. (1978) *Adv. Cyclic Nucleotide Res.* **9**, 285–303.
Wiesel, F.A., Farde, L. & Halldin, C. (1989) *Acta Psychiat. Scand.* **80** (Suppl. 352), 30–34.
Wilkinson, G.R. & Shand, D.G. (1975) *Clin. Pharmacol. Ther.* **18**, 377–390.
Wong, D.F., Wagner, H.N., Tune, L.E. *et al.* (1986) *Science* **234**, 1558–1563.

CHAPTER 2

THE PHARMACOLOGY OF CLOZAPINE-LIKE, ATYPICAL ANTIPSYCHOTICS

David M. Coward

Sandoz Pharma Ltd. Clinical Research & Development, CH-4002 Basle, Switzerland

Table of Contents

2.1 Introduction

The term 'atypical neuroleptic' originates from the clinical observation that the dibenzazepine clozapine (8-chloro-11-(4-methyl-1-piperazinyl)-5H-dibenzo]*b*,*e*]-[1,4]-diazepine; Table 1) exhibits antipsychotic activity in the absence of debilitating, short- (e.g. dystonia) or long-term (e.g. tardive dyskinesia) extrapyramidal side-effects (EPS) (Gross & Langer, 1966; Angst *et al.*, 1971). In addition to challenging the early dogma that EPS must accompany antipsychotic efficacy (see Stille & Hippius, 1971), these findings with clozapine led to a major search for other pharmacological agents showing similar differentiation. Despite the fact that these efforts have been continuing for more than 20 years, however, it must be acknowledged that they have

ANTIPSYCHOTIC DRUGS AND THEIR SIDE-EFFECTS
ISBN 0-12-079035-1

Table 1 Chemical structure and psychotropic classification of clozapine and several closely related structures.

Substance	X	R₁	R₂	Classification
Clozapine	NH	Cl	–	Atypical neuroleptic
HF-2046	NH	–	Cl	Classical neuroleptic
Fluperlapine	CH₂	F	–	Atypical neuroleptic
Perlapine	CH₂	–	–	Sedative/hypnotic
Clotiapine	S	–	Cl	Classical neuroleptic
Loxapine	O	–	Cl	Classical neuroleptic
Tilozepine	CH₂	Cl	(thiophene)	Atypical neuroleptic
RMI 81 582				Atypical neuroleptic

With the exception of clozapine's 2-chloro-isomer (HF-2046), where only preclinical data exist (see Table 2), the clinical profiles of the various agents are known.

resulted in only marginal success. Thus, while it is possible that several agents showing structural and pharmacological similarities to clozapine would have matched its EPS profile, notably fluperlapine, tilozepine and RMI 81582 (Young & Meltzer, 1980; Fischer-Cornelssen, 1984; Table 1), side-effects terminated their clinical development. To date, in fact, it appears that only the substituted benzamide sulpiride has gained some acceptance as an agent liable to produce only mild EPS (see Chapter 3).

More recently, findings have arisen with clozapine which require that the original definition of an atypical antipsychotic agent be reassessed or at least further qualified.

Thus, there is now irrefutable evidence that this drug exhibits additional clinical attributes which distance it from other known agents, and which are considered by many to represent a further milestone in the pharmacotherapy of this mental illness. The basis for this belief stems from the outcome of a large clinical study designed to address an opinion long held by many psychiatrists, namely, that clozapine's antipsychotic activity is superior to that of other neuroleptics in many schizophrenic subjects.

In order to examine this issue, Kane and collaborators (1988) selected subjects considered to be resistant to a variety of conventional neuroleptics, confirmed their therapy-resistant status by performing a prospective study of their response to haloperidol and then randomly allocated them to a double-blind treatment paradigm comparing clozapine to a combination of chlorpromazine and the antimuscarinic agent benztropine. The outcome of this study was unequivocal, showing that whereas a satisfactory reduction of psychosis occurred in less than 10% of patients receiving chlorpromazine, approximately one-third of those who received clozapine showed marked improvement. Moreover, negative symptoms such as blunted affect and social withdrawal were also improved to a much greater and significant extent in the clozapine treatment group. On this basis, therefore, a modern-day, clinical definition of atypicality would be the demonstration of antipsychotic activity associated with one or more of the following attributes, preferably in controlled trials:

(1) Low acute EPS liability (dystonia, parkinsonism)
(2) No tardive dyskinesia liability
(3) Efficacy in therapy-resistant subjects
(4) Significant improvement of negative symptoms.

The question as to whether a compound's effects or lack of effects on prolactin secretion are a critical factor in its classification as a typical or atypical neuroleptic is open to debate. While clozapine's failure to elevate serum prolactin levels contributed to its early designation as an atypical drug and also led its dopamine D_2 receptor blocking activity to be questioned (see Meltzer, 1990), sulpiride shows reduced EPS-liability in association with a strong elevation of prolactin levels. Thus, drug effects on this parameter alone are insufficient to justify the classification of new compounds as typical or atypical.

These new clinical findings with clozapine have understandably rekindled interest in how this drug acts within the CNS, clarification of this issue offering the possibility of developing similarly effective agents lacking clozapine's major drawback, namely, a propensity to cause a higher incidence of granulocytopenia and potentially fatal agranulocytosis than other antipsychotic drugs (see Krupp & Barnes, 1989). Despite the fact that many findings and hypotheses have been put forward during the last 25 years, however, a widely accepted, cohesive explanation has proved elusive. The following sections compare the pharmacological properties of clozapine to those of classical neuroleptics such as haloperidol and chlorpromazine, as well as to those of several structurally related, neuroleptic and non-neuroleptic agents showing varying degrees of overlap with this agent. These findings are then reviewed in relation to the various hypotheses that have been put forward in an attempt to explain clozapine's atypical properties.

2.2 Neuroleptic-like properties in animal studies

Clozapine belongs to a large series of tricyclic compounds with a 7-membered central ring (Table 1) that can, depending upon the type and degree of substitution, exhibit classical (loxapine) or atypical neuroleptic (clozapine), sedative/hypnotic (perlapine) or even antidepressant properties (e.g. amoxapine, a demethylated form of loxapine). Early pharmacological studies showed clozapine to exert general CNS-depressant activity in rodents, the similarity of this effect to that produced by chlorpromazine identifying it as a likely major tranquillizer. However, even in early studies showing that acutely administered clozapine caused dose-dependent suppression of spontaneous activity in the mouse (Table 2), it was noted that repeated administration led to tolerance development, a phenomenon not observed with classical neuroleptics (Stille et al., 1971). Despite this early difference, other test procedures revealed additional similarities between clozapine and conventional drugs which, by inference, may be relevant to the prediction of antipsychotic activity. The most widely used of these is the conditioned avoidance test, in which clinically effective antipsychotic drugs are reported to block the avoidance response of rats to a light and/or sound signal without impairing their ability to escape a subsequent electrical shock (Courvoisier et al., 1953; Janssen et al., 1966). Stille and co-workers (1971) showed that clozapine clearly inhibits conditioned avoidance responding of the rat, although its potency is very much lower than that of either haloperidol or

Table 2 Clozapine's ability to inhibit locomotor activity (LMA; mouse), conditioned avoidance responding (CAR; rat) and apomorphine-induced gnawing (APO; rat), as well as induce catalepsy (CAT; rat), in comparison with HF–2046, haloperidol and chlorpromazine.

Substance	ED_{50} LMA (mg/kg p.o.)	ED_{50} CAR (mg/kg p.o.)	ED_{50} APO (mg/kg s.c.)	ED_{50} CAT (mg/kg s.c.)
Clozapine	2.5	20.0	$>>20.0$	$>>20.0$
HF-2046	3.0	2.0	1.7	1.8
Haloperidol	0.3	0.4	0.1	0.2
Chlorpromazine	3.5	4.1	2.6	3.8

The data represent mg/kg doses and are derived from earlier studies of Stille and colleagues (Stille et al., 1971; Buerki et al., 1973).

chlorpromazine (Table 2). While this finding was considered to be 'an important factor in [clozapine's] classification as a psychotherapeutic agent' (Stille *et al.*, 1971), it must be tempered by the fact that tolerance develops to the action of clozapine, but not to that of, for example, chlorpromazine (White, 1979). Furthermore, the possibility that clozapine's antimuscarinic activity (Stille *et al.*, 1971; Snyder *et al.*, 1974) could contribute towards a neuroleptic-like profile in this test procedure cannot be ruled out (Fibiger *et al.*, 1975). Interestingly, the structurally and clinically similar agent fluperlapine (Table 1; Fischer-Cornelssen, 1984) is even weaker than clozapine as an inhibitor of conditioned avoidance responding in the rat ($ED_{50} = 39.0$ mg/kg p.o.), and also exhibits tolerance development (White, 1979).

Some of the most striking and consistent effects of clozapine in both animal and human studies relate to its effects on various types of EEG activity. For example, when drug effects on the basic EEG of the rabbit are examined, clozapine leads to a marked increase of spindling activity at a dose of 0.6 mg/kg i.v., which is greater than the effects produced by comparable doses of haloperidol, chlorpromazine, fluphenazine or loxapine (Stille *et al.*, 1971). Similarly, arousal reactions in the rabbit EEG produced by either stimulation of the ascending reticular formation or i.v. administration of the cholinergic agent arecoline are strongly and more readily suppressed by clozapine than by classical neuroleptics, and the drug significantly prolongs the rhythmic after-discharges known as caudate spindles which can be produced by single, short-lasting stimulation of the rat caudate nucleus (Stille *et al.*, 1971; Table 3). This latter action is shared with classical neuroleptics and other atypical, clozapine-like agents such as fluperlapine and tilozepine (Table 3), but not by the sedative/hypnotic agent perlapine (Stille *et al.*, 1971). Finally, studies on the sleep–wake cycle of the rat have shown clozapine to produce changes in dozing, slow wave and paradoxical sleep patterns which are qualitatively similar to those seen with neuroleptic butyro-phenones or phenothiazines. In common with haloperidol, chlorpromazine and the similarly atypical agent fluperlapine, for example, clozapine treatment results in increased dozing and marked reductions of both slow wave and paradoxical sleep (Table 3). Additionally, the dozing pattern resulting from administration of both classes of neuroleptics becomes atypical, visual inspection of the EEG revealing a basic 8–10 Hz rhythm punctuated by almost continuous spindles of 8–12 Hz (Sayers & Kleinlogel, 1974).

2.3 Atypical properties of clozapine

As mentioned earlier, the clinical testing of clozapine in the mid-1960s provided both a surprise and a dilemma. On the one hand, there was evidence for an excellent antipsychotic action in schizophrenic subjects (Gross & Langer, 1966; Angst *et al.*, 1971), on the other, there was a lack of accompanying EPS considered to be a

Table 3 Similarities between the actions of the atypical neuroleptics clozapine and fluperlapine and the classical neuroleptics chlorpromazine and haloperidol in preclinical tests examining the influence of drugs on various EEG parameters.

Substance	$ED_{150\%}$ Arousal	CS prolongation			%Δ Sleep phase duration				
		Dose	Max. ↗ (%)	Time (h)	Dose	I	II	III	IV
Clozapine	0.7	20.0	75	1.5	20.0	+13	+56	-44	-78
Fluperlapine	0.5	10.0	58	1.5	10.0	-58	+119	-47	-98
Haloperidol	>>20.0	5.0	37	6.0	5.0	-53	+154	-44	-96
Chlorpromazine	15.0	20.0	38	4.0	20.0	-43	+112	-71	-100

Studies were performed as described by Stille et al. (1971), using groups of four or more rabbits (arousal) or rats (caudate spindle, CS) and sleep/wake cycle studies. Sleep phases measured were (I) waking, (II) dozing, (III) slow wave sleep and (IV) paradoxical sleep. Drug effects shown represent statistically significant differences from vehicle-treated control groups (two-tailed).

prerequisite for the classification of a drug as a neuroleptic at that time. This latter finding was consistent with the lack of cataleptogenic activity of clozapine noted in animal studies (Table 3), however, and led to the first questioning of this supposed relationship (Stille & Hippius, 1971). Further confirmation of clozapine's atypicality was provided by the demonstration that (1) it causes only a short-lasting increase of serum prolactin levels (Meltzer *et al.*, 1975, 1986), (2) it does not antagonize apomorphine- or amphetamine-induced stereotypies in the rat (Stille *et al.*, 1971; Table 3), and (3) it fails to induce dopaminergic supersensitivity after chronic administration to the rat as judged by both a lack of sensitization to the behavioural effects of apomorphine and a failure to observe the development of tolerance towards its striatal homovanillic acid (HVA)-elevating action (Sayers *et al.*, 1975).

The conclusion that clozapine fails to exhibit marked antidopaminergic activity, stemming from the above studies, was subsequently questioned by feedback from radioligand-binding studies indicating that clozapine's relative affinity for the dopamine D_2 receptor was consistent with its clinical potency as an antipsychotic agent (Creese *et al.*, 1976; Seeman *et al.*, 1976). In addition, its low EPS liability was ascribed to its concomitant antimuscarinic activity (Snyder *et al.*, 1974; Miller & Hiley, 1974), an action known to obviate the induction of dystonias and parkinsonism associated with classical neuroleptic usage. This latter possibility was addressed in a series of studies by Sayers and colleagues (1976), who showed that anticholinergic activity fails to prevent the development of dopaminergic supersensitivity associated with classical neuroleptic treatment, and was further questioned by the emerging evidence that concomitant anticholinergic treatment does not appear to reduce the risk of tardive dyskinesia development (Klawans, 1973; Gerlach, 1977).

2.4 Neurotransmitter interactions of clozapine and related agents

Clozapine and structurally related agents are known to interact with many neurotransmitter systems. However, whereas classical neuroleptic agents show high affinity for the D_2 receptor, clozapine's strongest monoamine interactions on the basis of *in vitro* binding studies are with noradrenergic and serotoninergic receptors (Table 4). In addition, clozapine also shows high affinity for muscarinic and histamine H_1 receptors, properties shared to a large degree with classical neuroleptics of the phenothiazine class (see Eichenberger *et al.*, 1989). The low affinity of clozapine for D_2 receptors is reflected by both a weak ability to elevate dopamine metabolite levels within the rat striatum (Buerki *et al.*, 1973) and its failure to exhibit apomorphine or amphetamine antagonism at clinically relevant doses (Table 3).

Further support for a lack of pronounced D_2 receptor blockade with clozapine stems from chronic administration studies in which clozapine differs from classical

Table 4 Comparison of the affinity of various typical and atypical neuroleptics for D_1 (SCH 23390), D_2 (spiperone), α_1 (prazosin), α_2 (clonidine) and 5-HT$_2$ (ketanserin) binding sites *in vitro*.

Substance	Receptor affinity (IC$_{50}$, nmol/litre)					
	D_1	D_2	(Ratio)	α_1	α_2	5-HT$_2$
Typical						
Chlorpromazine	110	17	(6.5)	2	1329	5
Clotiapine	4	3	(1.3)	21	2440	2
Fluphenazine	17	0.2	(77)	0.5	2379	3
Haloperidol	365	10	(37)	7	7216	70
Loxapine	72	30	(2.4)	3	3435	1
Atypical						
Clozapine	279	834	(0.3)	2	225	8
Fluperlapine	96	1565	(0.06)	8	1791	11
(Perlapine)	198	1803	(0.1)	19	4945	70
RMI 81582	19	160	(0.1)	11	988	4
Tilozepine	94	273	(0.3)	8	197	6

Studies were performed as described elsewhere (Hoyer *et al.*, 1985; Ruedeberg *et al.*, 1986; Urwyler & Coward, 1987), with IC$_{50}$ values representing the means from two or more separate determinations. Findings with the sedative/hypnotic agent perlapine are included for structure–activity purposes.

neuroleptics in not leading to striatal supersensitivity, a factor that has been linked to its failure to produce tardive dyskinesia (Sayers *et al.*, 1975). Although a causative role of D_2 receptor supersensitivity in tardive dyskinesia development is being increasingly challenged (Casey & Keepers, 1988), recent findings suggest that its occurrence might nevertheless serve as a useful marker for such liability. For example, there is compelling evidence that D_2 receptor blockade within the basal ganglia leading to supersensitivity development also results in secondary changes in GABA function, and that these latter changes may be principal factors in relation to the emergence of tardive dyskinsia. GABA is a major neurotransmitter in many of the efferent pathways from dopamine-innervated areas such as the nucleus accumbens and corpus striatum, and also plays a central role within nigrothalamic and nigrotectal pathways (Nauta *et al.*, 1978; Redgrave *et al.*, 1980). In fact, most of the behavioural effects produced by dopamine promotion or blockade within the rat CNS can be mimicked by injecting GABA agonists or antagonists into the zona reticulata of the substantia nigra (Olianas *et al.*, 1978, Scheel-Kruger *et al.*, 1981), and nigral injections of GABA antagonists in the rat have been found to produce oral dyskinesias reminiscent of those seen after classical neuroleptic exposure in man (Arnt & Scheel-Kruger, 1980). The relevance of these findings to clozapine's lack of tardive dyskinesia liability is suggested by studies showing that whereas chronic administration of classical neuroleptics reduces GABA turnover within the rat substantia nigra (Mao *et al.*, 1977), resulting in GABAergic supersensitivity within this region (Gale, 1980; Coward, 1982; Frey *et al.*, 1987), chronic clozapine treatment increases rather than decreases striato-nigral GABA turnover (Marco *et al.*, 1976) and fails to result in increased GABA sensitivity (Coward, 1982). This inhibition of striato-nigral GABAergic function by classical neuroleptics, when continued on a long-term basis, may well underlie the eventual emergence of tardive dyskinesia-like phenomena as indicated by findings in both the rat (Gunne & Häggström, 1983) and monkey (Gunne *et al.*, 1984).

2.5 Mechanisms underlying clozapine's atypicality

While the reason(s) for clozapine's low EPS liability in the face of clear antipsychotic activity has been a central issue within the neuroleptic research area for many years, the situation has now been compounded by the demonstration of statistically superior efficacy of the drug in many schizophrenic subjects (Kane *et al.*, 1988; see earlier). Thus, any attempt to explain clozapine's clinical attributes must nowadays address the additional question of what unique properties of the drug might also explain these newer findings. To date, three hypotheses have been forwarded in an attempt to explain some or all of clozapine's atypical properties:

(1) 5-HT_2 and D_2 receptor blockade
(2) Selective blockade of mesolimbic dopamine function
(3) D_1 and D_2 receptor blockade.

The following sections review the evidence for each of these hypotheses.

2.5.1 5-HT_2 and D_2 receptor blockade

An examination of clozapine's relative affinities for 5-HT_2 and D_2 receptors shows the former to be greater than the latter (Table 4), suggesting that at the clinical doses producing the degree of D_2 blockade predicted by the correlation studies of, for example, Creese and co-workers (1976), most, if not all, central 5-HT_2 receptors must be blocked. The relevance of this situation was first considered in connection with acute EPS liability, preclinical studies having indicated an interaction between dopaminergic and serotoninergic mechanisms in relation to the induction or alleviation of catalepsy – a possible animal correlate of neuroleptic-induced acute EPS in man. The situation here is equivocal, some studies indicating a contributory role for serotonin in catalepsy production (Carter & Pycock, 1977; Balsara *et al.*, 1979), others finding no influence on neuroleptic-induced catalepsy after treatment with either *p*-chlorophenylalanine (Sarnek & Baran, 1975), metergoline

(Vidali & Fregnan, 1979) or the selective 5-HT$_2$ antagonist ketanserin (Arnt et al., 1986). Moreover, clozapine-related, classical neuroleptics such as clotiapine and loxapine, which exhibit high 5-HT$_2$ receptor affinity (Table 4), would be expected to show reduced EPS liability compared to other neuroleptics if this hypothesis were valid.

Other workers (Meltzer et al., 1989) have taken a different approach to the 5-HT$_2$ issue, employing multivariate analysis of in vitro receptor-binding data to distinguish between classical and non-classical neuroleptics. This led them to conclude that a reasonably accurate classification can be made upon the basis of 5-HT$_2$:D$_2$ receptor affinity ratios, with greater 5-HT$_2$ than D$_2$ blocking activity being a requirement for atypicality. While this would appear to solve the issue of, for example, clotiapine's classical nature (no separation between 5-HT$_2$ and D$_2$ blocking activity), this type of approach is also open to criticism. This stems from (1) the inclusion of several non-neuroleptic agents in the classification and analyses, (2) insufficient clinical feedback on several other compounds to warrant their designation as atypical agents, (3) the likelihood that some of the receptor affinities established in vitro do not reflect the compounds' absolute or relative activities at these sites in vivo (Andersen et al., 1986; Leysen et al., 1988) and (4) the incorrect classification of the EPS-inducing agent amoxapine (a demethylated form of the classical neuroleptic loxapine) as an atypical neuroleptic on this basis. Additionally, if downregulation of cortical 5-HT$_2$ receptors after acute, subacute or chronic administration is taken as a reflection of a drug's functional interaction with this receptor in vivo, the same workers have shown that there is sufficient overlap between clozapine and several classical neuroleptics (Matsubara & Meltzer, 1989) to further question the contribution of 5-HT$_2$ blockade to its atypical EPS profile. Clinical studies pertaining to this hypothesis are still rare, although the selective 5-HT$_2$ antagonist ritanserin has been reported to reduce extrapyramidal symptoms in patients receiving classical neuroleptics (Bersani et al., 1986). However, this study was of an open nature, baseline EPS severity was only mild to moderate and the greatest improvements occurred in relation to tremor and akathisia rather than rigidity and akinesia.

While the contribution of clozapine's 5-HT$_2$ receptor blockade to its low EPS liability is open to debate, there may be a better basis for considering this action in relation to its beneficial effects on negative symptoms. Thus, several studies have reported serotonin depletion to result in an improvement of this class of symptoms (Casacchia et al., 1975; De Lisi et al., 1982; Stahl et al., 1985), and there are reports of similar results after treatment with selective 5-HT$_2$ antagonists (Reyntjens et al., 1986). These findings, together with clear indications that clozapine influences central 5-HT function in man (Ackenheil, 1989), support the contention that the drug's 5-HT$_2$ antagonism could have a positive bearing on this aspect of its atypical profile. On the other hand, this would again appear to need to be associated with only weak D$_2$ blockade in order to explain the failure of loxapine and clotiapine to exhibit clozapine-like activity in this regard.

Clinical experience with the newly introduced antipsychotic agent risperidone (Janssen *et al.*, 1988), which shows a similar relative affinity for 5-HT_2 and D_2 receptors as clozapine, is also expected to shed more light on the contribution of serotonin blockade towards atypical neuroleptic activity.

2.5.2   Striatal versus mesolimbic actions of clozapine

Since it is generally reasoned that schizophrenia may reflect a primary or secondary disturbance of limbic as opposed to basal ganglia function (Stevens, 1973), with the opposite being the case in relation to motor disturbances, many studies have addressed the question of whether clozapine's atypical properties might be attributable to a preferential dopamine-blocking action of the drug within the mesolimbic system, particularly the nucleus accumbens (Anden & Stock, 1973; Waldmeier & Maitre, 1976). This region receives a major dopaminergic input from the ventral tegmental area and functions as a critical interface between limbic and motor structures (Nauta *et al.*, 1978; Stevens, 1973; Stevens *et al.*, 1974).

While some early biochemical turnover studies suggested that clozapine might indeed exhibit preferential inhibition of mesolimbic dopamine function (e.g. Anden & Stock, 1973; Zivkovic *et al.*, 1975), many others failed to reach this conclusion (Bartholini *et al.*, 1975; Westerink & Korf, 1975; Wiesel & Sedvall, 1975; Walters & Roth, 1976). In an attempt to overcome one of the major problems in many of these biochemical studies – the question of what altered tissue levels or ratios of HVA and DOPAC really reflect – several groups adopted an electrophysiological approach in order to address the 'mesolimbic issue'. On this basis, it would appear that clozapine does indeed produce proportionally greater suppression of mesolimbic as opposed to striatal dopamine function, at least after chronic administration. For example, while clozapine increases the firing rate of both nigrostriatal and mesolimbic dopamine neurons after acute administration, only the mesolimbic population exhibits chronic depolarization blockade after repeated exposure to the drug (Chiodo & Bunney, 1983; White & Wang, 1983). Comparable treatment with the classical neuroleptic haloperidol, in contrast, results in depolarization blockade of both populations of neurons. These findings are consistent with the biochemical finding that tolerance fails to develop to clozapine's elevation of striatal HVA levels in the rat (Bowers & Rozitis, 1976) and, to some extent, with voltametric studies examining the effects of chronic neuroleptic administration on striatal and accumbal DOPAC release (Maidment & Marsden, 1987). The clinical relevance of the above findings is suggested by the fact that the onset of depolarization blockade within the two systems correlates with the clinical emergence of both antipsychotic efficacy and EPS of the parkinsonian type.

Despite the reproducibility of the above-mentioned electrophysiological findings and their extrapolation to the clinical setting, such a preferential mesolimbic action of clozapine could only relate to its acute EPS liability. Thus, classical neuroleptics share clozapine's ability to reduce mesolimbic dopamine function in this manner, without matching its antipsychotic activity, and it is also known that a clozapine-like, differential effect on mesolimbic dopamine function, regardless of whether it is measured biochemically (Bartholini, 1976), behaviourally (Costall & Naylor, 1976) or electrophysiologically (Chiodo & Bunney, 1985), is shown by the classical neuroleptic agent thioridazine. Alternatively, a clozapine-like profile can be produced by combining haloperidol with an anticholinergic agent (Chiodo & Bunney, 1985). This finding refutes a possible link between the occurrence of depolarization blockade within the nigrostriatal system and the induction of tardive dyskinesia since it is known that combining classical neuroleptics with anticholinergic agents does not lower the risk for tardive dyskinesia development (Tarsy & Baldessarini, 1977).

What remains to be addressed in relation to a greater or more selective influence of clozapine on limbic or mesolimbic system function is the possibility that this agent might interact with dopamine receptor subtypes preferentially localized within these regions. Recent studies have shown that subtypes of both D_1 and D_2 receptors exist within the rat CNS, for example, and some of these show preferential localization within certain limbic and mesolimbic structures (Monsma et al., 1990; Undie & Friedman, 1990; Sokoloff et al., 1990). Whether or not clozapine will prove to be distinguishable from classical neuroleptics on this kind of basis remains to be seen.

2.5.3 D_1 and D_2 receptor blockade

Studies with the selective D_1 receptor antagonist SCH 23390 have shown it to influence many of the behavioural phenomena arising from D_2 receptor stimulation (see Waddington, 1986), raising questions about the clinical relevance of neuroleptic interactions with D_1 receptors. In fact, clozapine has long been recognized as a moderate inhibitor of D_1-linked adenylate cyclase activity, an effect consistent with its more recently demonstrated ability to displace tritiated SCH 23390 from D_1 binding sites (Table 4). However, the possibility of D_1 blockade contributing to clozapine's unique clinical profile has formerly been dismissed since many classical neuroleptics are stronger D_1 antagonists than clozapine in vitro (see Table 4), but are indistinguishable from other classical neuroleptics in the clinic. Several factors have now led to a reappraisal of this interpretation. First, an examination of the relative D_1 and D_2 receptor affinities of several structurally related, clinically tested compounds (Tables 1 and 4) shows that those agents considered to show similar preclinical and, at least as far as EPS liability goes, clinical characteristics to clozapine (such as fluperlapine, tilozepine and RMI 81582), show 3–16 times greater affinity for D_1 compared to D_2 receptors. This picture is reversed with classical neuroleptics such as butyrophenones, phenothiazines and thioxanthenes (Table 4), with the substituted benzamides showing no relevant D_1 affinity (see Coward et al., 1989). Secondly, there is strong evidence that clozapine and fluperlapine may be more potent D_1 antagonists in *vivo* than predicted from *in vitro* data (Andersen *et al.*, 1986; Chipkin & Latranyi, 1987; Saller *et al.*, 1989), whereas the reverse may be true for the strong *in vitro* D_1 blockers fluphenazine and *cis*-flupenthixol (Andersen, 1988; Hess *et al.*, 1988; Saller *et al.*, 1989).

Confirmation that the above-mentioned binding data with clozapine and the conclusions drawn from them are of functional relevance has been provided by studies employing the technique of trans-striatal dialysis in the conscious rat and, more recently, by behavioural studies designed to examine this particular issue (Murray & Waddington, 1990). Using the first approach, Imperato and co-workers were able to test and confirm the working hypothesis stemming from the binding studies, namely, that low doses of clozapine block striatal D_1 receptors whereas higher doses are required to block D_2 receptors. Evidence supporting this interpretation stems from the finding that s.c. administration of clozapine at doses of 1.0–5.0 mg/kg results in an increased recovery of dopamine and its metabolites HVA and DOPAC from the striatum, and that these effects are reduced or prevented by prior administration of selective D_1 agonists (Imperato & Angelucci, 1988; Coward *et al.*, 1989). Conversely, the same series of studies show that, after treatment with such low doses of clozapine, direct intrastriatal administration of the selective D_2 agonist LY 171555 results in a strong reduction of dopamine recovery via the dialysate, indicating that release-modulating D_2 receptors are not blocked. This picture changes when higher doses of clozapine are examined, and in a manner consistent with the notion that the onset of D_2 receptor blockade should become demonstrable. Thus, at 20.0 mg/kg s.c., clozapine elevates striatal HVA and DOPAC levels to a much greater extent than that of dopamine itself – a profile seen with conventional D_2 antagonists (Imperato & DiChiara, 1985), and also blocks the normal ability of intrastriatally applied LY 171555 to suppress dopamine release (Imperato & Angelucci, 1988; Coward *et al.*, 1989). The question of whether these findings relate to the clinical situation has also been addressed and the feedback, to date, is generally positive. Thus, while the database is still relatively small, positron emission tomography (PET) scan studies employing radiolabelled SCH 23390 and raclopride to examine apparent D_1 and D_2 receptor occupancy rates in schizophrenics responding to therapeutic doses of various neuroleptics show D_2 occupancy rates under clozapine to lie between 40 and 65%, and D_1 occupancy to be 35–40% (Farde *et al.*, 1988, 1989). The first figure is lower than that attained with a wide range of classical neuroleptics (70–85% D_2 occupancy), the second higher (no or very little D_1 occupancy with classical agents).

The hypothesis that clozapine's interaction with D_1 receptors might be a critical factor in relation to some aspects of its clinical profile is supported by a number of additional observations, these relating to both its superior antipsychotic activity and its neurological side-effect profile. Regarding efficacy, it is known that D_1 receptors are more numerous than D_2 receptors (Boyson *et al.*, 1986), particularly within the human cortex (De Keyser *et al.*, 1988), and may show increased coupling to adenylate cyclase in schizophrenic subjects (Memo *et al.*, 1983). Moreover, animal studies suggest that D_1-

linked mechanisms play a critical role in the expression of both reinforcing and aversive motivational processes (Shippenberg & Herz, 1988), a disturbance of such function possibly relating to the emergence of negative symptoms such as anergia and anhedonia. It is therefore possible that clozapine's D_1 blocking activity might contribute to both its usefulness in neuroleptic-resistant subjects and some of its beneficial effects on negative symptoms. Concerning EPS liability, there is now strong evidence that D_1 receptors are closely associated with striato-nigral pathways involved in both basal ganglia output and, after chronic treatment, the emergence of tardive dyskinesia-like phenomena (see above). Recent studies reporting the cloning and *in situ* hybridization of the D_1 receptor show, for example, that whereas little or no messenger RNA for this receptor occurs within the substantia nigra, large amounts are to be found within nigra-projecting, medium spiny neurons of the caudate nucleus (Dearry *et al.*, 1990; Sunahara *et al.*, 1990). These findings, together with those of earlier lesion studies (Spano *et al.*, 1977), indicate that the known high density of nigral D_1 receptors is attributable to their localization on the terminals of striatal efferents, many of which are GABAergic. By inference, a neuroleptic exhibiting functional blockade of the D_1 receptor might reasonably be expected to show different EPS liability to agents acting predominantly or exclusively via D_2 receptor blockade, particularly in the long term. This notion receives further support from the observation that whereas some striatal D_2 receptors are linked in an inhibitory fashion to D_1 receptor systems, this type of interaction does not appear to occur within the mesolimbic system (Stoof & Verheijden, 1986). This could contribute to clozapine's differential effects within the nigrostriatal and mesolimbic systems, since it would explain why combining classical neuroleptics with anticholinergic agents, which reverse drug-induced depolarization blockade of A9 neurons, still fails to mimic the long-term neurological profile of clozapine. On the other hand, the failure of clinically relevant doses of clozapine to induce dopaminergic supersensitivity in animal studies or tardive dyskinesia in man could be related to the degree of D_2 receptor occupancy never reaching a critical level (possibly $> 70\%$) beyond which compensatory mechanisms and, eventually, decompensation come in to play.

Despite the preclinical and clinical support available for the 'D_1 bias' hypothesis, it cannot be accepted until two major questions have been answered. First, why are structurally related agents such as loxapine and clotiapine so clearly classical, and, secondly, why does perlapine not exhibit atypical antipsychotic properties? The answer to the first question, notwithstanding the known possibility of differences in binding affinities between the *in vitro* and the *in vivo* situation, might lie in the strong D_2 blocking activity of these agents. This, as in the case of the 5-HT$_2$ issue, could conceivably mask the expression of D_1-related benefits. The second question is more difficult to answer, especially since the addition of a single fluorine atom to the 8-position of this structure gives rise to the atypical neuroleptic fluperlapine (Table 1) without, however, changing the *in vitro* binding profile (Table 4). On the other hand, perlapine fails to resemble fluperlapine or clozapine in some of the EEG-based tests mentioned earlier, particularly with regard to caudate spindle prolongation (Stille *et al.*, 1971). Taken together, these observations question the expression of perlapine's dopamine antagonistic activity *in vivo*, or indicate that this drug does not share a still undiscovered property of fluperlapine and clozapine.

2.6 Conclusions

Although clozapine remains unique more than 25 years after its clinical introduction, there are reasons to believe that many of its clinical attributes would have been shared by fluperlapine and, possibly, tilozepine and RMI 81582. Animal studies show that these agents are typified by a virtual lack of apomorphine-antagonistic and cataleptogenic activity, produce only weak and transient inhibition of conditioned avoidance behaviour, but show clear overlap with classical neuroleptics with regard to various EEG effects. Mechanistically, clozapine-like agents differ from classical neuroleptics in showing proportionally greater 5-HT_2 and D_1 receptor blockade than D_2 blockade, these factors possibly contributing towards reduced EPS liability, better negative symptom responsiveness and, in the latter case, antipsychotic efficacy in many therapy-resistant subjects. Despite the steadily increasing support for these conclusions, however, it is premature to conclude that this is the end of the 'clozapine story'. Thus, subtypes of both D_1 and D_2 receptors have now been identified (Monsma *et al.*, 1990; Undie & Friedman, 1990), and an explanation has to be found for the many reputable reports of clozapine's successful, often low dose usage in the treatment of both L-dopa-induced psychosis and tardive dyskinesia (Casey, 1989). It is to be hoped that the rekindled research interest in clozapine will help to answer these open questions and pave the way for still further progress in the drug treatment of schizophrenia.

2.7 Summary

The dibenzazepine clozapine represents the most significant advance in the pharmacotherapy of schizophrenia since the introduction of chlorpromazine, its attributes ranging from a failure to induce serious short- or long-term extrapyramidal motor disturbances (EPS) to a demonstrated ability to bring about significant improvement of both positive and negative symptoms in patients resistant to treatment with conventional neuroleptic agents. Pharmacologically, clozapine is a strong arousal inhibitor, shares several EEG effects with conventional neuroleptics, produces only weak and transient inhibition of conditioned avoidance responding however and, in further contrast to classical neuroleptics, fails to inhibit apomorphine-induced stereotypies or induce catalepsy. The latter properties, linked to its superior EPS profile, have been ascribed to a lack of strong D_2 receptor blockade, concomitant antiserotoninergic or anticholinergic activity, and/or a preferential action within the mesolimbic system. Current opinion, however, favours the first two possibilities. Clozapine's antipsychotic activity in therapy-resistant subjects may be linked to D_1 receptor blockade. Thus, preclinical studies show low doses of clozapine to preferentially block D_1 as opposed to D_2 receptors, while PET scan studies in patients show D_1 receptor occupancy within the caudate nucleus to be greater with clozapine treatment than with classical neuroleptics. Negative symptom improvement might also relate to this D_1 principle, or may stem from the drug's strong 5-HT_2 receptor blocking activity. It is to be expected that further clarification of these issues will lead to still better antischizophrenic drugs and also further our insights into the disease process of schizophrenia.

References

Ackenheil, M. (1989) *Psychopharmacology* **99**, S32–S37.
Anden, N.E. & Stock, G. (1973) *J. Pharm. Pharmacol.* **25**, 346–348.
Andersen, P.H. (1988) *Eur. J. Pharmacol.* **146**, 113–120.
Andersen, P.H., Nielsen, E.B., Gronvald, F.C. & Braestrup, C. (1986) *Eur. J. Pharmacol.* 120, 143–144.
Angst, J., Bente, D., Berner, P. *et al.* (1971) *Pharmakopsychiat.* **4**, 201–211.
Arnt, J. & Scheel-Kruger, J. (1980) *Eur. J. Pharmacol.* **62**, 51–61.
Arnt, J., Hyttel, J. & Bach-Lauritsen, T. (1986) *Acta Pharmacol. Toxicol.* **59**, 319–324.
Balsara, J.J., Jadhav, J.H. & Chandorkar, A.G. (1979) *Psychopharmacology* **62**, 67–69.
Bartholini, G. (1976) *J. Pharm. Pharmacol.* **28**, 429–433.
Bartholini, G., Keller, H.H. & Pletscher, A. (1975) *J. Pharm. Pharmacol.* **27**, 439–442.
Bersani, G., Grispini, A., Marini, S. *et al.* (1986) *Curr. Ther. Res.* **40**, 492–499.
Bowers, M.B. & Rozitis, A. (1976) *Eur. J. Pharmacol.* **39**, 109–115.
Boyson, S.J., McGonigle, P. & Molinoff, P.B. (1986) *J. Neurosci.* **6**, 3177–3188.
Buerki, H.-R., Ruch, W., Asper, H. *et al.* (1973) *Schweiz. med. Wschr.* **103**, 1716–1724.
Carter, C.J. & Pycock, C.J. (1977) *Br. J. Pharmacol.* **60**, 267P.
Casacchia, M., Casati, C. & Fazio, C. (1975) *Biol. Psychiat.* **10**, 109–110.
Casey, D.E. (1989) *Psychopharmacology* **99**, S47–S53.
Casey, D.E. & Keepers, G.A. (1988) In *Psychopharmacology: Current Trends* (eds Casey, D.E. & Christensen, A.V.), pp. 74–93, Berlin, Springer-Verlag.
Chiodo, L.A. & Bunney, B.S. (1983) *J. Neurosci.* **3**, 1607–1619.
Chiodo, L.A. & Bunney, B.S. (1985) *J. Neurosci.* **5**, 2539–2544.
Chipkin, R.E. & Latranyi, M.B. (1987) *Eur. J. Pharmacol.* **136**, 371–375.
Costall, B. & Naylor, R.J. (1976) *Eur. J. Pharmacol.* **40**, 9–19.
Courvoisier, S., Fournel, J., Ducrot, R. *et al.* (1953) *Arch. Int. Pharmacodyn.* **92**, 305–361.
Coward, D.M. (1982) *Psychopharmacology* **78**, 180–184.
Coward, D.M., Imperato, A., Urwyler, S. & White, T.G. (1989) *Psychopharmacology* **99**, S6–S12.
Creese, I., Burt, D.R. & Snyder, S. (1976) *Science* **192**, 481–483.
Dearry, A., Gingrich, J.A., Falardeau, P. *et al.* (1990) *Nature* **347**, 72–76.

De Keyser, J., Claeys, A., De Backer, J.-P. et al. (1988) Neurosci. Lett. 91, 142–147.
De Lisi, L.E., Freed, W.I., Gillin, J.C. et al. (1982) Biol. Psychiat. 17, 471–477.
Eichenberger, E., Herrling, P.L. & Loew, D.M. (1989) In Psychopharmaka. Physiologische, pharmakologische und pharmakokinetische Grundlagen fuer ihre klinische Anwendung (ed. Koella, W.P.), pp. 124–189, Stuttgart, Gustav Fischer.
Farde, L., Wiesel, F.-A., Halldin, C. & Sedvall, G. (1988) Arch. Gen. Psychiat. 45, 71–76.
Farde, L., Wiesel, F.-A., Nordstrom, A.-L. & Sedvall, G. (1989) Psychopharmacology 99, S28–S31.
Fibiger, H., Zis, A. & Phillips, A. (1975) Eur. J. Pharmacol. 30, 309–314.
Fischer-Cornelssen, K.A. (1984) Arzneim.-Forsch. 34(1a), 125–130.
Frey, J.M., Ticku, M.K. & Huffman, R.D. (1987) Brain Res. 425, 73–84.
Gale, K. (1980) Nature 283, 569–570.
Gerlach, J. (1977) Am. J. Psychiat. 143, 781–784.
Gross, H. & Langer, E. (1966) Wien med. Wschr. 116, 814–816.
Gunne, L.-M. & Häggström, J.-E. (1983) Psychopharmacology 81, 191–194.
Gunne, L.-M., Häggström, J.-E. & Sjoquist, B. (1984) Nature 309, 347–349.
Hess, E.J., Norman, A.B. & Creese, I. (1988) J. Neurosci. 8, 2361–2370.
Hoyer, D., Engel, G. & Kalkman, H.O. (1985) Eur. J. Pharmacol. 118, 13–25.
Imperato, A. & Angelucci, L. (1988) Psychopharmacology 96 (Suppl.: Abstracts of the XVIth C.I.N.P. Congress, Munich), 79.
Imperato, A. & DiChiara, G. (1985) J. Neurosci. 5, 297–306.
Janssen, P., Niemegeers, C. & Schellekens, K. (1966) Arzneim.-Forsch. 15, 104–117.
Janssen, P.A.J., Niemegeers, C.J.E., Awouters, F. et al. (1988) J. Pharmacol. Exp. Ther. 244, 685–693.
Kane, J., Honigfeld, G., Singer, J. & Meltzer, H.Y. (1988) Arch. Gen. Psychiat. 45, 789–796.
Klawans, H.L. (1973) Am. J. Psychiat. 130, 82–86.
Krupp, P. & Barnes, P. (1989) Psychopharmacology 99, S118–S121.
Leysen, J.E., Gommeren, W., Janssen, P.F.M. et al. (1988) In Psychopharmacology: Current Trends (eds. Casey, D.E. & Christensen, A.V.), pp. 12–26, Berlin, Springer-Verlag.
Maidment, N.T. & Marsden, C.A. (1987) Eur. J. Pharmacol. 136, 141–149.
Mao, C.C., Cheney, D.L., Marco, E. et al. (1977) Brain Res. 132, 375–379.
Marco, E., Mao, C.C., Cheney, D.L. et al. (1976) Nature 264, 363–365.
Matsubara, S. & Meltzer, H.Y. (1989) Life Sci. 45, 1397–1406.
Meltzer, H.Y. (1990) In Recent Advances in Schizophrenia (eds Kales, A., Stefanis, C.N. & Talbott, J.), pp. 237–256, New York, Springer-Verlag.
Meltzer, H.Y., Daniels, S. & Fang, V.S. (1975) Life Sci. 17, 339–342.
Meltzer, H.Y., Nash, J.F., Koenig, J.I. & Gudelsky, G.A. (1986) Clin. Neuropharmacol. 9 (Suppl. 4), 316–318.
Meltzer, H.Y., Matsubara, S. & Lee, J.-C. (1989) J. Pharmacol. Exp. Ther. 251, 238–246.
Memo, M., Kleinman, J.E. & Hanbauer, I. (1983) Science 221, 1304–1307.
Miller, R.J. & Hiley, C.R. (1974) Nature 248, 596–597.
Monsma, F.J., McVittie, L.D., Gerfen, C.R. et al. (1990) Nature 342, 926–929.
Murray, A.M. & Waddington, J.L. (1990) Eur. J. Pharmacol. 186, 79–86.
Nauta, W.H.J., Smith, G.P., Faull, R.L.M. & Domesick, V.B. (1978) Neuroscience 3, 385–401.
Olianas, M.C., De Montis, G.M., Mulas, G. & Tagliamonte, A. (1978) Eur. J. Pharmacol. 49, 233–241.
Redgrave, P., Dean, P., Donohoe, T.P. & Pope, S.G. (1980) Brain Res. 196, 541–546.
Reyntjens, A., Gelders, Y.G., Hoppenbrouwers, J.A. & Bussche, G.V. (1986) Drug Devel. Res. 8, 205–211.
Ruedeberg, C., Urwyler, S., Schulthess, C. & Herrling, P.L. (1986) Naunyn-Schmiedeberg's

Arch. Pharmacol. **332**, 354–357.

Saller, C.F., Kreamer, L.D., Adamovage, L.A. & Salama, A.I. (1989) *Life Sci.* **45**, 917–929.

Sarnek, J. & Baran, L. (1975) *Arch. Immunol. Ther. Exp.* **23**, 511–516.

Sayers, A.C. & Kleinlogel, H. (1974) *Arzneim.-Forsch.* **24**, 982–983.

Sayers, A.C., Buerki, H.-R., Ruch, W. & Asper, H. (1975) *Psychopharmacologia* **41**, 97–104.

Sayers, A.C., Buerki, H.-R., Ruch, W. & Asper, H. (1976) *Psychopharmacology* **51**, 15–22.

Scheel-Kruger, J., Magelund, G., Olianas, M. *et al.* (1981) *Adv. Biosci.* **31**, 31–41.

Seeman, P., Lee, T., Chau-Wong, M. & Wong, K. (1976) *Nature* **261**, 717–719.

Shippenberg, T.S. & Herz, A. (1988) *Eur. J. Pharmacol.* **151**, 233–242.

Snyder, S., Greenberg, D. & Yamamura, H.I. (1974) *Arch. Gen. Psyuchiat.* **31**, 58–61.

Sokoloff, P., Giros, B., Martres, M.-P. *et al.* (1990) *Nature* **347**, 146–151.

Spano, P., Trabucchi, M. & Di Chiara, G. (1977) *Science* **196**, 1343–1345.

Stahl, S.M., Uhr, S.B. & Berger, P.A. (1985) *Biol. Psychiat.* **20**, 1098–1102.

Stevens, J.R. (1973) *Arch. Gen. Psychiat.* **29**, 177–189.

Stevens, J.R., Wilson, K. & Foote, W. (1974) *Psychopharmacologia* **39**, 105–119.

Stille, G. & Hippius, H. (1971) *Pharmakopsychiat. Neuro-Psychopharmakol.* **4**, 182–191.

Stille, G., Lauener, H. & Eichenberger, E. (1971) *Il Pharmaco* **26**, 603–625.

Stoof, J.C. & Verheijden, P.F.H.M. (1986) *Eur. J. Pharmacol.* **129**, 205–206.

Sunahara, R.K., Niznik, H.B., Weiner, D.M. *et al.* (1990) *Nature* **347**, 80–83.

Tarsy, D. & Baldessarini, R.J. (1977) *Biol. Psychiat.* **12**, 431–450.

Undie, A.S. & Friedman, E. (1990) *J. Pharmacol. Exp. Ther.* **253**, 987–992.

Urwyler, S. & Coward, D.M. (1987) *Naunyn-Schmiedeberg's Arch. Pharmacol.* **335**, 115–122.

Vidali, M. & Fregnan, G.B. (1979) *Curr. Ther. Res.* **25**, 544–556.

Waddington, J.L. (1986) *Biochem. Pharmacol.* **35**, 3661–3667.

Waldmeier, P.C. & Maitre, L. (1976) *J. Neurochem.* **27**, 587–589.

Walters, J.R. & Roth, R.H. (1976) *Naunyn-Schmiedeberg's Arch. Pharmacol.* **296**, 5–14.

Westerink, B.H.C. & Korf, J. (1975) *Eur. J. Pharmacol.* **33**, 31–40.

White, F.J. & Wang, R.Y. (1983) *Life Sci.* **32**, 983–993.

White, T.G. (1979) The pharmacology and neurochemistry of 106–689. Data on file, Basle, Sandoz Ltd.

Wiesel, F.A. & Sedvall, G. (1975) *Eur. J. Pharmacol.* **30**, 364–367.

Young, M.A. & Meltzer, H.Y. (1980) *Psychopharmacology* **67**, 101–106.

Zivkovic, G., Guidotti, A., Revuelta, A. & Costa, E. (1975) *J. Pharmacol. Exp. Ther.* **194**, 37–46.

CHAPTER 3

PHARMACOLOGY AND CLINICAL PROPERTIES OF SELECTIVE DOPAMINE ANTAGONISTS WITH FOCUS ON SUBSTITUTED BENZAMIDES

Jes Gerlach

Research Institute of Biological Psychiatry, St Hans Hospital, Department P, Roskilde, Denmark

Table of Contents

3.1 Introduction

Despite beneficial effects in the individual patient and positive influences in psychiatry, the neuroleptics used in the treatment of schizophrenia have two conspicuous deficiencies:

(1) The therapeutic effect is insufficient. About 20% of the schizophrenic population is resistant, showing no or minimal improvement, while the rest, that is, the majority of schizophrenic patients, experience a variable degree of symptom reduction. In most cases the symptoms persist, though in a weakened form.

(2) All antipsychotics have side-effects, varying from subtle, often unrecognized impairment of mental functioning (such as anhedonia and reduced pleasure in life) to severe and potentially irreversible tardive dyskinesia and the fatal neuroleptic malignant syndrome (see Chapter 14).

The primary goal of current research into new antipsychotic drugs is to overcome these problems.

This chapter will deal with the different forms of existing and potential antipsychotic medications which act via a selective inhibition of dopaminergic mechanisms (Table 1). The discovery of the existence of a multitude of dopamine receptors, each with partially differentiated functions, has given new vitality to research into dopamine's role in schizophrenia and has also given the hope of developing better antidopaminergic antipsychotics, with respect to efficacy and side-effect potential.

Table 1 Established and potential antipsychotics with selective effects upon dopamine functions.

---

1. *Selective dopamine receptor blockade*
   Selective $D_2/D_3/D_4$ receptor blockers
      Substituted benzamides (see Table 3)
      Pimozide
   D_1 receptor antagonists
      SCH 39166
      NNC 756, NNC 687
      BW 737C

2. *Partial D_2 agonists – autoreceptor agonists*[a]
      SDZ HDC 912
      Terguride
      Roxindole
      3-PPP
      SND 919

3. *Inhibition of spontaneous firing in dopamine neurons (depolarization block) with a preferential effect in mesolimbic pathways*
      Sulpiride
      Remoxipride
      Sertindole
      Clozapine

---

[a]The partial agonists are placed according to increasing intrinsic activity.

3.2 Antagonisms of dopamine receptors

The dopamine receptors can be divided into two main categories: the 'D_1-like' receptors (D_{1a}, D_{1b} and D_5), and the 'D_2-like' receptors (D_{2long}, D_{2short}, D_3 and D_4) (Sibley & Monsma, 1992; see Chapter 4). All existing neuroleptics block 'D_2-like' receptors, but it is still unknown to what extent blockade of the different receptors contributes to an antipsychotic effect. Pure D_2, D_3 or D_4 antagonists have not yet been developed.

Some antipsychotics also block the 'D_1-like' receptors to some extent; this is especially true of the thioxanthines flupenthixol and zuclopenthixol, which have a relatively weak D_1 blockade compared to D_2 blockade, and the atypical neuroleptic clozapine, which has a weak, but equal blockade of D_1 and D_2 receptors (Farde *et al.*, 1992; see Chapter 2). In recent years, several selective D_1 antagonists have been developed, but their clinical potential has not yet been established (see below).

Two other dopamine mediated approaches to developing antipsychotic compounds include partial D_2 receptor agonists (autoreceptor agonists) and drugs acting through an inhibition of spontaneous activity in dopamine neurons (depolarization block) (Table 1).

3.2.1 Blockade of 'D_2-like' receptors. Substituted benzamides

The binding of neuroleptics to the three 'D_2-like' receptors (D_2, D_3, D_4) differs somewhat from neuroleptic to neuroleptic (Sokoloff *et al.*, 1990; Van Tol *et al.*, 1991). Haloperidol and other traditional neuroleptics have a strong affinity for D_2 receptors and somewhat less affinity for D_3 and D_4 (Table 2). The atypical neuroleptic clozapine, on the other hand, has a strong affinity for the D_4 receptor, less for D_2 and D_3. The substituted benzamides have a weaker affinity for 'D_2-like' receptors, but the relationship between the blockade of D_2, D_3 and D_4 receptors corresponds roughly to the blockade of haloperidol (Table 2).

These differences in the affinities of neuroleptics for the 'D_2-like' receptors may be of importance to their therapeutic effects, but it has hitherto not been possible, with any certainty to identify any clinical differences between neuroleptics which could be attributed to this differentiated dopamine receptor affinity. Clozapine's special effect may be associated with the preferential D_4 blockade, but the broad-spectrum effect of this drug, including its effects on D_1 receptors and perhaps 5-HT receptors may be of equal importance.

The substituted benzamides represent a group of neuroleptics with a specific therapeutic profile associated with the hitherto most specific affinity for certain 'D_2-like' receptors. These drugs have attracted increasing interest in recent years as atypical neuroleptics with relatively few side-effects, including fewer extrapyramidal symptoms (EPS) than other dopamine antagonists such as haloperidol. Some substituted benzamides (such as sulpiride) have been used for more than 20 years, while others (remoxipride) have been developed and marketed only recently. Originally,

Table 2 Ranking of $D_2/D_3/D_4$ receptor occupancy of classical and atypical neuroleptics.

	D_2	D_3	D_4
Haloperidol	++++	++	+
Pimozide	+++	+++	+
Clozapine	++	+	++++
Sulpiride	+++	++	+
Remoxipride	+++	+	+
Raclopride	+++	++	(+)
Amisulpride	+++	++	a
Sultopride	+++	++	a

Occupancy is shown in a semiquantitative ranking from (+) (1–5% occupancy) to ++++ (>80% occupancy). The occupancy estimation is based upon Sokoloff *et al.* (1990) and Van Tol *et al.* (1991).
[a]No values available.

sulpiride was used for treatment of gastrointestinal symptoms, and one substituted benzamide (metoclopramide) is still used exclusively for this indication. (Metoclopramide is not used in psychiatry, although it has some antipsychotic effect, Stanley *et al.*, 1980.)

Although the majority of substituted benzamides are relatively selective towards the D_2 receptors, they are heterogeneous pharmacologically and clinically. Some, such as sultopride and clobopride resemble traditional neuroleptics, while others, such as sulpiride and remoxipride are 'atypical', with less psychomotor inhibition and fewer EPS.

Figure 1 shows some of the best-known substituted benzamides and their chemical formulas, and Table 3 offers a tentative clinical classification of substituted benzamides into classical and atypical neuroleptics.

In the following sections, the pharmacological and clinical properties of substituted benzamides will be evaluated. Emphasis will be placed upon sulpiride and remoxipride, the two most well-established atypical members of the group.

3.2.1.1 Rodent data

As previously mentioned, the substituted benzamides bind relatively selectively to D_2 receptors and have little or no affinity for D_1, α- and β-adrenergic, 5-HT$_2$, histaminergic, GABAergic, muscarinic, opioid or phencyclidine receptors (Hall *et al.*, 1986; Köhler *et. al.*, 1990). However, remoxipride has high affinity for the sigma site, while sulpiride (and clozapine) has no affinity for this receptor (Köhler *et. al.*, 1990). The sigma receptor appears to be of no importance in the mediation of antipsychotic

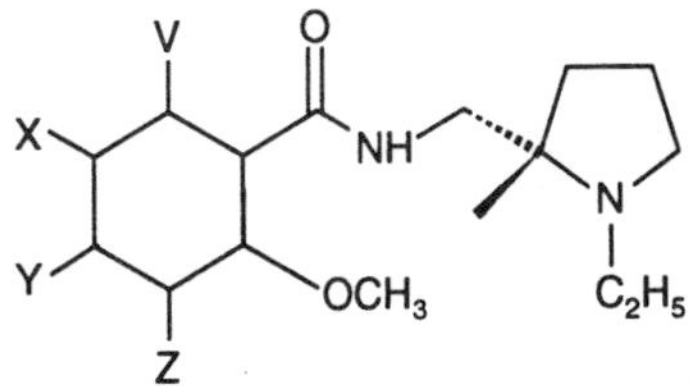

	V	X	Y	Z
Sulpiride	H	NH_2SO_2	H	H
Remoxipride	OCH_3	Br	H	H
Amisulpride	H	$C_2H_5SO_2$	NH_2	H
Eticlopride	OH	C_2H_5	H	Cl

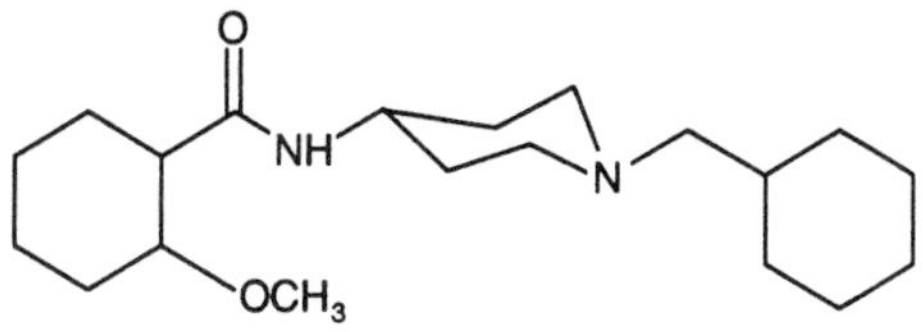

Clebopride

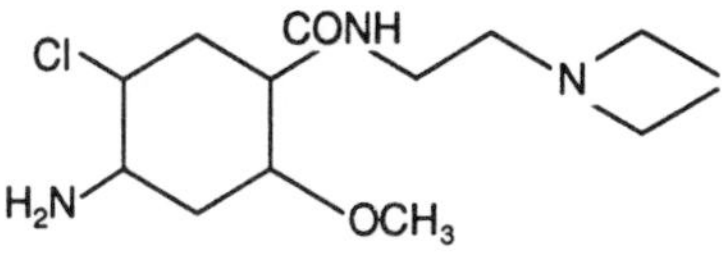

Metoclopramide

Figure 1 Formula of substituted benzamides with 'classical' and 'atypical' effects.

Table 3 Clinical classification of substituted benzamides.

'Atypical' neuroleptics
  Sulpiride
  Remoxipride
  Amisulpride

'Classical' neuroleptics
  Clebopride
  Emonapride
  Eticlopride
  Sultopride
  Tiapride

Use in gastroenterology
  Metoclopramide

effect. Clebopride and emonapride, having classical neuroleptic properties, also bind to the 5-HT and α_1 receptors (Jenner & Marsden, 1984).

Substituted benzamides have a receptor binding to D_2 receptors which is different from that of traditional neuroleptics in that it is especially sensitive to the presence of Na^+ (omission of sodium ions from the incubation buffer decreases the ability of substituted benzamides to displace the specific binding of [³H]spiperone, but does not affect the binding of other neuroleptics; Theodorou et al., 1980), the pH (Strange, 1992), and mutation of a conserved aspartic acid (Asp 80) residue in the second membrane-spanning region (Neve et al., 1991). Recently, it has been shown that substituted benzamides have a higher affinity for D_{2short} than for D_{2long} (Castro & Strange, 1993).

It is notable that the *in vitro* affinity for the D_2 binding sites differs widely between the substituted benzamides, with the following ranking: remoxipride < metoclopramide < sulpiride < raclopride < eticlopramide (Hall et al., 1986; Köhler et al., 1990).

Substituted benzamides displace [³H]spiperone *in vivo* in limbic and ventral tegmental structures, but not in striatal tissue, at doses that selectively block apomorphine-induced hyperactivity (Köhler et al., 1990). Blockade of [³H]spiperone in the striatum is observed only at high doses, which produce catalepsy. Moreover, sulpiride and remoxipride cause a low maximal dopamine receptor binding displacement in the striaturm compared to other terminal areas. Even at high doses, neither drug displaces striatal [³H]spiperone more than 40–50%, in contrast to the 80–90% displacement by chlorpromazine and haloperidol (Köhler et al., 1990).

In a study of the dopamine utilization in various brain areas, it has been found that remoxipride at doses which block apomorphine-induced hyperactivity and oral stereotypies exerts a selective action on the matrix dopamine terminals of the medial part of the caudate, while haloperidol increases dopamine utilization in both the matrix and the patchy dopamine terminals (Fuxe & Ögren, 1991). This means that remoxipride can discriminate between dopamine utilization within the diffuse (matrix) and the island (striatomes) dopamine innervation within the striatum. This may correspond to the receptor binding selectivity mentioned above.

In an electrophysiological model, sulpiride and remoxipride have been found to decrease the number of spontaneously active dopamine neurons in mesolimbic/mesocortical pathways, while the effect is limited in the nigrostriatal pathway, corresponding to clozapine (see Section 3.2.3.2).

In a behavioural rat model it has been shown that sulpiride and remoxipride inhibit apomorphine-induced locomotion at relatively small doses, while much higher doses are required to cause catalepsy (EPS model). Traditional neuroleptics such as haloperidol produce both effects at the same dose level (Ögren et al., 1990; Ögren & Hall, 1992). If this model is valid, it indicates that these substituted benzamides should have antipsychotic effects at dose levels far below the EPS level, while haloperidol should induce EPS at antipsychotic dose levels.

The potencies of substituted benzamides to bind to presynaptic D_2 receptors are of great interest in relation to the discussion of whether these drugs have a special beneficial effect upon negative symptoms. Sulpiride has been found to have a strong affinity to presynaptic D_2 receptors, corresponding to or stronger than that of haloperidol, while remoxipride is much weaker in this respect (Herrera-Marschitz et al., 1984; Ögren et al., 1990). This has been shown both in a biochemical model (γ-butyrolactone-induced increase of dopamine synthesis can be inhibited by a dopamine agonist, and this effect can be prevented by presynaptic receptor antagonists) and in a behavioural model (low doses of dopamine agonists, such as pergolide, reduce locomotor activity in rodents, presumably due to autoreceptor stimulation, and this effect can be prevented by presynaptic D_2 receptor antagonists). Also, amisulpride, another 'atypical' substituted benzamide, in low doses preferentially blocks presynaptic D_2 receptors (Maubrey et al., 1989).

Throughout the past 20 years, the dopamine supersensitivity idea has played a major role in the characterization of neuroleptic drugs, chiefly because it was thought that the risk of causing tardive dyskinesia could be predicted. The results have been contradictory and there has often been a divergence between biochemical and behavioural supersensitivity. Recent research into receptor mechanisms and the associated intraneuronal effector mechanisms (such as G-proteins, adenyl cyclase and second messengers) has shown that supersensitivity can develop at many different levels, and that receptor number, for example, may be a poor expression of supersensitivity. Behavioural supersensitivity is therefore a more useful concept, but its value is still limited as the clinical correlation is unknown. Tardive dyskinesia can only partially be ascribed to supersensitivity, and is more likely caused by a dysbalance between D_1 and D_2 receptor functions in favour of D_1 (Gerlach & Casey, 1988; Peacock et al., 1990; Lublin et al., 1993).

Following prolonged treatment with sulpiride (2-4 weeks) only a mild dopamine supersensitivity has been seen in the form of a small increase in stereotypical response (but not in locomotion) to apomorphine (Fuxe et al., 1980; Jenner et al., 1982; Rupniak et al., 1985) and quinpirole (Prosser et al., 1989). This effect of sulpiride is significantly weaker than the corresponding response to prolonged haloperidol exposure.

Receptor binding studies have yielded conflicting results. Some groups have found an increase in mesolimbic and striatal [^{3}H]spiroperidol B_{max} values after administration of high doses of (+/-)-sulpiride (100 mg/kg twice a day) for 3 weeks (Jenner et al. 1982) while other groups have found no changes after similar doses (Bannet et al., 1980; Rupniak et al., 1985). Prosser et al. (1989) demonstrated a relatively small increase in striatal B_{max} values, but no change in mesolimbic D_2 receptor density.

Remoxipride (10 μmol/kg orally for a period of 14 days) as well as haloperidol (1 μmol/kg) caused a 50% increase in the number of striatal D_2 receptors, while only haloperidol, and not remoxipride, caused an exaggeration of apomorphine-induced stereotypies (Ögren et al., 1990). However, the dose of remoxipride appears to have been relatively low in this study.

Taken together, it seems obvious that substituted benzamides, including sulpiride and remoxipride, can induce dopamine supersensitivity, although to a lesser degree than traditional neuroleptics. Once again, the clinical implication of such a difference is unknown.

In conclusion, most of the above mentioned points (molecular biology, dopamine receptor displacement, dopamine utility, behavioural parameters, supersensitivity) indicate that antipsychotics such as sulpiride and remoxipride differ from traditional neuroleptics in their binding to the D_2 receptor protein and by the induction of less catalepsy and less dopamine supersensitivity. Although some of the results may be attributed to a reduced bioavailability of these drugs due to a relatively low lipophilicity (Benakis *et al.*, 1984; Köhler *et al.*, 1990), the data from experiments on animals suggest that sulpiride and remoxipride possess more selective biochemical and behavioural effects than those of traditional neuroleptics. The question is whether this can be identified and utilized in the clinic.

3.2.1.2   Non-human primate data

The non-human primate model for studying neuroleptic-induced EPS has several advantages. Identical dystonic/dyskinetic syndromes occur in humans and monkeys (especially cebus monkeys) induced by the same drugs and doses, whereas rodents do not develop dystonia, only catalepsy (the relation of which to dystonia, parkinsonism or akathisia is less clear). Furthermore, acute and tardive dyskinesia can be developed and studied. While the primate model of EPS seems satisfactory and valid, the primate psychosis model is more uncertain. Apomorphine- and amphetamine-induced behaviour, especially increased arousal, reactivity and perhaps stereotypical body movements may be useful as a psychosis model, but is still artificial, being pharmacologically induced. In cebus monkeys it has been found that remoxipride (4 and 8 mg/kg) induces acute dystonia/dyskinesia which is identical with the syndrome induced by haloperidol (0.01 and 0.02 mg/kg), and that remoxipride (2 and 4 mg/kg) and haloperidol (0.005 and 0.01 mg/kg) have an equal antagonistic effect upon apomorphine- and amphetamine-induced increased arousal (psychosis model) (Gerlach & Casey, 1990). As can be seen, the doses for 'antipsychotic' effect and for induction of EPS overlapped, and no difference was found between remoxipride and haloperidol. This contrasts to the findings in the rat model where a wide separation was found between doses inducing catalepsy and doses counteracting apomorphine-induced locomotion (see Section 3.2.1.1). It should be added that the dose ratio between the two drugs (1:400) suggests that remoxipride in the doses used in the treatment of schizophrenia (150–900 mg/kg) may cause relatively fewer EPS (corresponding to haloperidol 0.5–2.0 mg daily). The effect of prolonged administration was not evaluated.

Raclopride has been used as a selective D_2 blocker in several monkey studies evaluating D_2 receptor functions. In all cases raclopride induced a typical acute dystonia/dyskinesia syndrome corresponding to haloperidol (Kistrup & Gerlach, 1987; Peacock *et al.*, 1990), and dose levels for EPS induction and the amphetamine antagonism were again overlapping (Peacock & Gerlach, 1993).

All classical neuroleptics can induce acute dystonia/dyskinesia, the substituted benzamides (sulpiride 25-50 mg/kg, sultopride 5-10 mg/kg, tiapride 12.5-50 mg/kg and metoclopramide 0.5-2 mg/kg), melperone and risperidone being no exception in spite of their 'atypicality' (Gunne & Barany, 1979; Liebman & Neale, 1980; Neale *et al.*, 1981; Porsholt & Jalfre, 1981; Casey, 1991). Thioridazine has a relatively weak effect, and clozapine is unable to produce dystonia; the monkeys become sedated without sleeping, laying down in drooping positions or sitting in bizarre positions, salivating, but never develop dystonia.

D_1 antagonists in long-term administration produce tolerance to dystonia so increasing doses can be given without induction of dystonia, only sedation and parkinsonism (see Section 3.2.2).

Only a few studies have examined the effect of withdrawal of substituted benzamides in monkeys, that is, the risk of developing tardive dyskinesia. Häggström (1984) found that sulpiride (20 mg/kg) in single-dose administration reduced dyskinesia in five dyskinetic cebus monkeys, although dystonia developed in four. No rebound dyskinesia developed. In contrast, metoclopramide (0.5 mg/kg) caused dystonia followed by rebound dyskinesia. Other studies have shown that raclopride (Lublin *et al.*, 1993), haloperidol and other classical neuroleptics can induce withdrawal dyskinesia (Gunne & Barany, 1979; Domino, 1985).

In conclusion, the monkey studies did not identify significant differences between the substituted benzamides and the classical neuroleptics, except with respect to doses, although a relatively mild withdrawal dyskinesia (tardive dyskinesia) was seen in a single study after sulpiride (20 mg/kg).

3.2.1.3 Human data

PET studies Studies using positron emission tomography (PET) have shown that sulpiride (800 mg/day), remoxipride (400 mg/day) and raclopride (6-8 mg/day) cause a D_2 receptor occupancy of 65-82% in the human brain, in all cases slightly lower than that of haloperidol (6-12 mg/day) (81-89%) (Farde *et al.*, 1988, 1992; Wiesel *et al.*, 1990). In these PET studies the substituted benzamides did not elicit EPS, while haloperidol caused EPS in four out of five cases. These studies indicate that EPS is related to the degree of D_2 receptor occupancy.

In a study by Farde *et al.* (1988) the time-course for receptor occupancy and drug levels was followed after withdrawal of sulpiride at 1200 mg/day. D_2 receptor occupancy remained above 65% for more than 27 h despite a reduction of serum drug concentration from approximately 5000 to 1000 nmol/litre. Following withdrawal of haloperidol (12 mg/day) the D_2 receptor occupancy decreased only by a few per cent over 54 h, while the serum drug concentration decreased from 23 to 8 nmol/litre. This discrepancy in the time-course for receptor occupancy and serum drug concentration is probably due to the hyperbolic relationship between receptor binding and serum drug concentration (at the higher dose level a marked drop in serum drug concentration is required to cause a decrease at the receptor level). Furthermore, the rate of receptor–drug dissociation is slower than the rate of reduction of free drug concentration (for discussion, see Farde *et al.*, 1988).

Therapeutic effect and side-effects   In clinical double-blind studies sulpiride (600–1800 mg/day) (Edwards *et al.*, 1980; Rao *et al.*, 1980; Gerlach *et al.*, 1985), remoxipride (150–900 mg/day) (Sedvall, 1990; Hebenstreit *et al.*, 1991; King *et al.*, 1992) and amisulpride (300–1200 mg/day) (Rüther *et al.*, 1989; Delcker *et al.*, 1990) have been shown to possess antipsychotic effects not significantly different from those of traditional neuroleptics such as haloperidol. However, this does not necessarily mean that the effect of substituted benzamides is identical to that of traditional neuroleptics. These drugs certainly have a beneficial effect in schizophrenia, but are not sufficiently effective in the treatment of psychotic agitation and aggression. Unfortunately, serious omissions in the research methodology in several clinical trials (with respect to patient selection, duration of treatment and incomparable doses) has resulted in uncertain conclusions as to therapeutic effects and side-effects, conclusions which have not been in agreement with subsequent practical clinical experience.

Over the years it has been claimed, especially by French psychiatrists, that certain substituted benzamides, especially sulpride and amisulpride, should have a 'disinhibitory effect' and should be beneficial in the treatment of negative schizophrenia symptoms (Bobon *et al.*, 1972; Deniker, 1978; Puech *et al.*, 1984). This claim is mainly based upon the observation that such drugs have a preferential presynaptic effect when used in low doses (see Section 3.2.1.1). However, there is a severe lack of definitional clarity and several methodological deficiencies in the clinical studies evaluating this question. Thus negative symptoms can be primary (related to the basic disease) or secondary (a consequence of positive symptoms, EPS, depression or social understimulation), and negative symptoms can be seen initially, that is, before the start of the illness, during the illness, or afterwards, as a postpsychotic defect state (Carpenter *et al.*, 1985). These factors have not been sufficiently clarified in the studies dealing with the potential anti-autistic effect of substituted benzamides.

When given in relatively high doses (for example, haloperidol 10–20 mg/day or sulpiride 800–1800 mg/day), all neuroleptics may improve negative symptoms together with positive symptoms in acute and chronic schizophrenia. Although it has been subject to discussion (Crow, 1985; Meltzer *et al.*, 1986), and although neuroleptics do not necessarily induce parallel reductions in positive and negative symptoms (Serban *et al.*, 1992), the effect upon negative symptoms is, at least in part, secondary to the effect upon positive symptoms (the postsynaptic effect), and not due to a special anti-autistic effect (presynaptic effect) (Van Kammen *et al.*, 1987; Möller 1991). At this high dose level, substituted benzamides do not appear to be more beneficial in the treatment of negative symptoms than traditional neuroleptics (De Leon & Simpson, 1991). In one controlled study (in young acute schizophrenic patients) it was found that, compared to chlorpromazine (400 mg/day), sulpiride (800 mg/day) had a significantly better effect upon autism (Härnryd et al., 1984). However, this difference may be due to the stronger sedative and psychomotor inhibitory effect of chlorpromazine compared to sulpiride.

When given in low doses, sulpiride (100–400 mg/day) may have some activating, anti-autistic effect in otherwise unmedicated schizophrenic patients without productive symptoms, patients who do not need the postsynaptic dopamine blockade. However, such patients are rare, and available documentation is limited (Elizur & Davidson, 1975; Niskanen et al., 1975; Peselow & Stanley, 1982). Remoxipride has not been tested in this condition.

In a recent French double-blind study in schizophrenic patients with pure negative symptoms, it was found that amisulpride (100 and 300 mg/day) equally improved negative symptoms by 40–50% as opposed to 20–25% with placebo (Boyer, 1989). No reactivation of productive symptoms was seen. In chronic schizophrenic patients with predominantly negative symptoms, Pichot & Boyer (1989) found that amisulpiride (mean 210 mg/day) yielded significantly better results on some Brief Psychiatric Rating Scale (BPRS) items (anergia items and anxiety–depression items) than fluphenazine (9.6 mg/kg). However a third of the patients in both groups dropped out, mainly due to an insufficient effect.

Adding sulpiride in low doses to a traditional neuroleptic therapy in chronic schizophrenic patients with suppressed productive symptoms and depression, anhedonia or apathy is without effect (personal unpublished data).

Taken together, available documentation on the activating/anti-autistic effect of the atypical substituted benzamides is limited. Although the hypothesis of a biphasic effect (activating at low doses, suppressing at high) is attractive and well-founded in rodent studies, it does not work in clinical practice.

The therapeutic advantage of sulpiride and remoxipride most likely lies in their low level of side-effects, including a limited suppression of general mental function. Because of the selective D_2 blockade, there are only few autonomic and cardiovascular reactions and only weak sedation. Furthermore, these drugs induce an apparently lower level of parkinsonism compared to haloperidol and similar neuroleptics (Edwards et al., 1980; Rao et al., 1980; Gerlach et al., 1985; Lewander et al., 1990; Hebenstreit et al., 1991).

In chronic schizophrenic patients with tardive dyskinesia, sulpiride (400–2100 mg/day) is able to suppress the dyskinesia score by a mean of 70%, corresponding to the effect of other dopamine antagonists such as haloperidol and pimozide (Gerlach & Casey, 1984; Schwartz et al., 1990). Only weak parkinsonism was induced. Following withdrawal, the dyskinesia returned to the baseline level, with no rebound aggravation. This suggests that sulpiride may have a low potential to induce tardive dyskinesia. No long-term studies, however, have been performed on this drug or any other substituted benzamide to document whether these drugs are less dyskinesia-inducing than traditional neuroleptics.

It seems reasonable to suggest that sulpiride and remoxipride produce a relatively selective suppression of psychotic symptoms, without a general inhibition of emotions and cognitive functions. This would undoubtedly lead to a higher quality of life and more patient satisfaction, but may also entail new demands, upon the patient, the family and the psychiatric team, because the patient may be more awake, responding to inner stimuli and feelings of any kind (Eriksson, 1992).

These observations raise the question of whether neuroleptics with affinity to a subpopulation of D_2 receptors can suppress schizophrenic symptoms in a more selective way than traditional D_2 blocking neuroleptics, without affecting other mental functions and with less parkinsonism and motor inhibition. The available evidence supports this view, but the advantage over existing neuroleptics seems marginal. It would probably not be possible to identify any difference between the atypical substituted benzamides described here and classical high-potency neuroleptics such as flupenthixol and pimozide given in the lowest effective dose. This question should be examined more closely in controlled cross-over studies using sensitive measures of subjective, emotional and cognitive functions and quality of life (see Collins *et al.*, 1991; Awad, 1992).

3.2.2 Blockade of 'D₁-like' receptors

Studies in rodents suggest that D_1 antagonists have antipsychotic effects (Andersen *et al.*, 1992; see Chapter 4). They are cataleptogenic, they antagonize locomotion and stereotypies induced by dopamine agonists, and they suppress conditioned avoidance response. In non-human primates, a D_1 antagonist (NNC 756) has been shown to have a stronger anti-amphetamine effect than a D_2 antagonist (raclopride) (Gerlach *et al.*, 1992).

Studies in primates suggest that D_1 antagonists have a more benign EPS profile than D_2 antagonists. Thus, in drug-naive monkeys, NNC 756 can be given in gradually increasing doses up to 1 mg/kg without producing dystonia, in contrast to raclopride which after an initial dose increase to 0.1 mg/kg has to be reduced and kept at a level of 0.01 mg/kg in order to avoid dystonia (Gerlach & Hansen, 1993). In another study in drug-naive cebus monkeys, Coffin *et al.* (1989) found that chronic weekly oral administration of the D_1 antagonist SCH 23390 (10–30 mg/kg) and clozapine (20 mg/kg) induced no abnormal movements, in contrast to haloperidol (1 mg/kg) and raclopride (10 mg/kg). However, when given subcutaneously in high *single* doses, the D_1 antagonist SCH 23390 can induce dystonia in drug-naive cebus monkeys (Casey, 1992).

When given to cebus monkeys which have previously received the D_2 antagonist raclopride, NNC 756 initially produces dystonia corresponding to D_2 antagonists.

Following prolonged treatment, however, tolerance develops, and the D_1 antagonist can be given in gradually increasing doses without causing dystonia (Gerlach & Hansen, 1993). Correspondingly, Coffin *et al.* (1991) found that SCH 39166, a D_1 antagonist, produced abnormal movements in monkeys which previously had received chronic treatment with haloperidol, but the movements completely disappeared after continued treatment with SCH 39166 for 5 days. Christensen (1990) has also shown a significant decrease in EPS during long-term administration of SCH 23390 to vervet monkeys previously exposed to D_2 antagonists.

D_1 antagonists can induce acute oral dyskinesia, but again, as with dystonia, during long-term treatment these dyskinesias tend to decrease, while they usually increase during treatment with a D_2 antagonist. The dyskinesia following withdrawal (tardive dyskinesia) of long-term treatment with a D_1 antagonist appears to be less than that after a D_2 antagonist (Gerlach & Hansen, 1993; Lublin, 1993; see also rat study by Glenthøj *et al.*, 1991).

Based on studies in primates, the side-effects of D_1 antagonists may be sedation, increasing during prolonged treatment, and slow movements (bradykinesia) (Christensen 1990; Gerlach & Hansen, 1993). Observations in humans treated with test doses of SCH 23390 in connection with PET studies have shown that this D_1 antagonist can cause akathisia (Farde, 1992).

The above-mentioned studies suggest that D_1 antagonists have antipsychotic effects, possibly superior to traditional D_2 antagonists, and a more favourable EPS profile with respect to dystonia and dyskinesia. They appear to induce sedation, parkinsonism and akathisia. The results of the first clinical trials are eagerly awaited.

3.2.3   Other antidopaminergic treatment principles

3.2.3.1   Partial dopamine receptor agonists – autoreceptor agonists

Partial D_2 agonists (also known as autoreceptor agonists because of their preferential affinity for presynaptic receptors) are substances which act both as agonists and antagonists at the D_2 receptors dependent upon their intrinsic activity. High intrinsic activity involves a high agonistic effect and no or minimal antagonistic effect, while low intrinsic activity means a low agonistic activity, that is, high antagonistic effect (Coward *et al.*, 1988; see Chapter 4). Table 1 lists some representative partial D_2 agonists.

Another factor determining the effect of partial agonists is the basal endogenous dopamine activity. When there is a high degree of endogenous activity (as there may be in some regions of the brain in schizophrenia), the compounds' antagonistic effects dominate. If there is a low endogenous activity, on the other hand (as there may be in some regions of the brain in schizophrenic patients characterized by negative symptoms), the agonistic effect predominates.

The partial D_2 agonist treatment principle is attractive. The hypothesis is that the antagonistic effect should diminish the dopamine hyperactive functions which may be associated with positive symptoms, while the agonistic effect should normalize the dopamine hypoactive areas which may be related to negative symptoms, with a concomitant lesser risk of EPS. The question is whether this theory works in practice.

Until now, the results have been disappointing. A partial D_2 agonist with low intrinsic activity (SDZ HDC 912) has been shown to have beneficial effects upon positive and negative symptoms, rather similar to traditional neuroleptics. Unfortunately, the drug also induced side-effects, not only traditional EPS (dopamine antagonistic effect), but also tachycardia (dopamine agonistic effect), while no special effect was seen upon negative symptoms (Naber *et al.*, 1992). On the other hand, partial agonists with higher intrinsic activity such as terguride and roxindole have had limited or no effects upon positive symptoms, but have caused psychomotor activation and (thereby) counteracted negative symptoms (Benkert *et al.*, 1990). For further discussion, see Gerlach (1991).

Will it be possible, using the partial agonist principle, to suppress positive symptoms and at the same time avoid EPS and improve negative symptoms? Probably not. The observations to date do not lead to much optimism, but other drugs with varying intrinsic activity should be tested in different psychiatric conditions. Thus, a recent monkey study has revealed that SND 919, a partial D_2 agonist with a relatively high intrinsic activity, has anti-amphetamine effect at 0.01–0.025 mg/kg (higher doses have no effect), and is unable to induce dystonia at any dose (Peacock & Gerlach, 1993).

It should also be noted that the hypothesis that positive symptoms are related to dopamine hyperactivity and negative symptoms to dopamine hypoactivity is probably wrong. The primary negative symptoms appear to be based upon the same pathophysiological process as the positive symptoms (cf. the previously mentioned observation that both positive and negative symptoms are ameliorated by neuroleptics, Section 3.2.1.3).

3.2.3.2 Selective dopamine depolarization block

Electrophysiological techniques have revealed that chronic treatment (more than 3 weeks) with a traditional neuroleptic such as haloperidol induces a so-called depolarization block, that is, an inhibition of spontaneous activity (firing rate) in dopamine neurons, both in the nigrostriatal pathway (A9, which is thought to be involved in the EPS effects) and in the mesolimbic and mesocortical pathways (A10, which is thought to be involved in the antipsychotic effects) (Bunney, 1984). In contrast, clozapine and thioridazine primarily antagonize the activity in A10. This corresponds to the clinical observations that haloperidol produces antipsychotic effects and EPS while clozapine and thioridazine produce effects with less EPS. However, it is still an open question whether an antipsychotic effect can be produced via depolarization block alone, without concomitant postsynaptic blockade of dopamine receptors.

A recent study has revealed that the substituted benzamides sulpiride and remoxipride inhibit the number of spontaneously active dopamine neurons in the mesolimbic pathways and cause much less inhibition in the striatal pathways (Skarsfeldt, 1992b). In contrast, the cataleptic benzamide, emonapride, had an effect in both areas.

A new drug, sertindole (1-[2-[4-[5-chloro-1-(4-fluorophenyl)-1H-indol-3-yl]-1-piperidnyl]ethyl]-2-imidazolidinone), also produces a selective inhibitory effect on limbic dopamine neurons. After 3 weeks of treatment, sertindole inactivates the number of spontaneously active dopamine neurons in the ventral tegmental area at doses more than a hundred times lower than those necessary for inactivation of dopamine neurons in the substantia nigra (A9) (Sanchez et al., 1991; Skarsfeldt, 1992a). In vitro, sertindole has a high affinity for 5-HT_2 receptors, D_2 receptors and α_1 receptors, while in vivo it is atypical, characterized by a remarkably weak or no effect in acute tests for dopamine antagonism, that is, no antistereotypic and cataleptogenic effects. Sertindole has also been shown to possess a low dystonia potential in primates. The ongoing clinical testing of this drug should clarify whether selective dopamine depolarization block is a useful treatment principle in schizophrenia.

3.3 Conclusion and future trends

Antidopaminergic treatment is still the only significant means of producing an antipsychotic effect. The new perspective is that an antidopaminergic treatment can be selective, antagonizing specific subgroups of dopamine receptors. The molecular identification of different dopamine receptors has made inroads towards the development of antipsychotics with selective effects upon 'D_1-like' ($D_{1a/b}$, D_5) and 'D_2-like' ($D_{2short/long}$, D_3, D_4) receptors.

Classical neuroleptics block the three 'D_2-like' receptors with decreasing occupancy: $D_2 > D_3 > D_4$ (Table 2). The same is true of substituted benzamides, although the affinities for the dopamine receptors are weaker. Despite their chemical likenesses (Figure 1), the substituted benzamides are a heterogeneous group of antipsychotics, some with classic neuroleptic properties (e.g. emonapride and sultopride), and others with atypical characteristics (sulpiride and remoxipride). Three substituted benzamides (sulpiride, remoxipride and amisulpride) have attracted great interest because of their atypical characteristics. In animal studies, these three have been found to be more selective (for example, they produce less catalepsy and dopamine supersensitivity) than classical neuroleptics such as haloperidol, and receptor molecular studies indicate that sulpiride and remoxipride have deviant receptor binding properties, including a special affinity for the D_{2short} receptor. In non-human primates, however, it has not been possible to establish any difference between these substituted benzamides and classical neuroleptics with respect to EPS and anti-amphetamine effects, except for the varying dosage levels and a potential lower risk for development of tardive dyskinesia following withdrawal. In the clinic, there are signs of some differences, but these are fewer than sometimes claimed. The chief clinical effects are as follows:

(1) Sulpiride (600–1800 mg/day), remoxipride (300–900 mg/day) and amisulpride (300–1200 mg/kg) have antipsychotic effects comparable to or slightly weaker than classical neuroleptics such as haloperidol (partially related to the milder sedation and other mental suppression produced by the substituted benzamides).

(2) All neuroleptics have a beneficial effect upon negative symptoms in schizophrenic patients presenting positive and negative symptoms, and it is doubtful whether the substituted benzamides are more anti-autistic than other neuroleptics. Whether substituted benzamides are more effective upon a *pure* negative symptomatology (seen in few drug-free schizophrenic patients) has not been documented.

(3) The advantage of the atypical substituted benzamides is that they produce relatively few side-effects, autonomic reactions, EPS, sedation and other forms of mental suppression. This is possibly a greater advantage than recognized at first glance: many patients complain about the subjective discomfort of neuroleptics, for example, the suppression of feelings, inability to experience pleasure and lack of initiative. A sufficient antipsychotic effect can be obtained with substituted benzamides, but the lower liability for side-effects is a valuable contribution towards a greater satisfaction, better quality of life and improved compliance. More clinical research is warranted in this area.

It must be concluded, however, that the therapeutic advantage of substituted benzamides compared to classical neuroleptics is relatively modest, especially as compared to D_2 selective, high-potency neuroleptics such as pimozide and flupenthixol. The difference in receptor affinities is simply too small. It would therefore be advantageous to attempt to develop new antipsychotics with new dopamine receptor profiles, for example, 'D_2-like' antagonists with a preference for D_4 receptors (such as clozapine). In rodents, D_1 receptor antagonists fulfil the criteria for antipsychotic effect, and in primate studies they produce less dystonia and dyskinesia, and also have a powerful anti-amphetamine effect. Such compounds might lead the treatment of schizophrenia to new paths.

The partial agonist principle is interesting, but has not yet met the expectations of a combined beneficial effect upon positive symptoms (antagonistic effect) and negative symptoms (agonist effect) and lack of EPS (limited D_2 blockade). Selective depolarization block, that is, inhibition of spontaneous firing in A10 (mesolimbic/mesocortical) dopamine neurons but not A9 (nigrostriatal) dopamine neurons is also an interesting treatment principle, the application of which has not yet been tested in the clinic.

Utilizing the different dopamine-mediated treatment principles, it should be possible to develop new antipsychotics with fewer side-effects, and hopefully also with additional therapeutic effects in negative symptoms and treatment-resistant patients.

References

Andersen, P.H., Gronvald, F.C., Hohlweg, R. *et al.* (1992) *Eur. J. Pharmacol.* **219**, 45-52.
Awad, A.G. (1992) *Hospital Community Psychiat.* **43**, 262-265.
Bannet, J., Gillis, S., Ebstein, R.P. & Belmaker, R.H. (1980) *Int. Pharmacopsychiat.* **15**, 334-337.
Benakis, A., Brown, J.P.H. & Benard, P. (1984) *Eur. J. Drug Metab. Pharmacokinet.* **9**, 365-370.
Benkert, O., Wetzel, H. & Wiedemann, K. (1990) In *Clinical Neuropharmacology: Proceedings from the 17th CINP Congress*, pp. 178-179, New York, Raven Press.
Bobon, J., Pinchard, A. & Collard, J. (1972) *Comp. Psychiat.* **13**, 123-131.
Boyer, P. (1989) In *Amisulpride* (eds Borenstein, P. *et al.*), pp. 11-123, Paris, Expansion Scientifique Francaise.
Bunney, B.S. (1984) *Trends Neurosci.* **6**, 212-215.
Carpenter, W.T., Henrichs, D.W. & Alphs, L.D. (1985) *Schizophrenia Bull.* **11**, 440-452.
Casey, D.E. (1991) *Psychopharmacol. Bull.* **27**, 47-50.
Casey, D.E. (1992) *Psychopharmacology* **107**, 18-22.
Castro, S.W. & Strange, P.G. (1993) *J. Neurochem.* **60**, 372-375.
Christensen, A.V. (1990) *Behav. Neurol.* **3**, 49-60.
Coffin, V.L., Latranyi, M.B. & Chipkin, R.E. (1989) *J. Pharmacol. Exp. Ther.* **249**, 769-774.
Coffin, V.L, Barnett, A. & McHugh, D.T. (1991) Abstract American Collegium Neuropsychopharmacologicum 30th Annual Meeting, Puerto Rico, December 1991.
Collins, E.J., Thomas, P.H. & Desai, H. (1991) *Schizophrenia Res.* **5**, 249-253.
Coward, D.M., Dixon, A.K., Urwyler, S. & Vigouret, J.-M. (1988) *Pharmacopsychiatry* **21**, 213-313.
Crow, T.J. (1985) *Schizophrenia Bull.* **11**, 471-486.
Delcker, A., Schoon, M.L., Oczkowski, B. & Gaertner, H.J. (1990) *Pharmacopsychiatry* **23**, 125-130.
De Leon, J.G. & Simpson, G.M. (1991) *Integr. Psychiat.* **7**, 39-47.
Deniker, P. (1978) *Am. J. Psychiat.* **135**, 923-927.
Domino, E.F. (1985) In *Dyskinesia. Treatment and Research* (eds Casey, D.E., Chase, T.N., Christensen, A.V. & Gerlach, J.), pp. 217-223, Berlin, Heidelberg, New York, Springer-Verlag.
Edwards, J.G., Alexander, J.R., Alexander, M.S. *et al.* (1980) *Br. J. Psychiat.* **137**, 522-527.
Elizur, A. & Davidson, S. (1975) *Curr. Ther. Res.* **18**, 578-584.
Eriksson, L. (1992) *Clin. Neuropharmacol.* **15** (Suppl. 1), 361B.
Farde, L. (1992) *Psychopharmacology* **107**, 23-29.
Farde, L., Wiesel, F.-A., Halldin, C. & Sedvall, G. (1988) *Arch. Gen. Psychiat.* **45**, 71-76.
Farde, L., Wiesel, F.-A., Nordström, A.-L. & Sedvall, G. (1989) *Psychopharmacology* **99**, 28-31.
Farde, L., Nordström, A.-L., Wiesel, F.-A., *et al.* (1992) *Arch. Gen. Psychiat.* **49**, 538-544.
Fuxe, K. & Ögren, S.O. (1991) *Acta Physiol. Scand.* **141**, 577-578.
Fuxe, K., Ögren, S.O., Hall, H. *et al.* (1980) *Adv. Biochem. Psychopharmacol.* **24**, 193-206.
Gerlach, J. (1991) *Schizophrenia Bull.* **17**, 289-309.
Gerlach, J. & Casey, D.E. (1984) *Acta Psychiat. Scand.* **69** (Suppl. 311), 93-102.
Gerlach, J. & Casey, D.E. (1988) *Acta Psychiat. Scand.* **77**, 369-378.
Gerlach, J. & Casey, D.E. (1990) *Prog. Neuro-Psychopharmacol. Biol. Psychiat.* **14**, 103-112.
Gerlach, J. & Hansen, L. (1992) *Br. J. Psychiat.* **160** (Suppl.), 34-37.
Gerlach, J. & Hansen, L. (1993) *J. Psychopharmacol.* (in press).
Gerlach, J., Behnke, K., Heltberg, J. *et al.* (1985) *Br. J. Psychiat.* **147**, 283-288.
Gerlach, J., Hansen, L. & Peacock, L. (1992) *Clin. Neuropharmacol.* **15** (Suppl. 1), 485B.

Glenthøj, B., Bowig, T.G. & Hemmingsen, R. (1991) In *Biological Psychiatry* (eds Racagni, I.G. *et al.*), Vol. 1, pp. 602-604, London, Elsevier Science.
Gunne, L.M. & Barany, S. (1979) *Psychopharmacology* **63**, 195-198.
Häggström, J.-E. (1984) *Acta Psychiat. Scand.* **69** (Suppl. 311), 103-108.
Hall, H., Sällemark, M. & Jerning, E. (1986) *Acta Pharmacol. Toxicol.* **58**, 61-70.
Härnryd, C., Bjerkenstedt, L., Björk, K. *et al.* (1984) *Acta Psychiat. Scand.* **69** (Suppl. 311), 7-30.
Hebenstreit, G.F., Laux, G., Schubert, H. *et al.* (1991) *Pharmacopsychiatry* **24**, 153-158.
Herrera-Marschitz, M., Ståhle, L., Tossman, U. *et al.* (1984) *Acta Psychiat. Scand.* **69** (Suppl. 311), 147-162.
Jenner, P. & Marsden, C.D. (1984) *Acta Psychiat. Scand.* **69** (Suppl. 311), 109-123.
Jenner, P., Hall, M.D., Murugaiah, K. *et al.* (1982) *Biochem. Pharmacol.* **31**, 325-328.
King, D.J., Blomqvist, M., Cooper, S.J. *et al.* (1992) *Psychopharmacology* **107**, 175-179.
Kistrup, K. & Gerlach, J. (1987) *Pharmacol. Toxicol.* **61**, 157-162.
Köhler, C., Hall, H., Magnusson, O. *et al.* (1990) *Acta Psychiat. Scand.* **82** (Suppl. 358), 27-36.
Lewander, T., Westerbergh, S.-E., Morrison, D. (1990) *Acta Psychiat. Scand.* **82**, 92-98.
Liebman, J. & Neale, R. (1980) *Psychopharmacology* **68**, 25-29.
Lublin, H. (1993) *Psychopharmacology* (in press).
Lublin, H., Gerlach, J. & Peacock, L. (1993) *Clin. Neuropharmacol.* **15**, 448-458.
Magnusson, O., Fowler, C.J., Mohringe, B. *et al.* (1988) *Arch. Pharmacol.* **337**, 379-384.
Maubrey, M.C., Jacquot, C., Gonidec, J. *et al.* (1989) In *Amisulpride* (eds Borenstein, P. *et al.*), pp. 3-23, Paris, Expansion Scientifique Francaise.
Meltzer, H.Y., Sommers, A.A. & Luchins, D.J. (1986) *J. Clin. Psychopharmacol.* **20**, 1098-1102.
Möller, H.J. (1991) In *Negative Versus Positive Schizophrenia* (eds Marneros, A., Andreasen, N.C. & Tsuang, M.T.), pp. 341-364, Berlin, Heidelberg, New York, Springer-Verlag.
Naber, D., Gaussares, C., Moeglen, J.M. *et al.* and the SDZ HDC 912 Collaborative Study Group (1992) In *Novel Antipsychotic Drugs* (ed. Meltzer, H.Y.), pp. 99-107, New York, Raven Press.
Neale, R., Fallon, S., Gerhardt, S. & Liebman, J. (1981) *Psychopharmacology* **75**, 254-257.
Neve, K.A., Neve, R.L., Fidel, S. *et al.* (1991) *Proc. Natl. Acad. Sci. USA* **88**, 2802-2806.
Nielsen, E.B. & Andersen, P.H. (1992) *Eur. J. Pharmacol.* **219**, 35-44.
Niskanen, P., Tamminen, T. & Viukari, M. (1975) *Curr. Ther. Res.* **17**, 281-284.
Ögren, S.O. (1992) In *Clinical Neuropharmacology* (eds Robert, P., Darcourt, G., Pringuey, D. & Mendlewicz, J.), pp. 462A-463A, New York, Raven Press.
Ögren, S.O. & Hall, H. (1992) In *Novel Antipsychotic Drugs* (ed. Meltzer, H.Y.), pp. 59-66, New York, Raven Press.
Ögren, S.O., Florvall, L., Hall, H. *et al.* (1990) *Acta Psychiat. Scand.* **82**, 21-26.
Peacock, L. & Gerlach, J. (1993) *Eur. J. Pharmacol.* (in press).
Peacock, L., Lublin, H. & Gerlach, J. (1990) *Eur.J. Pharmacol.* **186**, 49-59.
Peselow, E.D. & Stanley, M. (1982) *Adv. Biochem. Psychopharmacol.* **35**, 163-194.
Pichot, P. & Boyer, P. (1989) In *Amisulpride* (eds Borenstein, P. *et al.*), pp. 125-137, Paris, Expansion Scientifique Francaise.
Porsholt, R.D. & Jalfre, M. (1981) *Psychopharmacology* **75**, 16-21.
Prosser, E.S., Pruthi, R. & Csernansky, J.G. (1989) *Psychopharmacology* **99**, 109-116.
Puech, A.J., Lecrubier, Y. & Simon, P. (1984) *Acta Psychiat. Scand.* **311** (Suppl. 311), 139-145.
Rao, V.A.R., Bailey, J., Mirkin, A. & Coppen, A. (1980) *Psychopharmacology* **80**, 73-77.
Rupniak, N.M.J., Hall, M.D., Kelly, E. *et al.* (1985) *J. Neural Transm.* **62**, 249-266.
Rüther, E., Eben, E., Klein, H. *et al.* (1989) In *Amisulpride* (eds Borenstein, P. *et al.*), pp.

63–72, Paris, Expansion Scientifique Francaise.

Sanchez, C., Arnt, J., Dragsted, N. *et al.* (1991) *Drug Devel. Res.* **22**, 239–250.

Schwartz, M., Moguillansky, L., Lanyi, G. & Sharf, B. (1990) *J. Neurol. Neurosurg. Psychiat.* **53**, 800–802.

Sedvall, G. (ed.) (1990) *Acta Psychiat. Scand.* **82** (Suppl. 358).

Serban, G., Siegel, S. & Gaffney, M. (1992) *J. Clin. Psychiat.* **53**, 229–234.

Sibley, D.R. & Monsma, F.J. (1992) *Trends Pharmacol. Sci.* **13**, 61–69.

Skarsfeldt, T. (1992a) *Synapse* **10**, 25–33.

Skarsfeldt, T. (1992b) Abstract American Collegium Neuropsychopharmacologium Meeting, Puerto Rico, December 1992.

Sokoloff, P., Giros, B., Martres, M.-P. *et al.* (1990) *Nature* **347**, 146–151.

Stanley, M., Lautin, A., Rotrosen, J. *et al.* (1980) *Psychopharmacology* **71**, 219–225.

Strange, P.G. (1992) *Neurochem. Int.* **20** (Suppl.), 59S–62S.

Theodorou, A.E., Jenner, P. & Marsden, C.D. (1980) *J. Pharm. Pharmacol.* **32**, 229–233.

Van Kammen, D.P., Hommer, D.W. & Malas, K.L. (1987) *Neuropsychobiology* **18**, 113–117.

Van Tol, H.H.M., Bunzow, J.R., Guan, H.-C. *et al.* (1991) *Nature* **350**, 610–619.

Waddington, J.L. (1988) *Gen. Pharmacol.* **19**, 55–60.

Wiesel, F.-A., Farde, L., Nordström, A.-L. & Sedvall, G. (1990) *Prog. Neuropsychopharmacol. Biol. Psychiat.* **14**, 759–767.

CHAPTER 4

PRE- AND POSTSYNAPTIC D_1 TO D_5 DOPAMINE RECEPTOR MECHANISMS IN RELATION TO ANTIPSYCHOTIC ACTIVITY

John L. Waddington

Department of Clinical Pharmacology, Royal College of Surgeons in Ireland, St Stephen's Green, Dublin 2, Republic of Ireland

Table of Contents

ANTIPSYCHOTIC DRUGS AND THEIR SIDE-EFFECTS
ISBN 0-12-079035-1

4.1   Pharmacological characteristics of dopamine receptor subtypes

4.1.1   Historical perspective and original definition of D_1 and D_2 receptors

Receptors for the great majority of known or presumed transmitter substances, for example, those in adrenergic, cholinergic, histaminergic and, most recently, serotoninergic systems, exhibit heterogeneity. Because such receptor multiplicity is typically reflected in (and, indeed, usually derives from) differences in physiological function subserved, the identification of compounds acting selectively at one subtype has commonly led to new drugs of important clinical utility. In many cases, these have constituted critical therapeutic advances.

In relation to the neurotransmitter dopamine, though a number of schemes for dopamine receptor classification have been proposed, most have failed to achieve widespread acceptance and have fallen into disuse (see Waddington & O'Boyle, 1987). The scheme that survived, and that has evolved to become a progenitor for much contemporary work on dopamine receptor multiplicity and function, has its basis in biochemical anomalies rather than inconsistencies in physiological responses. When it was found that substituted benzamide neuroleptics such as sulpiride and metoclopramide failed to inhibit the stimulation of adenylyl cyclase by dopamine, a property previously thought to characterize essentially all known neuroleptic drugs, and that dopaminergic ergots such as lergotrile and lisuride failed to mimic such stimulatory activity of dopamine (Spano *et al.*, 1978; Kebabian, 1978), and noting complementary neuroanatomical data, Kebabian & Calne (1979) proposed that dopamine receptors linked to the stimulation of adenylyl cyclase and resultant cAMP production be designated D_1, while those unlinked to adenylyl cyclase be designated D_2. These basic concepts were reviewed and elaborated by Seeman (1980) and by Creese *et al.*, (1983).

Over subsequent years, this scheme has been subject both to temporary and to permanent revisions. Studies focusing on radioligand-binding techniques, largely excluding behavioural and other functional considerations, initially extended this scheme to four 'binding sites' (D_1 to D_4). Unfortunately, at this time differing research groups sometimes used this nomenclature in contradictory ways. However, the proposed quadruplet heterogeneity was subsequently resolved and subsumed within the original D_1/D_2 framework. More enduringly, it became apparent that though D_2 receptors are not linked to the stimulation of adenylyl cyclase, many are, in fact, linked to this enzyme system in an inhibitory manner (see Waddington & O'Boyle, 1989).

4.1.2 Molecular neurobiology of D_1, D_2, D_3, D_4 and D_5 receptors, and associated signal transduction mechanisms

Classically, receptor subtyping has its basis in physiological considerations. More recently, molecular biological techniques have provided an alternative approach to receptor multiplicity in terms of identifying distinct genes which encode such subtypes and their associated protein sequences.

Cloning of a rat D_2 receptor cDNA and characterization of the expressed protein has been followed by the putative localization of the human D_2 receptor gene to chromosome 11 (Bunzow *et al.*, 1988; Grandy *et al.*, 1989a). Subsequently, cloning of rat and human D_1 receptor cDNA and characterization of the expressed protein has been reported, with the human D_1 receptor gene having a putative location on chromosome 5 (Dearry *et al.*, 1990; Zhou *et al.*, 1990; Sunahara *et al.*, 1990; Monsma *et al.*, 1990). D_1 and D_2 receptor protein sequences both appear to exist as six loops (three extracellular and three intracellular) linking seven transmembrane domains, with an extracellular N-terminal section and an intracellular C-terminal tail. They are otherwise distinct, D_1 and D_2 sequences being intronless or interrupted by multiple introns, respectively, and they exhibit an overall amino acid identity of 29% (44% within transmembrane domains). Further evidence has now indicated the D_2 receptor to exist as long (D_{2long}) and short (D_{2short}) protein isoforms derived from a single gene but produced by alternative mRNA splicing (Eidne *et al.*, 1989; Giros *et al.*, 1989; Monsma *et al.*, 1989; Grandy *et al.*, 1989b; Chio *et al.*, 1990).

Recently, molecular biological studies have identified additional, distinct dopamine receptor cDNAs and expressed protein sequences: the D_3 receptor (Sokoloff *et al.*, 1990) exhibits 52% homology (75% within transmembrane domains) with the D_2 receptor, and shows a generally D_2-like pharmacological profile; similarly, the D_4 receptor (Van Tol *et al.*, 1991) exhibits 41% homology (36–78% within transmembrane domains) with the D_2 receptor, and also shows a generally D_2-like pharmacological profile; conversely, the D_5 receptor (Sunahara *et al.*, 1991) exhibits 50% homology (80% within transmembrane domains) with the D_1 receptor, and shows a generally D_1-like pharmacological profile. Most recently, the D_{1b} receptor (Tiberi *et al.*, 1991) has been identified as the rat homologue of the human D_5 receptor; this exhibits 50% homology (80% within transmembrane domains) with the 'classical' D_1 receptor (proposed designation, D_{1a}), and shows a generally D_1-like pharmacological profile. It should be emphasized that, with few exceptions (see Section 4.2.4.3), antipsychotic drugs in current clinical use and experimental agents under theoretical consideration are little able to distinguish between either D_1 and D_5 receptors or between D_2, D_3 and D_4 receptors. Thus, there appear to be at least two major families of dopamine receptor subtypes: the 'D_1-like' (D_{1a}, D_{1b}/D_5) and the 'D_2-like' (D_{2long}, D_{2short}, D_3 and D_4). For these reasons, the classical D_1/D_2 nomenclature will be retained in this chapter, bearing in mind that such designations actually encompass the 'D_1-like' and 'D_2-like' families, respectively (Sibley & Monsma, 1992).

The consequences of the interaction between a neurotransmitter and its receptor are transduced by a variety of second messenger and effector systems. Dopamine receptors interact with guanine nucleotide-binding regulatory proteins (G-proteins), which link them to their signal transduction pathways; indeed, the basic dopamine receptor topography of the seven transmembrane domains noted above is a general characteristic common to catecholamine and other receptors (e.g. α- and β-adrenergic, 5-HT_{1A} serotonergic and M1 muscarinic) linked to G-proteins. D_1 receptors are coupled to a stimulatory G_s regulatory protein activating adenylyl cyclase, and possibly to other second messenger systems and ion channels, while for D_2 receptors the situation appears yet more complex; they are coupled to an inhibitory G_i regulatory protein and inhibition of adenylyl cyclase, and may directly activate potassium (K^+) channels, influence phosphoinositide (PI) hydrolysis and/or calcium (Ca^{2+}) influx (Vallar & Meldolesi, 1989; Andersen *et al.*, 1990). The coupling of at least some D_2 receptors directly with the opening of K^+ channels has generated considerable recent interest, while effects on PI hydrolysis are as yet inconsistent. A combined molecular biological and neurochemical approach has indicated that the nature of D_2 receptor coupling appears to depend on the specific properties not only of the receptor molecule itself, but also of the cell type in which it is expressed (Vallar *et al.*, 1990). There is recent evidence that both D_1 and D_2 receptors can inhibit (Na^+, K^+)ATPase which couples the hydrolysis of ATP to the countertransport of Na^+ and K^+ ions across the plasma membrane (Bertorello *et al.*, 1990).

4.1.3 Initial presumptions on the role of D_2 antagonism in antipsychotic activity

The proposition that neuroleptic drugs block brain dopamine receptors goes back more than 25 years. However, the relationship of this property to therapeutic efficacy in schizophrenia and other psychoses received powerful support in the mid-1970s from data indicating that the *in vitro* affinities of a broad range of neuroleptic drugs for dopamine antagonist binding sites in the brain were correlated highly with their clinical potencies to control psychotic symptoms. Subsequent re-evaluation of this relationship in terms of the D_1/D_2 schema indicated very high correlations between affinity for the D_2 receptor and a wide range of pharmacological actions of neuroleptics, including antipsychotic activity, that were not evident in relation to affinity for the D_1 receptor; similarly, selective or preferential D_2 antagonists, such as the substituted benzamides or butyrophenones, reproduced the pharmacological and clinical effects of less selective or mixed antagonists of both D_1 and D_2 receptors, such as the phenothiazines and thioxanthenes. On this basis, the D_2 receptor was ascribed a prepotent or even exclusive role in the regulation of dopamine-mediated phenomena, including the antipsychotic action of neuroleptics, with the D_1 receptor relegated to an enzyme-linked entity of no known functional relevance. Seeman (1980) and Creese *et al.* (1983) have comprehensively reviewed contemporary thinking over that period. One critical line of evidence is lacking in the above analysis; that is, 'confirmatory' studies using selective D_1 antagonists. It may seem strange in retrospect that such a scheme for receptor subtyping and functional sequelae could evolve in the absence of a selective antagonist for one of the putative subtypes; however, so strong was the correlational and other indirect evidence for D_2 prepotence that the failure to identify any selective D_1 antagonist had little or no impact on such theorizing. By analogy with classical receptor systems, this view would predict these 'D_2-mediated' functions to show double dissociation in terms of insensitivity to a selective D_1 antagonist, were one to be identified. With the introduction in 1983/84 of SCH 23390 and its close homologue SKF 83566 as the first selective D_1 antagonists (see Waddington, 1986), it rapidly became all too apparent that behavioural and physiological processes were unexpectedly and powerfully influenced by such agents.

4.2 D_1 receptor antagonists as putative antipsychotic agents

4.2.1 Behavioural effects of selective D_1 antagonists in rodents

The notion that D_2 receptors play the fundamental role and that D_1 receptors play no evident role in dopamine-mediated behaviours carried with it the presumption that, when finally identified, selective D_1 antagonists would specifically inhibit the stimulation of adenylyl cyclase by dopamine but would be without activity in conventional models of dopaminergic function. However, it was soon demonstrated in rodent studies that SCH 23390 and SKF 83566 readily induced catalepsy and blocked stereotyped behaviour induced by the classical, non-selective dopamine agonists apomorphine and amphetamine, thus showing basic properties indistinguishable from those of typical neuroleptics having either preferential D_2 or non-selective dopamine antagonist activity.

Even more unexpected was the ability of these D_1 antagonists to block the behavioural stimulation induced by selective D_2 agonists. These 'paradoxical' findings were complemented by evidence that while compulsive stereotyped behaviour was not induced either by selective D_1 or selective D_2 agonists, such behaviour was evident on co-stimulation of both dopamine receptor subtypes by their current administration; thus, not only did these D_1 antagonists block responsivity to D_2 agonists, but D_1 agonists promoted synergistically such D_2 agonist responses.

Enigmatically, these phenomena were evident in intact animals, but not in animals with long-term disruption of ongoing dopaminergic activity. Following sustained dopamine depletion with reserpine and inhibition of its synthesis with α-methyl-p-tyrosine, or lesioning of dopaminergic pathways with 6-hydroxydopamine, animals then responded to agonists of *either* subtype, and these responses were blocked only by the antagonist of the particular receptor stimulated. The impact of such unexpected findings can be gauged by the dramatic increase in the literature on these topics, the initial years of which have been reviewed by Waddington (1986) and by Breese & Creese (1986).

4.2.2 D_1:D_2 receptor interactions

The explanation offered for such phenomena was that D_1 and D_2 receptors do not invariably act independently, but rather interact functionally in the regulation of typical dopamine-mediated behaviours. Thus, in the intact animal, tonic activity through D_1 receptors was proposed to exert a 'permissive' or 'enabling' role in the expression of D_2 receptor-stimulated events in a process of cooperative/synergistic D_1:D_2 interactions; such interactions appeared to be critically dependent on the functional integrity of dopaminergic neurons, being no longer evident following long-term disruption of their tonic activity (see Waddington, 1986, 1989a; Waddington & O'Boyle, 1987, 1989; Arnt, 1987; Clark & White, 1987). These cooperative/synergistic D_1:D_2 interactions in the regulation of typical dopaminergic behaviours were clearly at variance with the opposing roles of D_1 and D_2 receptors in the stimulation and inhibition of striatal adenylyl cyclase activity, respectively, and thus they appeared initially without mechanistic support. However, entirely compatible profiles of interaction were subsequently obtained for the effects of similar peripherally administered drug combinations on the firing rate of globus pallidus neurons; furthermore, while functionally independent effects of D_1 and D_2 agonists and antagonists have been sometimes reported to follow their iontophoretic application on to striatal cells, other iontophoretic studies in the striatum and accumbens continue to indicate cooperative D_1:D_2 interactions (see Waddington & O'Boyle, 1987, 1989; Clark & White, 1987; Walters *et al.*, 1987; Wachtel *et al.*, 1989; Waddington, 1989a). Though some authors have argued that D_1:D_2 interactions derive from effects on D_1 and D_2 receptors located at anatomically distinct sites (see Robertson & Robertson, 1987; LaHoste & Marshall, 1990), the most recently identified complementary interactions, at the levels of radioligand-binding sites (Seeman *et al.*, 1989) and striatal (Na^+, K^+)ATPase (Bertorello *et al.*, 1990), suggest a local effect.

4.2.3 Antipsychotic potential and side-effects liability of selective D_1 antagonists

It appears that selective D_1 antagonists can produce effects very similar to those of D_2 antagonists via blockade of discrete receptor subtypes through which initially distinct events readily come to influence a common and possibly local physiological process. In the above analysis, this was exemplified in terms of classical dopaminergic responses. However, the selective D_1 antagonists SCH 23390 and SKF 83566 not only inhibit dopamine agonist-induced motor behaviour, they also inhibit conditioned avoidance responding, intracranial self-stimulation and the amphetamine cue in drug discrimination responding, and are therefore active in those rodent behavioural models currently believed to predict clinical antipsychotic efficacy (Waddington, 1988). These properties do not appear to be idiosyncratic effects of the 1-phenylbenzazepine series from which both SCH 23390 and SKF 83566 derive, as they are also evident in preliminary studies with new selective D_1 antagonists (Daly & Waddington, 1992) that are chemically distinct: NNC 756 (a 1-benzofuranylbenzazepine; Andersen *et al.*, 1988), SCH 39166 (a benzonaphthazepine; Chipkin *et al.*, 1988) and A-69024 (a 1-benzyltetrahydroisoquinoline; Kerkman *et al.*, 1989).

An important related matter is whether such drugs might be more or less likely to induce the adverse effects that are encountered during therapy with classical or D_2 antagonist neuroleptics, and whether any different problems might be encountered. Selective D_1 antagonists can induce catalepsy in rodents, suggesting some likelihood of inducing extrapyramidal side-effects such as parkinsonism; however, they are active at very low doses in models predictive of antipsychotic efficacy, and these various properties might be readily dissociated by dose (see Waddington, 1988). Furthermore, in a new rodent model purporting to distinguish atypical neuroleptics with reduced acute extrapyramidal liabilities from typical agents, SCH 23390 more resembled clozapine and thioridazine than haloperidol or chlorpromazine (Ellenbroek *et al.*, 1987). Though selective D_1 antagonists readily inhibit spontaneous motility in rodents, the relationship of this crude index to likelihood of clinical sedation remains unclear; however, in view of effects on specific sleep parameters (Trampus & Ongini, 1990), this remains a possibility. As they show little affinity for cholinergic and generally modest affinity for adrenergic receptors, few prominent anticholinergic or hypotensive side-effects would be predicted. Also, selective D_1 antagonists do not induce the dramatic pituitary D_2-mediated elevations in prolactin level seen during treatment with typical neuroleptics, and their blockade of peripheral D_1 receptors would not be expected to induce major cardiovascular or other changes (see Waddington, 1988). Of critical importance is the extent to which such drugs might be more or less likely to induce tardive dyskinesia. In the opinion of the present author

(Waddington, 1989b), the weaknesses of the dopamine receptor supersensitivity hypothesis are so profound as to vitiate any attempt to predict such liability on the basis of their known interactions with brain dopaminergic systems, whether on acute or following 'chronic' administration; they have yet to be examined over prolonged periods in putative phenomenological models of tardive dyskinesia (Waddington, 1990). In the absence of any specific notion as to the pathophysiology of neuroleptic malignant syndrome, the likelihood of selective D_1 antagonists inducing this extremely rare but potentially fatal reaction is entirely unknown.

The vast bulk of our knowledge on selective D_1 antagonists derives from studies in rodents, and thus non-human primates have the potential to provide more sophisticated and phylogenetically relevant information on these issues. SCH 23390 has been shown to disrupt conditioned avoidance responding in monkeys at doses which produced few signs of any acute dyskinetic syndrome(s), while such reactions were common after a comparable dose of haloperidol; however, these studies were carried out in monkeys rendered susceptible to acute neuroleptic-induced dyskinesias by repeated prior administration of haloperidol. In other laboratories, SCH 23390 induced in previously haloperidol-treated monkeys an anticholinergic-reversible dystonic syndrome indistinguishable from that induced by typical neuroleptics and selective D_2 antagonists (see Waddington, 1988), and recent studies (Peacock et al., 1990) continue to report such events; again, the use of animals with a history of prior long-term exposure to haloperidol confounds any attempt to generalize such findings to the drug-naive state.

Studies by Coffin et al. (1989) indicated that neither acute nor prolonged oral administration of SCH 23390 to drug-naive monkeys resulted in any form of motor symptomatology, other than sedation, while comparable haloperidol treatment was associated with the emergence of a multifaceted dyskinetic/dystonic syndrome; conversely, Casey (1992) has noted that acute parenteral administration of SCH 23390 to drug-naive monkeys of another species induces a brief dystonic syndrome that was otherwise indistinguishable in form and intensity from that induced by D_2 antagonists. It will be essential to determine whether these studies are in contradiction or alternatively represent extremes along a continuum of response as determined by considerations of species, dose and route of administration. Stereotyped behaviour and social isolation induced by d-amphetamine in non-human primates have been proposed by some investigators to constitute symptomatological and pharmacological models of positive and of negative psychotic symptoms, respectively. While typical neuroleptic drugs can suppress stereotypy they have less effect on social isolation, in keeping with the controversial perspective that negative symptoms may be less responsive to such agents, and it may be of some significance that preliminary data indicate SCH 23390 to antagonize both phenomena; strong but brief catalepsy was noted in all animals, apparently drug-naive, who had received parenteral SCH 23390 (Ellenbroek et al., 1989).

Clearly, studies of selective D_1 antagonists have, over the past 8 years, resulted in a complete revision of contemporary views on the dopaminergic regulation of psychomotor behaviour and on the role of the D_1 receptor in such regulation. Because of their activity in those behavioural models believed currently to predict antipsychotic activity, and of more inconsistent data that they might be less liable to induce the major side-effects of typical neuroleptics, they represent a potentially new approach to the treatment of psychotic disorders (Waddington, 1988, 1989c). This prospect has generated considerable excitement and speculation among psychopharmacologists and psychiatrists over the past few years, but there has been little feedback from human subjects; pharmaceutical companies have yet to release formally their 'satisfactory' phase I data on oral administration to normal volunteers, though akathisia similar to that induced by D_2 antagonists has been reported in each of three volunteers who received 0.5–1.0 mg [^{11}C]SCH 23390 i.v. for positron emission tomographic studies (L. Farde, 1992). It is only recently that the first clinical trial in patients has been scheduled with SCH 39166 (Chipkin, 1990). If the results are positive (i.e. greater efficacy, or similar efficacy but with fewer side effects), then a novel and superior treatment may have been identified on the basis of preclinical concepts and data; if they are negative (i.e. no efficacy, or efficacy with serious adverse reactions), then we would have cause to question many of those preclinical concepts. Rarely can the outcome of clinical trials have been awaited with such intensity of interest.

4.2.4 Cautionary observations

4.2.4.1 More than one direction of D_1:D_2 interaction?

Though much of the reasoning that has led to clinical trials with selective D_1 antagonists is based on the role of cooperative/synergistic D_1:D_2 interactions in the regulation of typical unconditioned, conditioned and motivational behaviours in rodents, certain complexities and anomalies must be recognized. In drug discrimination paradigms, the cues of selective D_1 and D_2 agonists do not appear to involve comparable mechanisms; selective D_1 and D_2 antagonists essentially block the cue only of their respective agonist counterpart. This implies considerable functional independence of such D_1- and D_2-mediated processes (see Waddington, 1989a). Furthermore, not only does a selective D_1 antagonist block typical motor responses to a selective D_2 agonist in accordance with a 'permissive' role for D_1 tone via cooperative D_1:D_2 interactions. In such circumstances other atypical behaviour is concurrently released, which appears only to be evident on D_2 stimulation when normally 'inhibitory' D_1 tone is removed; a comparable profile is seen using a combination of D_1 agonist and D_2 antagonist (Murray & Waddington, 1989a, b). This suggests that certain rodent behaviours can have their genesis in oppositional D_1:D_2 interactions, which appear to have a biological correlate in the oppositional role of D_1 and D_2 receptors in the regulation of striatal (but not accumbal) adenylyl cyclase activity (see Waddington, 1989a; Waddington & O'Boyle, 1989). However, when considered in isolation, their potential clinical significance is not clear.

4.2.4.2 Species differences in D_1:D_2 interaction?

Though in a number of instances comparison of selective D_1 and D_2 antagonist drug effects in non-human primates with those in rodents has revealed what appear to be comparable phenomena (see Section 4.2.3), there is increasing recognition of a number of anomalies. For example, the synergistic interaction between D_1 and D_2 agonists described in intact or 6-hydroxydopamine-lesioned rodents was not evident in monkeys, at least in those rendered parkinsonian by prior injection of 1-methyl-4-phenyl-1,2,3,6-tetrahydropyridine (MPTP); in this model, D_1 agonist treatment alone failed to exert the motility-restoring effect of D_2 agonists and indeed appeared to reduce D_2 agonist responses on co-administration. Similarly, in monkeys withdrawn from long-term treatment with haloperidol, D_2 agonist responses were attenuated by concurrent D_1 agonist treatment, which caused some sedation when given alone. These results would suggest a form of D_1:D_2 interaction opposite to that occurring in rodents, yet they must be set against the similar action of D_1 and D_2 antagonists to induce dystonia in such neuroleptic-withdrawn monkeys (Waddington & O'Boyle, 1989; Waddington, 1989a). The most recent studies continue to indicate such anomalous effects of acute D_1 versus D_2 agonists in previously treated (Peacock et al., 1990; Boyce et al., 1990) and, critically, in normal (Bedard & Boucher, 1989) monkeys, though chronic co-administration of a D_1 and D_2 agonist to MPTP-treated monkeys did demonstrate some synergism in restoring motility (Rouillard et al., 1990).

What might be the basis of what appear to be species differences in response between rodents and (non-human and human) primates? If it is not an artefact of conducting studies usually on drug-naive rodents versus usually previously treated primates, it might reflect species differences in the cooperative/synergistic and oppositional D_1:D_2 interactions which appear to regulate distinct forms of behaviour in rodents (see Section 4.2.4.1); if the overall effect of D_1 and/or D_2 agents reflects some balance between those two forms of interaction, there may be phylogenetic differences in that balance between rodent and primate species. Alternatively, there may be more fundamental differences in D_1 and/or D_2 systems; for example, while the majority of rodent studies indicate a two- to fourfold greater density of D_1 than of D_2 receptors in the striatum, the most recent in vitro and in vivo studies in human caudate-putamen tissue indicate these two subtypes to have generally similar densities (Waddington, 1989a). In relation to anomalous agonist responses in primates, SKF 38393 and its analogues are far from ideal probes. Their partial D_1 agonist activity might fail to enhance (Braun et al., 1989) or even attenuate high levels of tonic activity through D_1 receptors, or they might exert differing actions according to the relative densities of (sometimes spare?) D_1 versus D_2 receptors; furthermore, this prototype compound shows additional anomalous properties unexpected of a selective D_1 agonist, acting to stimulate prolactin secretion in man (Fabbrini et al., 1988) and to sometimes induce emesis in monkeys (Close et al., 1990) and cats (Sweidan et al., 1990). While any one or combination of the above might contribute to such apparent differences in behavioural response between rodents and primates, until these issues are resolved it must remain a possibility that they are of clinical significance.

4.2.4.3 The roles of D_3, D_4, D_5 and other putative dopamine receptor subtypes?

We are familiar with further physiological subdivision of established receptor subtypes, for example α_1-, α_2-, β_1- and β_2-adrenergic, M1 and M2 cholinergic and 5-HT_{1A}, 5-HT_{1B} and 5-HT_{1C}, and a variety of lines of evidence now suggest that D_1 and D_2 receptors may each exhibit further multiplicity. D_1 binding sites have been found in brain regions where dopamine fails to stimulate adenylyl cyclase, and when associated they appear to have a different subcellular distribution; similarly, displacement of D_1 binding and inhibition of dopamine-stimulated adenylyl cyclase show some pharmacological differences, while in behavioural and electrophysiological studies some dopaminergic actions of selective D_1 agonists appeared unrelated to their efficacy to stimulate adenylyl cyclase. Taken together, such findings indicate that there may exist subtypes of D_1 receptor that are coupled and uncoupled to adenylyl cyclase (see Mailman et al., 1986; Waddington, 1989a). Recent studies reinforce this notion (Murray & Waddington, 1989a; De Keyser et al., 1989a) and suggest that at least some of those D_1 receptors which do not stimulate adenylyl cyclase may be linked to alternative (PI?) transduction mechanisms (Mahan et al., 1990; Undie & Friedman, 1990). Within the family of 'D_1-like' receptors (see Section 4.1.2), the regional distribution of the D_{1b}/D_5 receptor appears to differ from that of the classical D_{1a} receptor; D_{1b}/D_5 receptors may have a corticolimbic, including hippocampal, distribution (Sunahara et al. 1991; Tiberi et al. 1991). In the absence of any ability of known D_1 antagonists to distinguish reliably between these subtypes, the clinical significance of such differences in their regional distribution are unknown but may need to be considered.

Long-standing suspicions of D_2 receptor heterogeneity have received new sustenance from behavioural (Rubinstein et al., 1988) and radioligand binding (De Keyser et al., 1989b but see Leonard et al., 1988) studies; further data indicating D_2 receptors associated with more than one form of D_1:D_2 interaction (Murray & Waddington, 1989b) and with more than one form of transduction mechanism (Vallar & Meldolesi, 1989) would be consistent with such heterogeneity. Within the family of 'D_2-like' receptors (see Section 4.1.2), the D_{2long} and D_{2short} splice variants (Eidne et al., 1989; Giros et al., 1989; Monsma et al., 1989; Grandy et al., 1989b; Chio et al., 1990) differ at a region of the receptor protein that may be involved in G-protein coupling; it is possible that these isoforms may be linked to different pathways of signal transduction. Furthermore, Todd et al. (1989) have described a D_2 receptor that appears to be the product of a gene distinct from those reported above and which may be coupled to an increase in intracellular Ca^{2+} independent of G-protein coupling. The regional distributions of the D_3 and of the D_4 receptor appear to differ from that of the classical D_2 receptor. Thus, the D_3 receptor is localized mainly to limbic regions, where it may be unassociated with adenylyl cyclase (Sokoloff *et al.*, 1990), while D_4 receptors may have a primarily corticolimbic localization (Van Tol *et al.*, 1991). Curiously, typical neuroleptics tended to show some preferential affinity for the classical D_2 receptor while certain atypical neuroleptics appeared to exhibit reduced D_2 preference; additionally, the atypical neuroleptic clozapine tended to show some preferential affinity for the D_4 receptor. However, these putative variations in preference were of little more than one order of magnitude. The clinical significance of such relatively modest differences in affinity may prove to be considerable, but they should not be overinterpreted in the absence of functional studies with agents which exhibit considerably higher selectivities for D_3, for D_4 and indeed for each of the new dopamine receptor subtypes identified by molecular biology.

4.3 'Selective' D_2 autoreceptor agonists, antagonists and partial agonists as putative antipsychotic agents

4.3.1 D_2 autoreceptor agonists and antagonists

4.3.1.1 Concept of 'selective' D_2 autoreceptor agonists of antipsychotic potential

An alternative route to the reduction of central dopaminergic neurotransmission is the stimulation of so-called autoreceptors (Carlsson, 1975). Behaviourally, low doses of the classical dopamine agonist apomorphine, considerably below those inducing behavioural stimulation and stereotypy, act to suppress spontaneous locomotor activity in a manner qualitatively similar to that of neuroleptics, and to induce a syndrome of sedation and yawning in rodents (Strombom, 1976; Di Chiara *et al.*, 1976; Gower *et al.*, 1984). The explanation offered was that such low doses of apomorphine reduce dopaminergic function via preferential activation of autoreceptors on the cell bodies and dendrites and on the presynaptic terminals of dopamine neurons, which mediate respectively the inhibition of neuronal activity and of dopamine synthesis and release (see Wolf & Roth, 1987; Chiodo, 1988). Both the nigrostriatal and mesolimbic dopaminergic systems appear to possess such autoreceptors, while their role in the regulation of the mesocortical system is more complex; cortical dopaminergic terminals may have release- but not synthesis-modulating autoreceptors while, with the possible exception of dopaminergic neurons projecting to the piriform cortex, somatodendritic autoreceptors may be absent in this system (Drukarch & Stoof, 1990). Autoreceptors appear to be of the D_2 subtype, and to function in a manner independent of interactions with D_1 receptor activity (Chiodo, 1988; Wachtel *et al.*, 1989).

It was believed that dopamine autoreceptors were pharmacologically distinct from their postsynaptic counterparts, and were characterized by considerably greater sensitivity to dopamine agonists such as apomorphine and bromocriptine. On this basis, 3-PPP was introduced as the first 'selective' dopamine autoreceptor agonist with apparently little or no action at normosensitive postsynaptic dopamine receptors (Hjorth *et al.*, 1981; but see Hjorth *et al.*, 1983), and agents such as B-HT 920 and EMD 49980 were subsequently proposed to have similar properties. This seemingly 'selective' action was variously proposed to have its basis in pre- and postsynaptic D_2 receptors being distinct entities, or in such agents being D_2 agonists of low efficacy and thus interacting preferentially with presynaptic receptors because of their reduced tonic dopaminergic input or larger receptor reserve in comparison with postsynaptic sites (see Drukarch & Stoof, 1990). Independent of the precise mechanism involved, the effect of typical dopamine agonists at low doses or of 'selective' dopamine auroreceptor agonists should be to reduce endogenous dopaminergic neurotransmission through both D_1 and D_2 receptors; thus, by generalization from the actions of typical dopamine antagonists, such agonists should also exert antipsychotic activity, while their failure to induce catalepsy in animals might indicate a low liability to induce extrapyramidal side-effects.

4.3.1.2 Clinical evidence

Initial systematic clinical studies with low doses of apomorphine did indeed report significant acute antipsychotic activity (Corsini *et al.*, 1977; Tamminga *et al.*, 1978), with the short duration of action of intramuscular or subcutaneous apomorphine necessitating rapid assessment procedures. However, subsequent studies with apomorphine, its orally active analogue *N*-propylnorapomorphine and ergot derivatives such as bromocriptine have more commonly produced less impressive, more inconsistent or negative results, and have indicated that in those circumstances where antipsychotic activity is evident acutely, it appears to be subject to rapid tolerance thereafter. The side-effects encountered most commonly were nausea and hypotension (see Tamminga *et al.*, 1986).

In relation to putative 'selective' dopamine autoreceptor agonists, there was no significant overall reduction in Brief Psychiatric Rating Scale (BPRS) scores for ten patients suffering from an acute episode of paranoid schizophrenia who were given B-HT 920, with only four patients showing meaningful amelioration of psychotic symptoms over 21 days, though all patients responded subsequently to neuroleptics. While no extrapyramidal side-effects were encountered, 7 of 12 patients treated initially showed a marked increase in psychomotor activity, which required discontinuation from the trial in two instances (Wiedemann *et al.*, 1990). Similarly, there was no significant overall reduction in BPRS scores for seven patients with primarily positive schizophrenic symptoms, who were given EMD 49980, only two of whom showed meaningful amelioration of psychotic symptoms and three of whom showed exacerbation of their symptoms; three patients experienced marked psychomotor activation necessitating discontinuation from the trial. In ten neuroleptic-free patients with primarily negative schizophrenic symptoms there was no significant overall effect of EMD 49980, with only two patients showing meaningful amelioration of such features and two patients developing positive symptoms to an extent requiring withdrawal from the study; this agent was generally well tolerated and no extrapyramidal side-effects were evident (Benkert *et al.*, 1990).

4.3.1.3 Cautionary observations

Despite what appeared to be a sound theoretical basis for such clinical studies, results to date have been inconsistent; sometimes significant but often unimpressive or negative findings have been reported, against a background of considerable inter-patient variability in response. However, several lines of evidence now suggest that the theoretical basis for the 'selective' dopamine autoreceptor agonist strategy may be much more complex than originally envisaged.

First, it now appears that dopamine autoreceptors and postsynaptic D_2 receptors are similar if not identical entities (Drukarch & Stoof, 1990); pharmacologically, 'selective' dopamine autoreceptor agonists such as B-HT 920 can show postsynaptic effects in synergism with a D_1 agonist, given to replace tonic activity through D_1 receptors (see Section 4.2.1) that is lost via reduced dopamine release (see Waddington & O'Boyle 1989), or in animals with supersensitive dopamine receptors, and may be better considered as D_2 agonists of reduced efficacy (see Arnt & Hyttel, 1990).

Secondly, there is a body of data indicating that suppression of spontaneous motor activity and induction of yawning by low 'autoreceptor-selective' doses of apomorphine are dissociable from reductions in extracellular levels of dopamine, and that they may be mediated by a subtype of postsynaptic D_2 receptor (see Stahle & Ungerstedt, 1990, and Section 4.2.4.3). There is contradictory evidence as to whether at least one element of this putative 'autoreceptor' syndrome, yawning, might involve receptors with a particular postsynaptic D_2-like profile in terms of cooperative/ synergistic interaction with D_1 receptors (Serra *et al.*, 1987; Spina *et al.*, 1989; but see Yamada *et al.*, 1990).

Thirdly, there is apparently complementary behavioural and electrophysiological evidence that repeated treatment with low 'autoreceptor-selective' doses of apomorphine is associated both with tolerance to suppression of spontaneous motility (Masuda *et al.*, 1987) and with some desensitization to inhibition of dopaminergic neuronal activity (Jeziorski & White, 1989).

Despite the inconsistent clinical experience to date and the emergence of the caveats and new notions discussed above, there is still considerable interest in the autoreceptor strategy for antipsychotic drug design and thus in identifying a new generation of 'autoreceptor-selective' dopamine agonists. U-68553B (Piercey *et al.*, 1990) has recently been reported to act as a potent autoreceptor agonist and to show less tolerance on repeated administration, in comparison with apomorphine. Furthermore while earlier 'selective' autoreceptor agonists such as 3-PPP did not inhibit conditioned avoidance responding in rats (Arnt *et al.*, 1983), a behavioural test widely used to predict antipsychotic activity (see Section 4.2.3), the new autoreceptor agonist PD 128483 (Heffner *et al.*, 1990) appears to inhibit such behaviour in non-human primates. Clarification of any antipsychotic potential for these and other similar agents will require both further study of the relevant dopaminergic processes and feedback from appropriate clinical trials.

Putative preferential autoreceptor antagonists such as (+)-AJ76 and (+)-UH232 have also been described (Svensson *et al.*, 1986). The most recent studies (Svensson *et al.*, 1990) indicate such agents to stimulate activity in habituated animals but to inhibit both dopaminergic stimulant-induced hyperactivity and intracranial self-stimulation. While such preliminary findings have been interpreted as of potential relevance for the treatment of negative and positive schizophrenic symptoms, respectively, these preliminary notions have yet to be explored more systematically and there is as yet no clinical feedback.

4.3.2 D_2 partial agonists

4.3.2.1 Concept of partial D_2 agonists of antipsychotic potential

This strategy has its origins in classical pharmacological concepts and in the primary mechanism of action of typical neuroleptic drugs. Partial agonists show affinity for, but lower intrinsic activity at, a given class of receptor than do conventional, full agonists, and show a reduced maximal agonist response (efficacy).

The prototype partial D_2 agonist terguride (transdihydrolisuride; Wachtel & Dorow, 1983; Koller & Herbster, 1987) and the subsequent agents OPC 4392 (Kiuchi *et al.*, 1988), SDZ 208-911 and SDZ 208-912 (Coward *et al.*, 1990), and (+)N-0437 (Timmerman *et al.*, 1990) have been claimed to have some of the following general properties in animals: attenuation of dopamine agonist-induced behavioural stimulation and of conditioned avoidance and intracranial self-stimulation behaviour; questionable induction of catalepsy; evident D_2 agonist activity at supersensitive D_2 receptors and in the inhibition of prolactin secretion, but without induction of emesis. An agent with such properties at D_2 receptors might act as a D_2 antagonist under circumstances of high dopaminergic activity or as a limited D_2 agonist under circumstances of low dopaminergic activity, and thus exert therapeutic effects both on the positive and on the negative symptoms of schizophrenia; additionally, it might have less liability to induce acute extrapyramidal side-effects (Coward *et al.*, 1989).

4.3.2.2 Preliminary clinical evidence

In 11 neuroleptic-withdrawn patients with a predominance of negative schizophrenic symptoms, 4 weeks of treatment with terguride was associated with a significant (but not complete) reduction in overall negative symptom scores, amelioration being evident in eight of the cases; there was no indication of acute exacerbation of positive symptoms (Schanz et al., 1988). Similarly, administration of OPC 4392 for 6 weeks to eight schizophrenic patients resulted in significant overall amelioration of negative symptoms. Although extrapyramidal side-effects were not observed, nausea and vomiting were evident over the first days of treatment (Gerbaldo et al., 1988).

Of the agents studied to date, SDZ 208-912 is reported to show particularly low intrinsic activity at D_2 receptors, and has recently been administered to 48 schizophrenic patients for a 4-week period. In this study 75% of patients were found to show a 'moderate to very good' response, which included amelioration both of positive and of negative symptoms; this was at the expense of 'mild to moderate' extrapyramidal side-effects, which necessitated anticholinergic medication in 13% of patients (Naber et al., 1990).

4.3.2.3 Cautionary observations

A number of problems present themselves in relation to these concepts. First, some authors have questioned the use of the term partial agonists to describe drugs of this type. Rather than failing to elicit a maximal response comparable to that of full agonists in given test systems, these agents might be better described as showing the properties of a full agonist or antagonist depending upon the experimental procedure employed (Koller & Herbster, 1987). Furthermore, other authors have proposed D_2 autoreceptor agonists to be low efficacy, that is, partial, agonists (see Section 4.3.1.3); on this basis, D_2 autoreceptor agonist and D_2 partial agonist effects would be variants of the same pharmacological property, differing only in emphasis and descriptor employed.

Secondly, there are some contradictory data on the actions of these drugs; for example, as to whether they induce catalepsy (Wachtel & Dorow, 1983; Koller & Herbster, 1987) or are essentially devoid of such activity (Coward et al., 1990); as described (Section 4.3.2.1), acute extrapyramidal side-effects have been noted in initial clinical studies.

Clearly, further preclinical studies are necessary to define in more detail the pharmacological actions of such agents. However, despite these caveats, the available experimental evidence has justified proceeding to clinical trials. The limited but provocative data available to date should be a spur to more systematic, controlled studies in carefully defined patient groups to better specify their therapeutic effects in relation to side-effects liability.

4.4 Implications for the dopamine hypothesis of schizophrenia

It is important to distinguish between the dopamine hypothesis of schizophrenia and the dopamine hypothesis of antipsychotic drug action. The latter proposes that reduction of dopaminergic function via either blockade of postsynaptic receptors or attenuation of presynaptic neuronal activity underlays the therapeutic effect of most known antipsychotic agents. Conversely, the former takes this concept a stage further and from it proposes that dopaminergic hyperfunction, via either supersensitivity of postsynaptic receptors or elevated activity of presynaptic neuronal activity, is an important element in the pathophysiology of schizophrenia (Carlsson, 1988).

The notions discussed in this chapter concern variants of this long-standing dopamine hypothesis of antipsychotic drug action, in terms of differing roles for distinct receptor subtypes in regulating dopamine-mediated function. In themselves, they do not yet demand any fundamental revision to the dopamine hypothesis of schizophrenia, pending more extensive feedback from clinical trials, but there are other reasons for contemplating such revision. Philosophically, the one hypothesis need not follow necessarily from the other. Indeed the search for neurochemical correlates of putative dopaminergic hyperfunction, either in post-mortem brain tissue (see Reynolds, 1989) or *in vivo* by positron emission tomography (PET; see Waddington, 1989d, and Chapter 5), has produced insubstantial or contradictory findings. Furthermore, much current theory considers schizophrenia to be a neurodevelopmental disorder of early origin (Weinberger, 1987; Murray & Lewis, 1987; Waddington & Torrey, 1991), with an emerging focus from recent neuropathological and magnetic resonance imaging studies on dysplasia of temporal lobe and related structures (Roberts, 1990; Waddington *et al.*, 1990; Waddington & Torrey, 1991). Curiously, one of the temporal lobe regions implicated more consistently in these processes, the parahippocampal gyrus/entorhinal cortex, shows in animals not only the high ratio of D_1 to D_2 receptor densities characteristic of several cortical regions but also an unusually high endogenous dopamine content (Dewar & Reader, 1989); the significance of these associations is unclear, but may repay further study.

Regarding the dopamine hypothesis of antipsychotic drug action at D_1 versus D_2 receptors, new insights have been suggested by several recent findings. Fundamentally, there is a widely perceived discrepancy between the acute dopamine receptor-blocking activity of neuroleptics and their delayed therapeutic effects; this has been approached by considering secondary effects consequent to primary dopamine receptor blockade (Pickar, 1988), or by questioning the substance of the perceived discrepancy (Keck *et al.*, 1989). In relation to the problems of extrapyramidal side-effects and/or lack of therapeutic efficacy, direct studies of neuroleptic action have been made possible by PET techniques: patients with parkinsonism or akathisia tend to have higher neuroleptic occupancies of D_2 receptors (Farde *et al.*, 1989), suggesting the possibility of defining on an individual basis a threshold occupancy for therapeutic efficacy with versus without such side-effects. Patients who show little or no therapeutic response have neuroleptic occupancies of D_2 receptors indistinguishable from those of responders (Wolkin *et al.*, 1989), suggesting that non-responders and responders might differ in pathophysiology. Provocatively, the atypical neuroleptic clozapine, which not only appears to induce fewer extrapyramidal side-effects but may be efficacious in some patients unresponsive to typical neuroleptics (Kane *et al.*, 1988), shows the highest occupancy of D_1 and lowest occupancy of D_2 receptors among all neuroleptics examined so far (Farde *et al.*, 1989). Indeed, in animal studies, clozapine appears to exert preferential attenuation of D_1 receptor-mediated function (see Murray & Waddington, 1990; also Chapter 2).

Though it remains important not to overlook the possible role(s) of non-dopaminergic systems in the pathophysiology of schizophrenia and in antipsychotic drug action (Reynolds, 1989; Kerwin, 1989; Carlsson & Carlsson, 1990; Itzhak & Stein, 1990; Waddington & Torrey, 1991), it should be emphasized that clarification of whether selective D_1 antagonists do or do not show therapeutic efficacy in this disorder will be a watershed in the evolution of these concepts (Waddington & Daly, 1992). Furthermore, the putative roles of individual, molecular biologically defined members of the 'D_1-like' (D_{1a}, D_{1b}/D_5) and of the 'D_2-like' (D_{2long}, D_{2short}, D_3 and D_4) families of dopamine receptor in mediating antipsychotic activity remain enigmatic, but may in the future challenge further our present perspectives.

Acknowledgements

The author's studies are supported by the Wellcome Trust, the Health Research Board and the Royal College of Surgeons in Ireland.

References

Andersen, P.H., Groenvald, F.C., Hohlweg, R. *et al.* (1988) *Soc. Neurosci. Abstr.* **14**, 935.

Andersen, P.H., Gingrich, J.A., Bates, M.D. *et al.* (1990) *Trends Pharmacol. Sci.* **11**, 231–236.

Arnt, J. (1987) In *Dopamine Receptors* (eds Creese, I. & Fraser, C.M.), pp. 199–231, New York, Alan R. Liss.

Arnt, J. & Hyttel, J. (1990) *J. Neural Transm.* **80**, 33–50.

Arnt, J., Christensen, A.V., Hyttel, J. *et al.* (1983) *Eur. J. Pharmacol.* **86** 185–198.

Bedard, P.J. & Boucher, R. (1989) *Neurosci. Lett.* **104**, 223–228.

Benkert, O., Wetzel, H. & Wiedemann, K. (1990) *Clin. Neuropharmacol.* **13** (Suppl. 2), 178–179.

Bertorello, A.M., Hopfield, J.F., Aperia, A. & Greengard, P. (1990) *Nature* **347**, 386–388.

Boyce, S., Rupniak, N.M.J., Steventon, M.J. & Iversen, S.D. (1990) *Neurology* **40**, 927–933.

Braun, A., Mouradain, M.M., Mohr, E. *et al.* (1989) *J. Neurol. Neurosurg. Psychiat.* **52**, 631–635.

Breese, G. & Creese, I. (1986) *Neurobiology of Central D-1 Dopamine Receptors*, New York,

Plenum Press.

Bunzow, J.R., Van Tol, H.H., Grandy, D.K. *et al.* (1988) *Nature* **336**, 783–787.

Carlsson, A. (1975) In *Pre- and Post-synaptic Receptors* (eds Usdin, E. & Bunney, W.E.), pp. 49–65, New York, Marcel-Dekker.

Carlsson, A. (1988) *Neuropsychopharmacology* **1**, 179–186.

Carlsson, M. & Carlsson, A. (1990) *Trends Neurosci.* **13**, 272–276.

Casey, D.E. (1992) *Psychopharmacology* **107**, 18–220.

Chio, C.L., Hess, G.F., Graham, R.S. & Huff, R.M. (1990) *Nature* **343**, 266–269.

Chiodo, L.A. (1988) *Neurosci. Biobehav. Rev.* **12**, 49–91.

Chipkin, R.E. (1990) *Trends Pharmacol. Sci.* **11**, 185.

Chipkin, R.E., Iorio, L.C., Coffin, V.L. *et al.* (1988) *J. Pharmacol. Exp. Ther.* **247**, 1093–1102.

Clark, D. & White, F.J. (1987) *Synapse* **1**, 347–388.

Close, S.P., Elliott, P.J., Hayes, A.G. & Marriott, A.S. (1990) *Psychopharmacology* **102**, 295–300.

Coffin, V.K., Latranyi, M.B. & Chipkin, R.E. (1989) *J. Pharmacol. Exp. Ther.* **249**, 769–774.

Corsini, G.U., Del Zompo, M., Manconi, S. *et al.* (1977) *Adv. Biochem. Psychopharmacol.* **16**, 645–649.

Coward, D., Dixon, K., Enz, A. *et al.* (1989) *Psychopharmacol. Bull.* **25**, 393–397.

Coward, D., Dixon, A.K., Urwyler, S. *et al.* (1990) *J. Pharmacol. Exp. Ther.* **252**, 279–285.

Creese, I., Sibley, D.R., Hamblin, M.W. & Leff, S.E. (1983) *Ann. Rev. Neurosci.* **6**, 43–71.

Daly, S.A. & Waddington, J.L. (1992) *Eur. J. Pharmacol.* **213**, 251–258.

Dearry, A., Gingrich, J.A., Falardeau, P. *et al.* (1990) *Nature* **347**, 72–76.

De Keyser, J., Walraevens, H., Ebinger, G. & Vauquelin, G. (1989a) *J. Neurochem.* **53**, 1096–1102.

De Keyser, J., Walraevens, H., de Backer, J.-P. *et al.* (1989b) *Brain Res.* **484**, 36–42.

Dewar, K.M. & Reader, T.A. (1989) *Synapse* **4**, 378–386.

Di Chiara, G., Porceddu, M.L., Vargiu, L. *et al.* (1976) *Nature* **264**, 564–567.

Drukarch, B. & Stoof, J.C. (1990) *Life Sci.* **47**, 361–376.

Eidne, K.A., Taylor, P.L., Zabavnik, J. *et al.* (1989) *Nature* **342**, 865.

Ellenbroek, B.A., Peeters, B.W., Honig, W.M. & Cools, A.R. (1987) *Psychopharmacology* **93**, 343–348.

Ellenbroek, B.A., Willemen, A.P. & Cools, A.R. (1989) *Neuropsychopharmacology* **2**, 191–199.

Fabbrini, G., Bran, A., Mouradian, M.M. *et al.* (1988) *J. Neural Transm.* **71**, 155–163.

Farde, L. (1992) *Psychopharmacology* **107**, 23–29.

Farde, L., Wiesel, F.A., Nordstrom, A.-L. & Sedvall, G. (1989) *Psychopharmacology* **99** (Suppl.), S28–S31.

Gerbaldo, H., Demisch, L. & Bochnik, H.J. (1988) *Psychopharmacology* **96** (Suppl.), S238.

Giros, B., Sokoloff, P., Martres, M.-P. *et al.* (1989) *Nature* **342**, 923–926.

Gower, A.J., Berendsen, H.H., Princen, M.M. & Broekkamp, C.L. (1984) *Eur. J. Pharmacol.* **103**, 81–89.

Grandy, D.K., Litt, M., Allen, L. *et al.* (1989a) *Am. J. Hum. Genet.* **45**, 778–785.

Grandy, D.K., Marchionni, M.A., Makam, H. *et al.* (1989b) *Proc. Natl. Acad. Sci., USA* **86**, 9762–9766.

Heffner, T.G., Christoffersen, C.L., Cooke, L.W. *et al.* (1990) *Soc. Neurosci. Abstr.* **16**, 589.

Hjorth, S., Carlsson, A., Wilkstrom, H. *et al.* (1981) *Life Sci.* **28**, 1225–1238.

Hjorth, S., Carlsson, A., Clark, D. *et al.* (1983) *Psychopharmacology* **81**, 89–99.

Itzhak, Y. & Stein, I. (1990) *Life Sci.* **47**, 1073–1081.

Jeziorski, M. & White, F.J. (1989) *Synapse* **4**, 267–280.

Kane, J., Honigfeld, G., Singer, J., Meltzer, H.Y. & the Clozaril Collaborative Study Group

(1988) *Arch. Gen. Psychiat.* **45**, 789-795.

Kebabian, J.W. (1978) *Life Sci.* **23**, 479-483.

Kebabian, J.W. & Calne, D.B. (1979) *Nature* **277**, 93-96.

Keck, P.E., Cohen, B., Baldessarini, R.J. & McElroy, S.L. (1989) *Am. J. Psychiat.* **146**, 1289-1292.

Kerkman, D.J., Ackerman, M., Artman, L.D. *et al.* (1989) *Eur. J. Pharmacol.* **166**, 481-491.

Kerwin, R.W. (1989) *Psychol. Med.* **19**, 563-567.

Kiuchi, K., Hirata, Y., Minami, M. & Nagatsu, T. (1988) *Life Sci.* **42**, 343-349.

Koller, W.C. & Herbster, G. (1987) *Neurology* **37**, 723-727.

LaHoste, G.J. & Marshall, J.F. (1990) *Behav. Brain Res.* **38**, 233-242.

Leonard, M.N., Halliday, C.A., Marriott, A.S. & Strange, P.G. (1988) *Biochem. Pharmacol.* **37**, 4335-4339.

Mahan, L.C., Burch, R.M., Monsma, F.J. & Sibley, D.R. (1990) *Proc. Natl. Acad. Sci., USA* **87**, 2196-2200.

Mailman, R.B., Schulz, D.W., Kilts, C.D. *et al.* (1986) In *Neurobiology of Central D-1 Dopamine Receptors* (eds Breese, G. & Creese, I.), pp. 53-72, New York, Plenum Press.

Masuda, Y., Murai, S., Saito, H. *et al.* (1987) *Pharmacol. Biochem. Behav.* **28**, 35-37.

Monsma, F.J., McVittie, L.D., Gerfen, C.R. *et al.* (1989) *Nature* **342**, 926-929.

Monsma, F.J., Mahan, L.C., McVittie, L.D. *et al.* (1990) *Proc. Natl. Acad. Sci., USA* **87**, 6723-6727.

Murray, A.M. & Waddington, J.L. (1989a) *Eur. J. Pharmacol.* **160**, 377-384.

Murray, A.M. & Waddington, J.L. (1989b) *Psychopharmacology* **98**, 245-250.

Murray, A.M. & Waddington, J.L. (1990) *Eur. J. Pharmacol.* **186**, 79-86.

Murray, R.M. & Lewis, S.W. (1987) *Br. Med. J.* **295**, 681-682.

Naber, D., Macher, J.-P., Gerlach, J. *et al.* (1990) *Abstracts of the XVIIth Congress of the Collegium Internationale Neuro-Psychopharmacologicum* **2**, 252.

Peacock, L., Lubin, H. & Gerlach, J. (1990) *Eur. J. Pharmacol.* **186**, 49-59.

Pickar, D. (1988) *Schizophrenia Bull.* **14**, 255-268.

Piercey, M.F., Broderick, P.A., Hoffman, W.E. & Vogelsang, G.D. (1990) *J. Pharmacol. Exp. Ther.* **254**, 369-374.

Reynolds, G.P. (1989) *Br. J. Psychiat.* **155**, 305-316.

Roberts, G.W. (1990) *Trends Neurosci.* **13**, 207-211.

Robertson, G.S. & Robertson, H.A. (1987) *Trends Pharmacol. Sci.* **8**, 295-299.

Rouillard, C., Bedard, P.J. & Di Paulo, T. (1990) *Eur. J. Pharmacol.* **185**, 209-215.

Rubinstein, M., Gershanik, O. & Stefano, F.J. (1988) *Naunyn-Schmiedeberg's Arch. Pharmacol.* **337**, 115-117.

Schanz, H., Olbrich, R. & Aufdembrinke, B. (1988) *Psychopharmacology* **96** (Suppl.), S239.

Seeman, P. (1980) *Pharmacol. Rev.* **32**, 229-313.

Seeman, P., Niznik, H.B., Guan, H.-C. *et al.* (1989) *Proc. Natl. Acad. Sci., USA* **86**, 10156-10160.

Serra, G., Collu, M. & Gessa, G.L. (1987) *Psychopharmacology* **91**, 330-333.

Sibley, D.R. & Monsma, F.J. (1992) *Trends Pharmacol. Sci.* **13**, 61-69.

Sokoloff, P., Giros, B., Martres, M.-P. *et al.* (1990) *Nature* **347**, 146-151.

Spano, P.F., Govoni, S. & Trabucci, M. (1978) *Adv. Biochem. Psychopharmacol.* **19**, 155-165.

Spina, L., Longoni, R., Mulas, A. & Di Chiara, G. (1989) *Psychopharmacology* **98**, 567-568.

Stahle, L. & Ungerstedt, U. (1990) *Pharmacol. Biochem. Behav.* **35**, 201-209.

Strombom, U. (1976) *Naunyn-Schmiedeberg's Arch. Pharmacol.* **292**, 167-176.

Sunahara, R.K., Niznik, H.B., Weiner, D.M. *et al.* (1990) *Nature* **347**, 80-83.

Sunahara, R.K., Guan, H.-C., O'Dowd, B.F. *et al.* (1991) *Nature* **350**, 614-619.

Svensson, K., Johansson, A.M., Magnusson, T. & Carlsson, A. (1986) *Naunyn-

Schmiedeberg's Arch. Pharmacol. **334**, 234-245.

Svensson, K., Kling-Petersen, T., Waters, N. *et al.* (1990) *Abstracts of the XVIIth Congress of the Collegium Internationale Neuro-Psychopharmacologicum* **2**, 311.

Sweidan, S., Edinger, H. & Siegel, A. (1990) *Pharmacol. Biochem. Behav.* **36**, 491-499.

Tamminga, C.A., Schaffer, M.H., Smith, R.C. & Davis, J.M. (1978) *Science* **200**, 567-568.

Tamminga, C.A., Gotts, M.D., Thaker, G.K. *et al.* (1986) *Arch. Gen. Psychiat.* **43**, 398-402.

Tiberi, M., Jarvie, K.R., Silvia, C. *et al.* (1991) *Proc. Natl. Acad. Sci., USA* **88**, 7491-7495.

Timmerman, W., Tepper, P.G., Bohus, B.G. & Horn, A.S. (1990) *Eur. J. Pharmacol.* **181**, 253-260.

Todd, R.D., Khurana, T.S., Sajovic, P. *et al.* (1989) *Proc. Natl. Acad. Sci., USA* **86**, 10134-10138.

Trampus, M. & Ongini, E. (1990) *Neuropharmacology* **29**, 889-893.

Undie, A.S. & Friedman, E. (1990) *J. Pharmacol. Exp. Ther.* **253**, 987-992.

Vallar, L. & Meldolesi, J. (1989) *Trends Pharmacol. Sci.* **10**, 74-77.

Vallar, L., Muca, C., Magni, M. *et al.* (1990) *J. Biol. Chem.* **265**, 10320-10326.

Van Tol, H.H.M., Bunzow, J.R., Guan, H.-C. *et al.* (1991) *Nature* **350**, 610-614.

Wachtel, H. & Dorow, R. (1983) *Life Sci.* **32**, 421-432.

Wachtel, S.R., Hu, X.-T., Galloway, M.P. & White, F.J. (1989) *Synapse* **4**, 327-346.

Waddington, J.L. (1986) *Biochem. Pharmacol.* **35**, 3661-3667.

Waddington, J.L. (1988) *Gen. Pharmacol.* **19**, 55-60.

Waddington, J.L. (1989a) *J. Psychopharmacol.* **3**, 54-63.

Waddington, J.L. (1989b) *Int. Rev. Neurobiol.* **31**, 297-353.

Waddington, J.L. (1989c) *Curr. Opinion Psychiat.* **2**, 89-92.

Waddington, J.L. (1989d) *Br. J. Psychiat.* **154**, 433-436.

Waddington, J.L. (1990) *Psychopharmacology* **101**, 431-447.

Waddington, J.L. & Daly, S.A. (1992) In *Novel Antipsychotic Drugs* (ed. Meltzer, H.Y.), pp. 109-115, New York, Raven Press.

Waddington, J.L. & O'Boyle, K.M. (1987) *Rev. Neurosci.* **1**, 157-184.

Waddington, J.L. & O'Boyle, K.M. (1989) *Pharmacol. Ther.* **43**, 1-52.

Waddington, J.L. & Torrey, E.F. (1991) *Arch. Gen. Psychiat.* **48**, 271-273.

Waddington, J.L., O'Callaghan, E., Larkin, C. *et al.* (1990) *Br. J. Psychiat.* **157**, (Suppl. 9), 56-65.

Walters, J.R., Bergstrom, D.A., Carlson, J.H. *et al.* (1987) *Science* **236**, 719-722.

Weinberger, D.R. (1987) *Arch. Gen. Psychiat.* **44**, 660-669.

Wiedemann, K., Benkert, O. & Holsboer, F. (1990) *Pharmacopsychiatry* **23**, 50-55.

Wolf, M.E. & Roth, R.H. (1987) In *Dopamine Receptors* (eds Creese, I. & Fraser, C.M.), pp. 45-96, New York, Alan R. Liss.

Wolkin, A., Barouche, F., Wolf, A.P. *et al.* (1989) *Am. J. Psychiat.* **146**, 905-908.

Yamada, K., Nagashima, M., Kimura, H. *et al.* (1990) *Psychopharmacology* **100**, 141-144.

Zhou, Q.-Y., Grandy, D.K., Thambi, L. *et al.* (1990) *Nature* **347**, 76-80.

CHAPTER 5

PREDICTION OF ANTIPSYCHOTIC ACTIVITY

Nadia M.J. Rupniak and Susan D. Iversen

Merck Sharp and Dohme Research Laboratories, Neuroscience Research Centre, Terlings Park, Harlow, Essex

Table of Contents

5.1 Introduction

Accurate prediction of a drug's therapeutic potential requires an understanding of the pathophysiology of the disease and convincing preclinical screens. For some CNS diseases, neuropathology is well defined and can be mimicked in experimental animals. Thus, neurological conditions closely resembling stroke and parkinsonism can be produced in animals, enabling the efficacy of new test drugs to be assessed using quantifiable end-points. However, as argued by Kumar (1977), our ability to reproduce human *psycho*pathology in animal models more often resembles an act of faith.

No specific lesion or neurochemical abnormality has yet been identified in schizophrenia against which drugs may be directed in animal screens. In the absence of a clear biochemical target one way to approximate the disease could be to develop

ANTIPSYCHOTIC DRUGS AND THEIR SIDE-EFFECTS
ISBN 0-12-079035-1

models of abnormal behaviour in animals. However, although the effects of psychotomimetic agents in man have been argued to resemble schizophrenia, interpretation of the effects of such drugs in animals is controversial. Psychopathology is arguably a uniquely human disturbance of thought, language, perception and beliefs to which abnormal behaviours in animals (such as head-weaving, sniffing and hyperactivity) bear a tenuous relationship.

The ability of certain drugs to control psychosis was first discovered fortuitously in man; sadly, this method may remain the best way to identify new treatments. Modern drug therapy to control schizophrenia has its origins in the use of reserpine (Sen & Bose, 1931) and the subsequent discovery of the antipsychotic activity of chlorpromazine (Delay et al., 1952). The neuroleptic effects of these agents in man provided a major breakthrough for psychiatry. However, innovative approaches to drug therapy for schizophrenia have since remained virtually stagnant for almost four decades.

This impasse does not reflect the success of existing treatments. Rather, the lack of progress reflects the absence of a convincing animal model of schizophrenia combined with the introduction of strict ethical controls over drug trials in man which make it less likely that novel antipsychotic agents will be discovered in the clinic by accident.

There is an urgent need for effective antipsychotic medications which do not cause the extrapyramidal disturbances which were recognized as a serious side-effect of neuroleptic drugs as soon as 2 years after their introduction (Steck, 1954). Drug-induced involuntary movements were estimated to affect up to 88% of schizophrenics treated for 6 months or longer with classical neuroleptic drugs (Knights et al., 1979). Moreover, a significant proportion of patients fail to respond adequately to neuroleptic drugs (eapecially those with 'negative' symptoms such as social withdrawal and flattened affect).

5.2 Preclinical screens for antipsychotic drugs

Faced with these constraints, pharmaceutical screens have often been based on characterizing the in vitro and in vivo profiles of known antipsychotic drugs, all of which share the ability to block dopamine receptors (see Chapter 1). Using this 'criterion drug' approach the effects of new drug candidates on cerebral dopamine function may be quantified and their likely antipsychotic activity inferred from the similarity of this profile with that of existing drugs. This strategy has the advantage that new compounds can be directly compared with existing treatments regarding efficacy, potency and side-effect profile. Although it might be expected that antipsychotic activity is likely to be present in compounds with dopamine antagonist activity and that such screens therefore have good predictive utility, there are serious drawbacks to this approach. The first is that such screens, by definition, generate 'me too' drugs. It is no accident that new antipsychotic drugs introduced into routine clinical use since 1952 are all dopamine receptor antagonists. It is therefore hardly surprising that there is an extremely good correlation between antipsychotic potency in man and displacement of tritiated ligands from brain dopamine receptors *in vitro* (Seeman, 1980). This unremarkable correlation appears to lend credence to the use of dopamine receptor antagonism as a specific screen for antipsychotic activity. However, no convincing abnormality of cerebral dopamine function has been established in unmedicated schizophrenics (see Rupniak *et al.*, 1983 for review). Similarly, it is not established that antidopamine activity is a necessary prerequisite for antipsychotic activity. Indeed, it has been argued that such screens are more predictive of a drug's propensity to induce unwanted extrapyramidal side-effects than of antipsychotic activity (Greenblatt *et al.*, 1980). Equally stifling for drug discovery is the possibility that antipsychotic drugs with *novel* mechanisms of action might not be detected using conventional screens.

5.3 Desirable preclinical profile using dopamine antagonist screens

Dopamine receptor antagonists will, by definition, exhibit 'antipsychotic' profiles in screens designed to reflect the pharmacology of neuroleptic drugs (see Chapter 1). Since the atypical neuroleptics sulpiride and clozapine exhibited selective profiles in such screens (Chapters 2 and 3), particular emphasis has been given to tests of mesolimbic dopamine function as predictors of antipsychotic activity.

Although sulpiride and clozapine are unrelated structurally and have markedly different pharmacological spectra, both have been suggested to act selectively on the mesolimbic dopamine system and appear less likely than other neuroleptics to induce motor disturbances in patients. Like classical neuroleptics, these drugs inhibit hyperactivity induced by systemic administration of apomorphine (Ljundberg & Ungerstedt, 1978) or bilateral intra-accumbens injection of dopamine (Costall & Naylor, 1976). Unlike other dopamine antagonists, sulpiride and clozapine show weak activity in inducing catalepsy (Stille *et al.*, 1971; Costall & Naylor, 1975) or antagonizing apomorphine-induced stereotypy (Costall & Naylor, 1975). These latter behaviours are thought to be striatally mediated (Costall *et al.*, 1975). Moreover, chronic treatment for up to 12 months with sulpiride or clozapine, unlike haloperidol, did not induce striatal dopamine receptor supersensitivity (Rupniak *et al.*, 1984). These observations were in agreement with electrophysiological data in rodents demonstrating a selective depolarization block of neurons in the ventral tegmental area, but not the substantia nigra, following treatment for 21 days with sulpiride or clozapine. In contrast, classical neuroleptics like haloperidol did not exhibit a regionally selective effect (White & Wang, 1983). Lack of activity in assays of striatal dopamine function was considered a desirable profile likely to indicate a low risk for extrapyramidal side-effects because these observations were compatible with early clinical reports that clozapine did not induce extrapyramidal disturbances in man, even after chronic treatment (Matz et al., 1974; Claghorn et al., 1983).

However, there are several weaknesses in this argument. First, the lack of effect of clozapine using pharmacologically relevant doses in numerous antipsychotic screens led Burki et al. (1975) to doubt that dopamine receptor blockade was a plausible explanation for its antipsychotic effects. Secondly, a recent report indicates that sulpiride does indeed induce tardive dyskinesias in man (Achiron et al., 1990), despite its selective profile as a 'mesolimbic' dopamine antagonist in animal screens. Thirdly, there is no evidence that antagonism of mesolimbic dopamine function is maintained during continuous chronic treatment with neuroleptic drugs for many months in rodents (Clow et al., 1980; Rupniak et al., 1985). In contrast, the antipsychotic effect of neuroleptic drugs in man takes several weeks to emerge (Johnstone et al., 1978) and is maintained chronically. None the less, the notion that an ideal antipsychotic drug would be a selective mesolimbic dopamine antagonist on acute administration continues to receive widespread acceptance.

5.4 Preclinical profiles of novel agents suggesting antipsychotic activity

In the following sections we shall review the evidence proposed to indicate a neuroleptic-like profile for agents which do not act directly on cerebral dopamine receptors. These include compounds which antagonize cerebral dopamine function via interactions with other neurotransmitter systems (CCK or 5-HT), and compounds interacting with a putative receptor (sigma site) for which a subgroup of known antipsychotic agents show high affinity. Where possible these profiles will be compared with clinical evidence for antipsychotic efficacy.

5.4.1 CCK (cholecystokinin) agonists

CCK-like immunoreactivity coexists with dopamine in mesolimbic neurons (Hokfelt et al., 1980) where microiontophoretic application of dopamine or CCK have functionally antagonistic effects on neuronal firing rates (White & Wang, 1984). There is considerable evidence for a functional interaction between cerebral CCK and dopamine systems, which implicated possible alterations in mesolimbic peptides in the antipsychotic activity of neuroleptic drugs. For example, repeated administration of haloperidol to rodents induced functional supersensitivity to the electro-physiological effects of CCK and increased CCK binding sites in the nucleus accumbens (Chang et al., 1983; Debonnet et al., 1990).

Evidence from behavioural paradigms further indicated that CCK possessed neuroleptic-like properties which appeared specific for mesolimbic dopamine-mediated behaviours. Numerous reports indicated that intra-accumbens injection of CCK could antagonize the locomotor stimulation induced by dopamine agonists given systemically or by direct microinjections into the nucleus accumbens (Hoh & Katsuura, 1981; van Ree et al., 1983; Schneider et al., 1983; Weiss et al., 1988). However, interpretation of these findings is complicated by other observations that intra-accumbens injection of CCK may *potentiate* dopamine agonist-induced hyperactivity (Crawley et al., 1985; Vaccarino & Rankin, 1989). These conflicting findings appear to depend on rostral–caudal differences in accumbens CCK function (Vaccarino & Rankin, 1989) and may be mediated via distinct populations of CCK receptors. Thus, in slices of posterior nucleus accumbens tissue application of CCK-8 stimulated endogenous dopamine release, and this effect was blocked by the selective CCK-A receptor antagonist devazepide. Conversely, in slices of anterior nucleus accumbens, CCK-8 inhibited potassium-evoked dopamine release and this effect was blocked selectively by the CCK-B receptor antagonist L-365, 260 (Marshall et al., 1990).

Given these opposite effects on dopamine function within the nucleus accumbens it would not be expected that systemic administration of CCK should necessarily cause antipsychotic effects. To date there is no conclusive evidence for a beneficial effect of CCK or the non-selective agonist ceruletide either given alone or as an adjunct to neuroleptics in studies involving over 500 schizophrenics (see Montgomery & Green, 1988, for review). Moreover, the clinical potential for a CCK agonist in schizophrenia is clouded by likely gastrointestinal side-effects and the possibility of triggering panic attacks (de Montigny, 1989). In addition, systemic administration of a CCK agonist would also be expected to influence dopamine function at extrapyramidal sites and hence possible disturbances in motor control cannot be excluded. Indeed, ceruletide and CCK-8 (like classical neuroleptic drugs) are able to suppress drug-induced dyskinesias in schizophrenic patients (Nishikawa et al., 1988) and in primates (Boyce et al., 1990).

5.4.2 5-HT (5-hydroxytryptamine) antagonists

Successful treatment of depression and, more recently, anxiety with antagonists of 5-HT receptors raises the possibility of a similar beneficial effect in other psychiatric conditions including schizophrenia. There is considerable evidence for a regulatory role of 5-HT in dopamine-mediated behaviours. For example, direct intra-accumbens injections of 5-HT blocked hyperactivity induced by dopamine (Costall et al., 1976) and apomorphine-induced stereotyped behaviours were modified in a complex manner by 5-HT agonists and antagonists in rats (Carter & Pycock, 1981). The ways in which different subtypes of 5-HT receptor are involved in these behaviours is not yet known. At present, interest has focused on the possible use of selective 5-HT_2 and 5-HT_3 receptor antagonists as antipsychotics.

5.4.2.1   5-HT$_2$ receptor antagonists

Interest in this field originated from a series of 5-HT$_2$ antagonists of which setoperone was a member. Interestingly, the hallucinogenic effects of lysergic acid diethylamide (LSD) and phenylisopropylamines appear to be mediated through stimulation of brain 5-HT$_2$ receptors (Titeler *et al.*, 1988). At present there is no direct evidence that selective 5-HT$_2$ antagonists possess antipsychotic activity, but setoperone was initially thought to have antipsychotic potential because of its combined dopamine and 5-HT$_2$ antagonist activity (indicated by displacement of [^{3}H]spiperone and [^{3}H]ketanserin binding *in vitro*). Other agents with similar pharmacological profiles were able to antagonize stereotypy, hyperactivity and climbing induced by dopamine agonists in rodents (see Lowe *et al.*, 1988, for review). In rats treated for 28 days and then withdrawn from setoperone a marked increase in striatal [^{3}H]spiperone-binding sites was observed, identical to that induced by repeated treatment with classical neuroleptic drugs. Unlike this upregulation of dopamine receptors, 5-HT$_2$ binding sites were decreased following repeated treatment with setoperone (Leysen *et al.*, 1986). Interestingly, we also observed a downregulation of cortical 5-HT$_2$ receptors following treatment of rats for 12 months with clozapine (Reynolds *et al.*, 1983). This action is not typical for neuroleptic drugs, but has been proposed as a mechanism of action of antidepressants. In a single, open, pilot study, the effect of setoperone was examined in schizophrenics with predominantly negative symptoms withdrawn from neuroleptics. Impressive improvements in autism, dysphoria, hallucinations and extrapyramidal symptoms were reported (Ceulemans *et al.*, 1985). Similar effects were reported using risperidone, also a mixed dopamine/5-HT$_2$ antagonist (Castelao *et al.*, 1989; Marder, 1992). However, it is not possible to conclude that the beneficial effects of setoperone or risperidone are attributable to 5-HT$_2$, rather than dopamine, receptor antagonism. Further investigations using more selective 5-HT$_2$ antagonists in controlled, double-blind clinical trials are clearly required.

One agent claimed to be a pure 5-HT$_2$ antagonist is ritanserin. Although this agent did not block amphetamine-induced hyperactivity in rodents at doses up to 0.2 mg/kg (Goodwin & Green, 1985) this may merely indicate relatively poor brain penetration since, like setoperone, ritanserin is an antagonist at both dopamine and 5-HT$_2$ receptors *in vitro* (Leysen *et al.*, 1986). The clinical efficacy of ritanserin in alleviating negative symptoms was reported by Reyntjens *et al.* (1986) in schizophrenics receiving concurrent neuroleptic medication.

5.4.2.2   5-HT$_3$ receptor antagonists

An antipsychotic profile for selective 5-HT$_3$ antagonists including ondansetron and zacopride has recently been proposed. Ondansetron has no known affinity for other neurotransmitter receptors (Butler *et al.*, 1988) but appears able to modulate limbic dopamine overactivity. In rats and marmosets, focal or systemic administration of ondansetron was able to inhibit hyperactivity induced by either acute intra-accumbens injection of amphetamine or by chronic infusion of dopamine into the nucleus accumbens for 13 days (Costall *et al.*, 1988). Ondansetron also antagonized the hyperactivity and increase in dopamine turnover induced by injection of the neurokinin agonist di-MeC7 into the ventral tegmental area (Hagan *et al.*, 1987). However, using a similar treatment regime for ondansetron which was active in the chronic intra-accumbens dopamine infusion model in rats, Koulu *et al.* (1990) found no evidence for any alteration in dopamine or 5-HT metabolism in mesolimbic areas. Clinical trials with ondansetron in schizophrenia are currently underway to determine whether this agent has antipsychotic activity or not.

5.4.3 Sigma antagonists

Several agents developed recently as potential antipsychotics were thought to act as selective sigma receptor antagonists. The prototypic sigma ligand is the benzo-morphan (+)-SKF 10047. In man, narcotic antagonists such as this are psychoto-mimetic (Keats & Telford, 1964) and induce a syndrome of 'delerium' in chronic spinal dogs (Martin *et al.*, 1976) and a motor syndrome comprised of head-weaving, locomotor stimulation and ataxia in rodents and primates (Brady *et al.*, 1982). Existing compounds acting at sigma sites lack pharmacological selectivity and many cause alterations in dopamine, noradrenaline, 5-HT, opiate and N-methyl-D-aspartate (NMDA) systems (see Jurien & Leonard, 1989). However, the identification of the novel sigma binding site for (+)-SKF 10047 and the ability of certain neuroleptic drugs (including haloperidol and pimozide) to displace [^{3}H](+)-SKF 10047 from these binding sites (Su, 1982) led to the proposal that antagonists of the sigma receptor might possess antipsychotic activity without inducing extrapyramidal side-effects.

Compounds thought to possess sigma antagonist activity include rimcazole and BMY 14802. Rimcazole was first identified using classical neuroleptic screens and was described as a selective antagonist of mesolimbic dopamine function (Ferris *et al.*, 1986). However, the evidence upon which this claim was based (inhibition of dopamine agonist-induced climbing and hyperactivity induced by intra-accumbens infusion of dopamine) has not been published in full. In a single published study, Ferris *et al.* (1982) reported that rimcazole was able to antagonize apomorphine-induced aggression in rats, but not stereotypy or hyperactivity induced by intrastriatal infusion of dopamine. Unfortunately, aggressive behaviour is not known as a specific model for mesolimbic dopamine function. Rimcazole had low affinity for known neurotransmitter binding sites *in vitro* and these behavioural effects were therefore considered to be mediated indirectly. Subsequently, it was discovered that rimcazole binds with high affinity to brain sigma sites labelled by [^{3}H](+)-SKF 10047 *in vitro* (Ferris *et al.*, 1986) and that the activation of dopamine neurons in the ventral tegmental area by (+)-SKF 10047 could be blocked by rimcazole (Ceci *et al.*, 1988). The antipsychotic potential of rimcazole has been investigated in several open clinical trials using small numbers of patients (reviewed by Deutsch *et al.*, 1988). In some cases promising findings were obtained, but a significant number of patients failed to complete the studies owing to lack of efficacy or induction of adverse effects. The outcome of double-blind placebo-controlled trials with rimcazole is awaited.

A second agent not yet evaluated in schizophrenia thought to act as a sigma receptor antagonist is BMY 14802. Like rimcazole this agent is a potent displacer of [^{3}H](+)-SKF 10047 binding *in vitro* but has low affinity for other neurotransmitter receptors, including dopamine (Taylor & Dekleva, 1987). Unlike rimcazole, BMY 14802 was reported to antagonize conditioned avoidance behaviour and inhibit apomorphine-induced stereotypy (see Taylor & Dekleva, 1987).

Unfortunately, even if these agents are shown to possess antipsychotic activity in man, evidence is accumulating which makes it unlikely that this could be attributed to a selective inhibition of sigma receptors. In drug discrimination studies using pigeons, the effects of BMY 14802 generalized to the 5-HT$_{1A}$ agonists buspirone and 8-hydroxy-dipropylaminotetralin, but not to a range of sigma ligands including haloperidol (Vanecek *et al.*, 1989). Recently the failure to demonstrate a membrane-bound sigma receptor has raised serious doubts about the function of this binding site (McCann *et al.*, 1989). Moreover, the psychotomimetic effects of certain benzomorphan sigma ligands have been incorrectly attributed to the (+) enantiomer, which has greatest affinity for the sigma site. In fact, psychotomimetic effects were most common using the (−) enantiomer and may therefore be mediated via *opiate* receptors (see Connick *et al.*, 1990). Moreover, the induction of head-weaving and other behaviours in rodents and primates by these compounds does not correlate with their affinity for sigma binding sites *in vitro*; rather these effects appear attributable to interactions with phencyclidine receptors (McCann *et al.*, 1989; Boyce *et al.*, 1991). Finally, it is unlikely that sigma antagonists would be antipsychotic agents devoid of unwanted motor side-effects since a number of sigma ligands, including haloperidol, induced dystonic posturing (torticollis) in rats following microinjection into the red nucleus (Walker *et al.*, 1988).

5.5 Discussion and targets for future research

Considerable efforts have been directed towards discovery of a safe and novel pharmacotherapeutic approach for schizophrenia. To date, these attempts have failed to identify a treatment of comparable efficacy to neuroleptic drugs. Lack of pharmacological specificity of development compounds, poor definition of receptor function and apparently unpredictive preclinical screens are factors contributing to this failure. Without establishing that antipsychotic activity can be achieved by a novel mechanism there is still no proof that antipsychotic activity can be dissociated from dopamine receptor antagonism. How then might we discover new leads in this area?

One way to break this deadlock might be to examine more closely other types of treatment successfully employed to control schizophrenia. Prior to the introduction of neuroleptic drugs, schizophrenia was treated using carbon dioxide inhalation, insulin coma, pentylenetetrazol-induced convulsions and electroconvulsive therapy (ECT). With the exception of ECT these techniques became obsolete with the advent of drug therapy and detailed investigation of whether they produced genuine symptomatic relief or had any common mechanism of action was not undertaken. ECT was first introduced to treat psychosis following anecdotal reports of the antithetical relationship between seizure incidence and psychosis subsequently confirmed in temporal lobe epileptics by Flor-Henry (1969). Surgical relief of temporal lobe epilepsy may even cause the *onset* of psychosis in some patients (Stevens, 1966). The efficacy of ECT in the treatment of acute schizophrenia has been clearly established in double-blind controlled studies (Taylor & Fleminger, 1980; Brandon *et al.*, 1985). Although ECT has been used for over 60 years, its mechanism of action remains unknown. Numerous studies in rodents suggested alterations in monoamine neurotransmission, but this has not yet been confirmed in patients (Slade & Checkley, 1980). Interestingly, inhibition of dopamine (and noradrenaline) function using reserpine or 6-hydroxydopamine in rodents increases susceptibility to seizure activity (Corcoran *et al.*, 1974), whilst dopamine agonists protect against seizures (Anlezark *et al.*, 1978). Thus the possibility exists that the antipsychotic effects of both ECT and neuroleptic drugs could be linked to seizure activity. (However, there is no direct evidence for a marked effect of neuroleptic drugs on seizure threshold.)

Over the last decade converging lines of evidence have implicated an abnormality in glutamate function in schizophrenia. This hypothesis could perhaps account for the beneficial effects of ECT and neuroleptic drugs in psychosis. The glutamate hypothesis was first advanced following the discovery of low CSF glutamate levels in schizophrenics which could not be attributed to neuroleptic medication (Kim *et al.*, 1980). Post-mortem abnormalities in glutamate receptors in the frontal and temporal lobes of schizophrenics have also been reported (for example, Nishikawa *et al.*, 1983). Cerebral glutamate-induced excitotoxicity might explain the beneficial effects of seizure activity in psychosis (Carlsson & Carlsson, 1990). NMDA receptor agonists are proconvulsant in mice (Czuczwar & Meldrum, 1982), suggesting that such agents might possess antipsychotic activity, provided they could be used safely. Conversely, agents which antagonize NMDA receptor function, such as phencyclidine (PCP) are potent anticonvulsants (Czuczwar & Meldrum, 1982; Leander *et al.*, 1988). The psychotomimetic effect of PCP in man and its similarity to schizophrenia have long been recognized (Luby *et al.*, 1962).

An abnormality in glutamate transmission might also explain the therapeutic efficacy of dopamine receptor antagonists. Since stimulation of dopamine receptors inhibits glutamate release from cortico-striate terminals *in vitro* (Rowlands & Roberts, 1980), it may be expected that neuroleptic drugs would enhance the release of glutamate (Kim *et al.*, 1980). A glutamate deficiency might lead to psychosis indirectly by increasing dopamine release. There is ample evidence for a functional opposition between glutamate and dopamine systems *in vivo*. In rodents the non-competitive NMDA receptor antagonist MK-801 causes marked locomotor stimulation (Clineschmidt *et al*., 1982) and could potentiate the effects of dopamine agonists (Carlsson & Carlsson, 1989). Conversely, MK-801 was able to reverse catalepsy induced by haloperidol (Schmidt & Bubser, 1989).

Recently, Carlsson & Carlsson (1990) argued that schizophrenia might also result from a primary glutamate abnormality *independently* of altered dopamine function. This proposal was based in part on the observation that MK-801 could stimulate locomotor activity in mice depleted of monoamines by treatment with reserpine and α-methyl-p-tyrosine; this activation was resistant to blockade by neuroleptic drugs (Carlsson & Carlsson, 1989). These findings warrant detailed investigation in higher species. Several studies using primates have failed to demonstrate locomotor stimulation by MK-801 or potentiation of the effects of dopamine agonists (Crossman *et al*., 1989).

Further research to establish whether excitatory amino acid neurotransmission can be enhanced in a safe manner may provide a key to unlock the mechanism of antipsychotic activity.

Acknowledgements

We thank Eleanor Brawn for typing this manuscript.

References

Achiron, A., Zoldan, Y. & Melamed, E. (1990) *Clin. Neuropharmacol.* 13, 248–252.

Anlezark, G.M., Horton, R.W. & Meldrum, B.S. (1978) *Adv. Biochem. Psychopharmacol.* 19, 383–388.

Boyce, S., Rupniak, N.M.J., Steventon, M. & Iversen, S.D. (1990) *Neurology* 40, 717–718.

Boyce, S., Rupniak, N.M.J., Steventon, M.J. *et al.* (1991) *Behav. Brain Res.* 42, 115–121.

Brady, K.T., Balster, R.L. & May, E.L. (1982) *Science* 215, 178–180.

Brandon, S., Cowley, P., McDonald, C. *et al.* (1985) *Br. J. Psychiat.* 146, 177–183.

Burki, H.R., Eichenberger, E., Sayers, A.C. & White, T.G. (1975) *Pharmakopsychiatry* 8, 115–121.

Butler, A., Hill, J.M., Ireland, S.J. *et al.* (1988) *Br. J. Pharmacol.* 94, 397–412.

Carlsson, M. & Carlsson, A. (1989) *J. Neural Transm.* 77, 65–71.

Carlsson, M. & Carlsson, A. (1990) *Trends Neurosci.* 13, 272–276.

Carter, C.J. & Pycock, C.J. (1981) *Neuropharmacology* 20, 261–265.

Castelao, J.F., Ferreira, L., Gelders, Y.G. & Heylen, S.L.E. (1989) *Schizophrenia Res.* 2, 411–415.

Ceci, A., Smith, M. & French, E.D. (1988) *Eur. J. Pharmacol.* 154, 53–57.

Ceulemans, D.L.S., Gelders, Y.G., Hoppenbrouwers, M.-L.J.A. *et al.* (1985) *Psychopharmacology* **85**, 329-332.

Chang, R.S.L., Lotti, V.J., Martin, G.E. & Chen, T.B. (1983) *Life Sci.* **32**, 871-878.

Claghorn, J.L., Abuzzahab, F.S., Wang, R. *et al.* (1983) *Psychopharmacol. Bull.* **19**, 138-140.

Clineschmidt, B.V., Martin, G.E., Bunting, P.R. & Papp, N.L. (1982) *Drug Devel. Res.* **2**, 135-145.

Clow, A., Theodorou, A.E., Jenner, P. & Marsden, C.D. (1980) *Psychopharmacology* **69**, 227-233.

Connick, J., Fox, P. & Nicholson, D. (1990) *Trends Pharmacol. Sci.* **11**, 274-275.

Corcoran, M.E., Fibiger, H.C., McCaughran, J.A. & Wada, J.A. (1974) *Exp. Neurol.* **45**, 118-133.

Costall, B. & Naylor, R.J. (1975) *Psychopharmacology* **43**, 69-74.

Costall, B. & Naylor, R.J. (1976) *Eur. J. Pharmacol.* **35**, 161-168.

Costall, B., Naylor, R.J. & Neumeyer, J.F. (1975) *Eur. J. Pharmacol.* **31**, 1-16.

Costall, B., Naylor, R.J., Marsden, C.D. & Pycock, C.J. (1976) *J. Pharm. Pharmacol.* **28**, 523-526.

Costall, B., Naylor, R.J. & Tyers, M.B. (1988) *Rev. Neurosci.* **2**, 41-65.

Crawley, J.N., Stivers, J.A., Blumstein, L.K. & Paul, S.M. (1985) *J. Neurosci.* **5**, 1972-1983.

Crossman, A.R., Peggs, D., Boyce, S. *et al.* (1989) *Neuropharmacology* **28**, 1271-1273.

Czuczwar, S.J. & Meldrum, B. (1982) *Eur. J. Pharmacol.* **83**, 335-338.

Debonnet, G., Gaudreau, P., Quirion, R. & de Montigny, C. (1990) *J. Neurosci.* **10**, 469-476.

Delay, J., Deniker, P. & Harl, J.M. (1952) *Ann. Medico-Psychol.* **110**, 112-117.

de Montigny, C. (1989) *Arch. Gen. Psychiat.* **46**, 511-517.

Deutsch, S.I., Weizman, A., Goldman, M.E. & Morihisa, J.M. (1988) *Clin. Neuropharmacol.* **11**, 105-119.

Ferris, R.M., Harfenist, M., McKenzie, G.M. *et al.* (1982) *J. Pharm. Pharmacol.* **34**, 388-390.

Ferris, R.M., Tang, F.L.M., Chang, K.-J. & Russel, A. (1986) *Life Sci.* **38**, 2329-2337.

Flor-Henry, P. (1969) *Epilepsia* **10**, 363-395.

Goodwin, G.M. & Green, A.R. (1985) *Br. J. Pharmacol.* **84**, 743-753.

Greenblatt, E.N., Coupet, J., Rauh, E. & Szucs-Myers, V.A. (1980) *Arch. Int. Pharmacodyn.* **248**, 105-119.

Hagan, R.M., Butler, A., Hill, J.M. *et al.* (1987) *Eur. J. Pharmacol.* **138**, 303-305.

Hoh, S. & Katsuura, G. (1981) *Eur. J. Pharmacol.* **75**, 313-316.

Hokfelt, T., Rehfeld, J.F., Skirboll, L. *et al.* (1980) *Nature* **285**, 476-478.

Johnstone, E.C., Crow, T.J., Frith, C.D. *et al.* (1978) *Lancet* **i**, 848-851.

Jurien, J.L. & Leonard, B.E. (1989) *Clin. Neuropharmacol.* **12**, 353-374.

Keats, A.S. & Telford, J. (1964) *Adv. Chem. Series* **45**, 170-176.

Kim, J.S., Kornhuber, H.H., Schmid-Burgk, W. & Holzmuller, B. (1980) *Neurosci. Lett.* **20**, 379-382.

Knights, A., Okasha, M.S., Salih, M.A. & Hirsch, S.R. (1979) *Br. J. Psychiat.* **135**, 515-523.

Koulu, M., Lappalainen, J., Hietala, J. & Sjoholm, B. (1990) *Psychopharmacology* **101**, 168-171.

Kumar, R. (1977) In *Principles of Behavioural Pharmacology* (eds Iversen, L.L., Iversen, S.D. & Snyder, S.H.), Vol. 7, pp. 231-261, New York, Plenum Press.

Leander, J.D., Lawson, R.R., Ornstein, P.L. & Zimmerman, D.M. (1988) *Brain Res.* **448**, 115-120.

Leysen, J.E., van Gompel, P., Gommeren, W. *et al.* (1986) *Psychopharmacology* **88**, 434-444.

Ljundberg, T. & Ungerstedt, U. (1978) *Psychopharmacology* **56**, 239-247.

Lowe, J.A., Seeger, T.F. & Vinick, F.J. (1988) *Med. Res. Rev.* **8**, 475-497.

Luby, E.D., Gottlieb, J.C., Cohen, B.C. *et al.* (1962) *Am. J. Psychiat.* **119**, 61-67.

McCann, D.J., Rabin, R.A., Rens-Domiano, S. & Winter, J.C. (1989) *Pharmacol. Biochem.*

Behav. **32**, 87–94.

Marder, S.R. (1992) *Clin. Neuropharmacol.* **15** (suppl. 1, part A), 92–93.

Marshall, F.H., Barnes, S., Pinnock, R.D. & Hughes, J. (1990) *Br. J. Pharmacol.* **99**, 845–848.

Martin, W.R., Eades, C.G., Thompson, J.A. *et al.* (1976) *J. Pharmacol. Exp. Ther.* **197**, 517–532.

Matz, R., Rick, W., Oh, D. *et al.* (1974) *Curr. Ther. Res.* **16**, 687–695.

Montgomery, S.A. & Green, M.C.D. (1988) *Psychol. Med.* **18**, 593–603.

Nishikawa, T., Takashima, M. & Toru, M. (1983) *Neurosci. Lett.* **40**, 245–250.

Nishikawa, T., Tanaka, M., Tsuda, A. *et al.* (1988) *Prog. Neuropharmacol. Biol. Psychiat.* **12**, 803–812.

Reynolds, G.P., Garret, Rupniak, N. *et al.* (1983) *Eur. J. Pharmacol.* **89**, 325–326.

Reyntjens, A.J.M., Gelders, Y.G., Hoppenbrouwers, M.-L.J.A. & Vanden Bussche, G. (1986) *Drug Devel. Res.* **8**, 205–211.

Rowlands, G.J. & Roberts, P.J. (1980) *Eur. J. Pharmacol.* **52**, 241–242.

Rupniak, N.M.J., Jenner, P.G. & Marsden, C.D. (1983) In *Theory in Psycho-pharmacology* (ed. Cooper, S.J.), Vol. 2, pp. 196–237, London, Academic Press.

Rupniak, N.M.J., Mann, S., Hall, M.D. *et al.* (1984) In *Catecholamines: Neuro-pharmacology and Central Neurons System-Therapeutic Aspects*, pp. 91–98, New York, Alan Liss.

Rupniak, N.M.J., Hall, M.D., Kelly, E. *et al.* (1985) *J. Neural Transm.* **62**, 249–266.

Schmidt, W.J. & Bubser, M. (1989) *Pharmacol. Biochem. Behav.* **32**, 621–623.

Schneider, L.H., Alpert, J.E. & Iversen, S.D. (1983) *Peptides* **4**, 749–753.

Seeman, P. (1980) *Pharmacol. Rev.* **32**, 230–313.

Sen, G. & Bose, K.C. (1931) *Indian Med. World* **2**, 194–201.

Slade, A.P. & Checkley, S.A. (1980) *Br. J. Psychiat.* **137**, 217–221.

Steck, H. (1954) *Ann. Medico-Psychol.* **112**, 737–743.

Stevens, J.R. (1966) *Arch. Gen. Psychiat.* **14**, 461–472.

Stille, G., Lauener, H. & Eichenberger, E. (1971) *Il Farmaco Ed. Pract.* **26**, 603–625.

Su, T.P. (1982) *J. Pharmacol. Exp. Ther.* **223**, 284–290.

Taylor, D.P. & Dekleva, J. (1987) *Drug. Devel. Res.* **11**, 65–70.

Taylor, P.J. & Fleminger, J.J. (1980) *Lancet* **i**, 1380–1382.

Titeler, M., Lyon, R.A. & Glennon, R.A. (1988) *Psychopharmacology* **94**, 213–216.

Vaccarino, F.J. & Rankin, J. (1989) *Behav. Neurosci.* **103**, 831–836.

Vanecek, S., Essman, W. & Woods, J.H. (1989) *FASEB J.* **3**, A442.

van Ree, J.M., Gaffori, O. & de Wied, D. (1983) *Eur. J. Pharmacol.* **93**, 63–78.

Walker, J.M., Matsumoto, R.R., Bowen, W.D. *et al.* (1988) *Neurology* **38**, 961–965.

Weiss, F., Tanzer, D.J. & Ettenberg, A. (1988) *Pharmacol. Biochem. Behav.* **30**, 309–317.

White, F.J. & Wang, R.Y. (1983) *Science* **221**, 1054–1057.

White, F.J. & Wang, R.Y. (1984) *Brain Res.* **300**, 161–166.

EFFECTS OF NEUROLEPTICS ON NEURONAL AND SYNAPTIC STRUCTURE

Paul J. Harrison

University Department of Psychiatry, Warneford Hospital, Oxford, UK and Department of Neuropathology, Radcliffe Infirmary, Oxford, UK

Table of Contents

The neurochemical effects of neuroleptics have been extensively investigated, as summarized elsewhere in this volume (see also Baker & Greenshaw, 1989). Less attention has been paid to the structural changes which these drugs may produce in the brain, even though the understanding of such processes is important for several reasons. First, the time-course of antipsychotic effects of neuroleptics suggests that structural reorganization may be required for their therapeutic action. Secondly, structural changes are thought to underlie the long-term side-effects of neuroleptics, notably tardive dyskinesia. Together, these factors indicate that neuropathological studies must complement neurochemical investigations if the beneficial and undesired actions of neuroleptics are to be understood. In addition to these considerations, awareness of the structural consequences of neuroleptics is also of value for neuropathological research into schizophrenia: since the large majority of schizophrenic patients have been treated with neuroleptics, it is necessary to be able to distinguish changes likely to be due to the drugs from those which characterize the disease (Harrison, 1993).

ANTIPSYCHOTIC DRUGS AND THEIR SIDE-EFFECTS
ISBN 0-12-079035-1

6.1 Neuroleptic effects on neurons

Given the large number of studies on the neurochemical effects of neuroleptics and the frequency with which pathological changes have been predicted to accompany them, there has been relatively little research addressing this question. It is only recently that well-conducted studies have been carried out. These are summarized in Table 1.

Neuroleptic treatment in rodents does not cause major or widespread alterations in the number or size of neurons. Neither is there consistent evidence of morphologically abnormal neurons nor of a gliotic response which would suggest ongoing neuronal damage and degeneration. However, a number of localized changes in other neuronal parameters have been identified following neuroleptic administration, although the changes are generally modest and not all have been replicated.

In the striatum, there is at most a modest (roughly 10%) loss of neurons after long-term use of neuroleptics (Pakkenberg *et al.*, 1973; Nielsen & Lyon, 1978; Jeste et al., 1992). There is some evidence that this change affects predominantly the subpopulation of large neurons in the ventrolateral quadrant. This specificity of neuroleptic effect may provide some indication as to the characteristics of the cell types involved. First, the sensorimotor cortex projects topographically upon the striatum, with the ventrolateral region being involved most closely with the representations of the head and mouth. Efferent subcortical connections of the striatum are also subject to a dorsoventral gradient. Moreover, the behavioural effects of ventrolateral striatal lesions are different to those in other striatal areas (see Nielsen & Lyon, 1978). These factors may be relevant to understanding the clinicopathological profile of tardive dyskinesia. Large cells in the striatum are primarily cholinergic interneurons (Kimura *et al.*, 1980) and are in direct synaptic contact with terminals of dopaminergic nigrostriatal neurons (Kubota *et al.*, 1987). Thus, it may be that blockade of dopaminergic transmission by neuroleptics has long-term toxic effects on the cholinergic neurons, in keeping with evidence for decreases in striatal cholinergic function seen after similar periods (Mahadik *et al.*, 1988). It is uncertain whether the reduced number of large neurons reflects cell loss or shrinkage; this has potential significance in that the latter might be a reversible phenomenon. However, the reduction in number of striatal cells (not classified by size) found by Nielsen & Lyon (1978) occurred in rats not killed until 16 weeks after cessation of neuroleptic injections, suggesting that at least part of the change is irreversible.

In summary, there is evidence that chronic neuroleptic treatment causes modest reductions in cell density within the striatum, affecting neurons which are postsynaptic upon the nigrostriatal projection and which express the D_2 dopamine receptor (Najlerahim *et al.*, 1989). In contrast, there are no changes in these parameters in neurons of the prefrontal cortex, which also receives dopaminergic innervation; thus the presence of dopaminergic afferents cannot be a sufficient criterion for a neuron to undergo neuroleptic-induced structural change (see Sections 6.2.3 and 6.2.4). No alterations in neuronal number or size are observed in the substantia nigra, implying that dopaminergic neurons themselves are not affected by neuroleptics in this way.

Table 1 Neuroleptic effects on neuronal number and size.

Reference	Drug, dose and duration	Parameters measured	Significant changes in neuroleptic-treated animals
1	Perphenazine enanthate, 3.4 mg/kg i.m. 2 weekly for 12 months	Number of neurons in cortex and basal ganglia[a]	20% reduction in basal ganglia; no change in cortex[b]
2	Group 1: as above[c]. Group 2: 40 mg/kg i.m. 2 weekly for 6 months	Number of neurons in substantia nigra pars compacta and reticulata	No changes in either group[b]
3	Flupenthixol decanoate, 4 mg/kg i.m. weekly for 36 weeks; killed 14–18 weeks later	Number of neurons in striatum	10% cell loss in ventrolateral striatum
4	Haloperidol 3 mg/kg i.m. daily for 16 weeks	Neuronal density and size in substantia nigra pars compacta	No changes
5	Haloperidol 3 mg/kg i.m. daily for 16 weeks[d]	Neuronal density and size in striatum	13% increase in neuronal size; no change in density
6	Haloperidol 3 mg/kg i.m. daily for 16 weeks[d]	Neuronal density and size in medial prefrontal cortex	No changes
7	Fluphenazine decanoate, 5 mg/kg i.m. 2 weekly for 4, 8 or 12 months	Neuronal density in striatum	Decreased density of large neurons after 8 months. No other changes[b]

References: 1: Pakkenberg *et al.* (1973); 2: Gerlach (1975); 3: Nielsen & Lyon (1978); 4: Benes *et al.* (1983); 5: Benes *et al.* (1985a); 6: Benes *et al.* (1985b); 7: Jeste *et al.* (1992).

The table only includes studies with appropriate control groups and statistical analyses. All studies were performed on rats.

[a]Region of cortex and basal ganglia not specified.
[b]Comment also made on morphology and arrangement of neurons and glia; no differences in treated animals were observed.
[c]The same animals as were used in ref. 1.
[d]Apparently the same animals as were used in ref. 4.

Table 2 Neuroleptic effects on synapses.

Reference	Drug, dose and duration	Parameters measured	Significant changes in neuroleptic-treated animals
1	Haloperidol 3 mg/kg i.m. daily for 16 weeks	Substantia nigra: number and area of axon terminals and dendrites; density of synaptic vesicles	Increased axon terminals per dendrite. No other changes
2	Haloperidol 3 mg/kg i.m. daily for 16 weeks	As above, in striatum	Increase in size of axon terminals. No changes in other parameters
3	Haloperidol 3 mg/kg i.m. daily for 16 weeks[a]	As above, in layer VI of medial prefrontal cortex	Loss of dendritic spines and associated axon terminals with asymmetrical postsynaptic membrane specializations (PMS); increase in other axon terminals. No other changes
4	Haloperidol 0.1 mg/kg i.m. daily for 3 weeks	Layer VI of prefrontal cortex: number of axodendritic and axospinous synapses; number, area and mitochondrial content of axon terminals; number and density of synaptic vesicles	Increase in axodendritic but decrease in axospinous synapses. Axodendritic synapses: reduced axon terminal area and mitochondria; postsynaptic densities longer. Axospinous synapses: minor changes
5	Haloperidol 0.5 mg/kg i.m. daily for 2 weeks (group 1). Group 2 killed 2 weeks after last dose	Caudate and nucleus accumbens: number of synapses and those with perforated postsynaptic densities (PPD); area of axon terminals	Increase in number of synapses with PPDs in caudate nucleus in group 1 only. No other changes

6	Haloperidol 1 mg/kg i.m. daily for 3 weeks	Caudate and hippocampus (CA1): parameters as in ref. 4 above	Caudate: increased axodendritic and axospinous synapses. Axospinous synapses have larger axon terminals with more mitochondria, size of postsynaptic density. Axodendritic synapses: smaller axon terminals with less mitochondria. No other changes or any in hippocampus
7	Haloperidol 1.3 mg/kg per day or clozapine 27 mg/kg per day orally for 12 months	Layer VI of prefrontal cortex: size of dendrites, spines and axon terminals; density of synaptic vesicles; presence of symmetrical, asymmetrical or absent PMS	Haloperidol: reduced calibre of dendrites. Both groups: fewer axodendritic synapses had asymmetric PMS. Clozapine: axospinous synapses had same PMS shift. No other changes
8	Haloperidol 0.5 mg/kg or clozapine 35 mg/kg i.m. daily for 2 weeks	Caudate nucleus, nucleus accumbens and layer VI of prefrontal cortex: number of synapses and those with PPD	Caudate nucleus: increased number of synapses with PPD after haloperidol. No changes with clozapine or in other areas
9	Haloperidol or raclopride, 7 mg/kg i.m. weekly for 7 months	Caudate nucleus: number of PPD synapses	Increased number of PPD synapses after haloperidol or raclopride

References: 1: Benes *et al.* (1983); 2: Benes *et al.* (1985a); 3: Benes *et al.* (1985b); 4: Klintzova *et al.* (1989); 5: Meshul & Casey (1989); 6: Uranova *et al.* (1991); 7: Vincent *et al.* (1991); 8: Meshul *et al.* (1992); 9: See *et al.* (1992).

The table only includes studies with appropriate control groups and statistical analyses. All experiments were performed on rats.

[a]Apparently the same animals as used in ref. 1, and in refs 4-6 of Table 1.

6.2 Neuroleptic effects on synapses

In parallel with morphometric studies of neurons, there have been a series of electron microscopic investigations to determine whether the number, distribution or morphological characteristics of synapses are altered following neuroleptic administration. Many parameters of synaptic structure are known to be affected by synaptic activity and environmental influences (see Meshul & Casey, 1989; Shepherd, 1990), allowing neuroleptic-induced changes to be interpreted with reference to these other factors in order to draw conclusions as to their likely origins and significance. The data are summarized in Table 2 and some of the key points are discussed here.

6.2.1 Substantia nigra

In this region there is an increased number of axon terminals per dendrite in a subpopulation of axons following treatment with haloperidol (Benes *et al.*, 1983). The finding was interpreted as evidence for collateral sprouting of axon terminals. The neurochemical identity of the affected synapses could not be determined, but on morphological grounds they are unlikely to be inhibitory.

6.2.2 Striatum (caudate nucleus)

It is in the caudate nucleus that synaptic alterations are most prominent, in line with the neuronal changes mentioned above. An increase in the size of axon terminals in the striatum occurs (Benes *et al.*, 1985a). The density of synaptic vesicles per terminal did not change, meaning that the total number of synaptic vesicles doubled in the enlarged terminals; unlike in the substantia nigra, the number of axon terminals per dendrite was unaltered. It was hypothesized that these changes are a counterpart of the increased firing and activity of nigrostriatal neurons induced by neuroleptics; however, it has not been established whether the affected axons are indeed dopaminergic. Meshul, Casey and colleagues (Meshul & Casey, 1989; Meshul *et al.*, 1992) have concentrated on different synaptic parameters, notably the number of synapses and the proportion which contain perforated postsynaptic densities (PPD). The rationale for measuring PPDs is that they are thought to reflect a more efficient or heavily used synapse. A significant increase of striatal synapses with PPDs after 2 weeks haloperidol treatment was found (Meshul & Casey, 1989); the pattern reverted to normal after 2 weeks off the drug. They did not replicate the increase in size of axon terminals reported previously (Benes *et al.*, 1985a), possibly due to the differences in drug dosage and duration between the studies (Table 2). The neuronal type containing the PPD and the axons which synapse on them remain unknown, but it is suggested that they may be glutamatergic corticostriate terminals which are affected as a correlate of the development of tolerance to neuroleptics (Meshul & Casey, 1989). Treatment with clozapine using a similar protocol was not accompanied by any effect on PPD synapses (Meshul *et al.*, 1992). This finding was interpreted with regard to the different pharmacological characteristics and absence of tardive dyskinesia associated with clozapine (see Chapters 2 and 14). The most recent study by this group demonstrates that increases in PPD synapse number are also observed after longer-term (7 month) haloperidol or raclopride administration (See *et al.*, 1992). Klintzova and colleagues (1989) reported on a large number of synaptic parameters in caudate nucleus after haloperidol treatment. They found an increased density of synapses, both axospinous (53%) and axodendritic (83%). Parameters of pre- and postsynaptic structure which reflect synaptic activity were also increased, probably in response to the elevated dopaminergic activity caused by haloperidol. Together, the data indicate that haloperidol and raclopride, but not clozapine, produce significant effects on synaptic plasticity with formation of new synapses and structural modifications to other synapses in the striatum.

6.2.3 Nucleus accumbens

The ventral part of the striatum (nucleus accumbens) receives a dopaminergic input from the ventral tegmental area. It therefore shares with the rest of the striatum a dopaminergic innervation, but differs from it in the source of these neurons. No changes in the number of synapses or proportion with PPDs were found in the nucleus accumbens after treatment (Meshul & Casey, 1989; Meshul *et al.*, 1992). The differential effect of neuroleptics in the nucleus accumbens compared to the striatum proper may relate to the differing properties of dopaminergic neurons arising from the substantia nigra as compared to the ventral tegmentum. It emphasizes that the neuropathological effects of neuroleptics cannot be explained purely by reference to the presence or absence of dopaminergic input; other relevant factors which need to be borne in mind may include the transmitter phenotype and non-dopaminergic connections of the neurons in question.

6.2.4 Prefrontal cortex

Lamina VI of the medial prefrontal cortex has been investigated ultrastructurally as it is another site of termination of dopaminergic afferents from the ventral tegmental area. In the prefrontal cortex, neuroleptics result in a selective loss of synapses with asymmetric postsynaptic membrane specializations (PMS) upon dendritic spines; there is also a concomitant increase in axon terminals associated with synapses with symmetric or absent PMS (Benes *et al.*, 1985b). The functional importance of PMS type is that asymmetric synapses are excitatory in action whereas symmetric ones are inhibitory. These data together suggest a remodelling of excitatory synaptic connections on dendrites and their spines (Benes *et al.*, 1985b; Vincent *et al.*, 1991) and are in keeping with data showing overall reductions in axospinous synapses and increases in axodendritic synapses in the same region (Klintzova *et al.*, 1989). The initial study (Benes *et al.*, 1985b) also reported losses of dendritic spines, a finding which was not observed when lower doses of haloperidol given over a longer time-course were used, nor when clozapine was administered (Vincent *et al.*, 1991; Table 2).

6.2.5 Hippocampus

The hippocampus (CA1 field) has been studied as an example of an area lacking significant dopaminergic input. It is unaffected by haloperidol with regard to multiple parameters of synaptic number and structure (Uranova *et al.*, 1991).

In summary, haloperidol causes changes in the number and features of synapses which are likely to be correlates of significant changes in functional properties of the affected synapses and neurons which form them. It is also clear that these alterations depend on many factors, including the precise area of brain, the neuronal phenotype, duration, dose and type of neuroleptic. The latter point is illustrated by the apparent absence of effect of clozapine on synaptic structure. Some of the changes which haloperidol induces are known to be reversible if it is stopped, but this important issue has not been addressed for most of the reported changes. It also remains difficult to integrate the basis for, and consequences of, the neuroleptic-induced morphological changes with the neurochemical effects of similar treatment protocols. This is a goal for future studies and may be accomplished in tandem with the gene expression work outlined in Section 6.4.

6.3 Neuroleptic effects in human brain

Extrapolation from rodent data on the structural effects of neuroleptics to humans must be guarded because of species differences in neuronal organization and drug sensitivity. From the earliest days of their use there have been case reports and small series claiming a variety of histological changes in the brains of people treated with neuroleptics. As with the initial animal studies, however, these were poorly controlled, if at all. The only point worthy of mention is that several studies found damage to large neurons in the caudate nucleus after long-term use of neuroleptics or after persistent dyskinesias (see Jellinger, 1977), which is of note given the animal data mentioned above and the possible relationship between striatal pathology and tardive dyskinesia.

The most valuable human neuropathological data come from Jellinger (1977), who studied the neuropathological changes in brains from 28 patients treated chronically with neuroleptics, most of whom had a diagnosis of schizophrenia. Fourteen had had significant dyskinesia, the other 14 had not. Comparisons were made between these two subgroups, and also between the 28 cases as a whole and a series of unmedicated schizophrenics and a series of neurologically normal, age-matched controls. Thus, the likely main confounding variables (age, presence of underlying psychosis, occurrence of dyskinesia) were controlled for. Although the presentation of the data is not entirely clear, several important conclusions can be drawn.

Changes were only observed in the caudate nucleus. They comprised abnormal and swollen large neurons and sometimes a mild surrounding gliotic reaction. Small neurons were unaffected. No morphometric analysis (for example, to count numbers of large neurons) was performed. These striatal alterations were found in 13 out of 28 (46%) of the neuroleptic-treated group compared to 4% of the untreated schizophrenics and 2% of the normal controls. Neuroleptic-treated cases with dyskinesia had a slightly greater incidence of pathology than the non-dyskinetic subgroup (57% versus 37.5%), possibly being commoner in those with tardive dyskinesia than parkinsonism. The occurrence of pathological changes did not relate to diagnosis or mode of death. These changes were specific to the caudate nucleus, especially the rostral part. No consistent neuropathological effects of neuroleptics were found in the rest of the basal ganglia, substantia nigra, or any other brain region, although the extent of the search is not stated. No gliosis was found in any other area. These latter findings are in contrast to the only other significant study of human material (Christensen *et al.*, 1970): in the brains of patients dying with tardive dyskinesia-like syndromes which had been induced by neuroleptics in most of the cases, Christensen and colleagues found a much higher incidence of gliosis (25 out of 28) and neuronal degeneration (25 out of 28) in the substantia nigra and brainstem than in controls (7 out of 28 and 4 out of 28, respectively). However, the control series was poorly matched, and in the light of other negative studies (see Jellinger, 1977), the significance of these nigral and brainstem changes after neuroleptics is uncertain.

Jellinger (1977) also reports on the electron microscopic appearance of the striatum in two dyskinetic neuroleptic-treated patients. Slightly enlarged axons were found together with increased mitochondria (cf. ref. 6 in Table 2), abnormal organelles, multigranular bodies with glycogen accumulations, membranous whorls and concentric multilamellar bodies. These features were interpreted as resembling the changes seen in degenerating or dystrophic neurons, though their significance is unclear given the small number of cases and the major limitations of electron microscopy on post-mortem tissue. The latter constraint also precludes autopsy studies of synaptic structure and number equivalent to those in rat brain (see Section 6.2). Investigation of synaptic effects of neuroleptics in human material may, however, become possible with newer approaches such as immunocytochemical detection of synaptic proteins.

Overall, given the problems of acquiring human neuropathological data in this field, it is noteworthy that the findings of Jellinger share key elements with those observed in the animal work. In particular, pathological changes in the caudate nucleus, primarily affecting the large neurons, are seen in both situations after chronic neuroleptic treatment. Future research needs to include development of techniques for analysis at the synaptic level, and must also consider the acute effects of neuroleptic toxicity, an issue not discussed in this chapter; at present there is virtually no information as to the neuropathological correlates of fatal neuroleptic overdose or neuroleptic malignant syndrome (see Jellinger, 1977; Factor & Singer, 1992).

6.4 Neuroleptics and gene expression

It remains difficult to relate the neurochemical alterations produced by neuroleptics to their structural effects. This difficulty reflects partly the lack of appropriate collaborative studies and partly the complexity of the relationship between these two aspects of neuroleptic actions (Uranova *et al.*, 1991; Vincent *et al.*, 1991; Meshul *et al.*, 1992). Some progress may be made by the study of gene expression, since not only do neuroleptics exert their actions via receptor blockade and other effects at the protein level, but also by virtue of being potent regulators of gene expression and protein synthesis. It is through their selective promotion or repression of gene transcription, and possibly at post-transcriptional levels too, that long-term structural (and neurochemical) effects may result. An indication of the influence of neuroleptics in this respect is given by the finding that the expression of approximately 0.5% of all rat brain genes is altered by flupenthixol (S.A. Whatley, personal communication).

There are several pathways by which neuroleptics may affect neuronal and synaptic organization via altered gene expression. For example, neuroleptics cause increases in expression of the messenger RNA encoding cellular proto-oncogenes such as c-*fos* (Miller, 1990; Rogue & Vincendon, 1992); oncogene products then change the transcription and processing of multiple other genes and affect neuronal properties (Hanley, 1988). In addition, neuroleptics alter the expression of a wide variety of neuropeptide genes (see Morris *et al.*, 1988; Ding & Mocchetti, 1992; Merchant *et al.*, 1992) and other genes (see Caboche *et al.*, 1992; Mercugliano *et al.*, 1992). These alterations are likely to be accompanied by changes in the amount and functional activity of these proteins, in turn leading to changes in the properties and organization of the affected neurons and synapses. Some of these processes may be signalled through nuclear effects of G-protein-linked receptors including the D_2 receptor (Collins *et al.*, 1992). Finally, altered synaptic activity regulates neuronal gene expression (Ginty *et al.*, 1992), completing the circuit between initial effects of neuroleptics on expression of receptors and other neuronal genes, and their ultimate structural and synaptic consequences. The main gap in such putative pathways lies at the point of identifying which specific gene products are responsible for this neuroleptic-induced plasticity. Candidates include the synapsins and synaptophysin, microtubule-associated proteins, and growth-associated proteins such as GAP-43, but as yet there are no data regarding the influence of neuroleptics on expression of their genes.

The neuroanatomical and gene specificity of the changes which neuroleptics produce can be explained by a combination of factors which differ between neuronal populations. These include the receptor subtypes which neurons express, their associated second messengers, and their differential connectivity. Moreover, the gene expression response is influenced by developmental stage, ageing and concurrent disease (Harrison & Pearson, 1989) as well as by the neuroleptic which is used (see Merchant *et al.*, 1992; Mercugliano *et al.*, 1992). Such factors together probably contribute to the variability in response to neuroleptic medication which is observed both clinically and in terms of the experimental effects discussed above. With suitable techniques now available, it is feasible to integrate the data regarding the neurochemical and neuropathological effects of neuroleptics. It may prove that these processes converge through the neuroleptic-induced expression of particular genes in specific neuronal populations.

References

Baker, G.B. & Greenshaw, A.J. (1989) *Cell. Molec. Neurobiol.* **9**, 1-44.

Benes, F.M., Paskevich, P.A. & Domesick, V.B. (1983) *Science* **221**, 969-971.

Benes, F.M., Paskevich, P.A., Davidson, J. & Domesick, V.B. (1985a) *Brain Res.* **329**, 265-274.

Benes, F.M., Paskevich, P.A., Davidson, J. & Domesick, V.B. (1985b) *Brain Res.* **348**, 15-20.

Caboche, J., Vernier, P., Rogard, M. *et al.* (1992) *Eur. J. Neurosci.* **4**, 438-447.

Christensen, E., Moller, J. & Faurbye, A. (1970) *Acta Psychiat. Scand.* **46**, 14-23.

Collins, S., Caron, M.C. & Lefkowitz, R.J. (1992) *Trends Biochem. Sci.* **17**, 37-39.

Ding, X.-Z. & Mocchetti, I. (1992) *Molec. Brain Res.* **12**, 77-83.

Factor, S.A. & Singer, C. (1992) In *Drug-induced Movement Disorders* (eds Lang, A.E. & Weiner, W.J.), pp. 199-230, Mt Kisco, New York, Futura.

Gerlach, J. (1975) *Psychopharmacol. (Berl.)* **45**, 51-54.

Ginty, D.D., Bading, H. & Greenberg, M.E. (1992) *Curr. Opin. Neurobiol.* **2**, 312-316.

Hanley, M.R. (1988) *Neuron* **1**, 175-182.

Harrison, P.J. (1993) In *The Neuropathology of Dementia* (eds Esiri, M.M. & Morris, J.H.), Cambridge, Cambridge University Press (in press).

Harrison, P.J. & Pearson, R.C.A. (1989) *Psychol. Med.* **19**, 813-819.

Jellinger, K. (1977) In *Neurotoxicology* (eds Roizin, L., Shiraki, H. & Grcevic, N.), pp. 25-42, New York, Raven Press.

Jeste, D.V., Lohr, J.B. & Manley, M. (1992) *Psychopharmacology* **106**, 154-160.

Kimura, H., McGeer, P.L., Peng, I. & McGeer, E.G. (1980) *Science* **208**, 1057-1059.

Klintzova, A.J., Haselhorst, U., Uranova, N.A. *et al.* (1989) *J. Hirnforsch.* **30**, 31-37.

Kubota, Y., Inagaki, S., Shimada, S. *et al.* (1987) *Brain Res.* **413**, 179-184.

Mahadik, S.P., Laev, H., Korenovsk, A. & Karpik, S.E. (1988) *Biol. Psychiat.* **24**, 199-217.

Merchant, K.M., Dobner, P.R. & Dorsa, D.M. (1992) *J. Neurosci.* **12**, 652-663.

Mercugliano, M., Saller, C.F., Salama, A.I. *et al.* (1992) *Neuropsychopharmacology* **6**, 179-187.

Meshul, C.K. & Casey, D.E. (1989) *Brain Res.* **489**, 338-346.

Meshul, C.K., Janowsky, A., Casey, D.E. *et al.* (1992) *Psychopharmacology* **106**, 45-52.

Miller, J.C. (1990) *J. Neurochem.* **54**, 1453-1455.

Morris, B.J., Hollt, V. & fHerz, A. (1988) *Neuroscience* **25**, 525-532.

Najlerahim, A., Barton, A.J.L., Harrison, P.J. *et al.* (1989) *FEBS Lett.* **255**, 335-339.

Nielsen, C.B. & Lyon, M. (1978) *Psychopharmacologia* **59**, 85-89.

Pakkenberg, H., Fog, R. & Nilakantan, B. (1973) *Psychopharmacologica (Berl.)* **29**, 329-336.

Rogue, P. & Vincedon, G. (1992) *Brain Res. Bull.* **29**, 469-472.

See, R.E., Chapman, M.A. & Meshul, C.K. (1992) *Synapse* **12**, 147-154.

Shepherd, G.M. (ed.) (1990) *The Synaptic Organization of the Brain*, New York, Oxford University Press.

Uranova, N.A., Orlovskaya, D.D., Apel, K. *et al.* (1991) *Synapse* **7**, 253–259.
Vincent, S.L., McSparren, J., Wang, R.Y. & Benes, F.M. (1991) *Neuropsychopharmacology* **5**, 147–155.

BRAIN IMAGING AND ANTIPSYCHOTIC DRUGS

Peter F. Liddle

*Department of Psychiatry, Royal Postgraduate Medical School,
Hammersmith Hospital, London, UK*

Table of Contents

7.1   Introduction

Antipsychotic drugs have been in use for four decades, but investigation of the action of these drugs has been hampered by the fact that until recently the presumed site of action was inaccessible to examination in the living human being. At last, a range of newly developed brain-imaging techniques offers the prospect of providing not only visual images of the structure and the function of the hitherto inaccessible living human brain, but also quantitative measurement of the interaction of pharmacological agents with brain tissue in life. However, this promise of new understanding of the brain must be accompanied by a note of caution. The complexity of brain physiological processes and of the techniques required to produce images of these processes gives rise to many potential pitfalls in the interpretation of brain images.

This is perhaps most clearly illustrated by the controversy that followed the initial reports by Wong and his colleagues at Johns Hopkins Hospital, Baltimore, of evidence for an increased number of D_2 receptors in the basal ganglia in untreated schizophrenic patients. Wong et al. (1986) employed positron emission tomography (PET) using the ligand N-methylspiperone labelled with the positron-emitting isotope ^{11}C to measure the density of D_2 dopamine receptors. Because N-methylspiperone binds so strongly, the rate of dissociation is very low and equilibrium between bound and unbound ligand is not achieved during the time-course of a PET study. Therefore, Wong and colleagues developed a technique for determining binding characteristics under non-equilibrium conditions, assuming that binding is effectively irreversible within the time-scale of the study. To permit measurement of binding across a range of levels of receptor occupancy, they employed predosing with haloperidol to achieve high levels of receptor occupancy. Their complex technique makes many assumptions, including the assumptions that the rate constant for binding is the same for haloperidol as for N-methylspiperone, and that the rate constant for dissociation of haloperidol and the partitioning of haloperidol between blood and brain is the same in schizophrenic patients as in normal individuals.

Meanwhile Farde, Sedvall and colleagues at the Karolinska Institute in Stockholm used the highly specific D_2 ligand raclopride, labelled with ^{11}C, to measure D_2 receptor density in schizophrenic patients. Equilibrium between bound and unbound raclopride can be achieved within the time-course of a PET study, making it possible to employ a relatively simple mathematical model to determine receptor density from the observed distribution of radiolabelled ligand. The Karolinska group did not find evidence of a generalized increase in the density of D_2 receptors in the basal ganglia in untreated patients, though they did find that the patients tended to have greater receptor density in the left putamen than in the right putamen (Farde et al., 1990).

The model employed by the Karolinska group ignores the possible influence of endogenous dopamine on the binding of the raclopride, and critics have suggested that differences between patients and controls in levels of endogenous dopamine might effectively conceal true differences in receptor numbers. It can readily be shown, by solving the simultaneous equations which describe the equilibrium binding of several different ligands, that failure to allow for endogenous dopamine will result in an incorrect estimate of the strength of binding, but not of B_{max} (the concentration of receptor sites), under circumstances where the concentration of endogenous dopamine is constant. Under circumstances in which endogenous dopamine increased with increasing level of D_2 blockade by raclopride there would be a tendency to underestimate B_{max}. Under such circumstances, a Scatchard plot (bound/free ligand concentration against bound ligand concentration) would deviate from linearity. In normal individuals in whom binding has been measured at multiple points over an adequate range of concentrations of raclopride, there is no evidence of departure of linearity in the Scatchard plots. The situation in schizophrenia has yet to be clarified. Gjedde & Wong (1991) proposed that the conflicting PET findings might be reconciled if schizophrenic patients have an increase in D_2 receptor density together with an increased tendency for endogenous dopamine levels to rise in response to dopamine blockade. It would be more parsimonious to assume that the differences between the reported findings arise either from differences in the patients studied or from differences in technique.

The balance of current evidence favours the conclusion that there is no generalized increase in D_2 receptor density in the basal ganglia in untreated schizophrenic patients. None the less, the controversy has served to emphasize that quantitative measurement of receptor binding characteristics in living subjects is a complex task, and none of the existing techniques addresses all of the potentially confounding factors adequately.

Evaluation of the evidence provided by brain-imaging techniques requires some knowledge of the physical processes of image generation, and also an understanding of the mathematical models used to describe the relationship between the quantity that is measured (for example, the number of radioactive decay events per unit volume of tissue) and the underlying physiological process of interest (for example, the binding of a ligand to a particular type of receptor). In this chapter, we begin with a brief account of the techniques of brain imaging, with emphasis on PET and single photon emission tomography (SPET). We discuss techniques for measuring changes in brain activity produced by antipsychotic drugs, and techniques for measuring ligand binding. In particular, we examine the models used to describe the distribution of radioactively labelled ligands in the brain. We then review the progress made so far in delineating the effects that antipsychotic drugs have on brain activity, and in quantifying the binding of antipsychotic drugs to receptors in the brain.

7.2 Brain-imaging techniques

The various attributes of brain structure and function accessible to current imaging techniques include the spatial distribution of grey and white matter; regional energy metabolism and blood flow; the characteristics of neuroreceptors; electrical activity; magnetic activity; and the distribution of metabolites and cell membrane components that can be identified by their magnetic resonance spectra. While the main focus of this chapter is on PET and SPET studies, recent developments of magnetic resonance imaging (MRI) offer the prospect of imaging the effects of antipsychotic drugs without exposure to radioactivity. If a paramagnetic tracer substance is administered, it is possible to use MRI to measure cerebral perfusion. This technique has been used to map the changes in brain activity associated with processing visual stimuli (Belliveau *et al.*, 1991), and might in principle be used to measure regional changes in brain activity produced by antipsychotic drugs.

7.2.1 Positron emission tomography (PET)

PET provides quantitative images of the distribution of positron-emitting isotopes which are distributed in the brain according to a physiological process of interest, such as cerebral perfusion, metabolism or binding to neuroreceptors. When radioactive decay of the isotope occurs, the emitted positron is annihilated by interaction with an electron in the adjacent brain tissue, generating two gamma-ray photons that travel in opposite directions, and that can be detected by detector crystals arranged in a circular array around the head. Whenever two photons are detected simultaneously in different detectors, it can be concluded that a positron–electron annihilation event has occurred along the straight line joining the two detectors. Measurement of coincidence events in a large number of pairs of detectors provides an estimate of the concentration of radioactivity averaged along a large number of straight-line paths through the brain. The technique of tomographic reconstruction is used to generate a quantitative image of the spatial distribution of radioactivity. An image of the underlying physiological processes that determine the distribution of the tracer in the brain can then be derived by applying a suitable mathematical model describing these physiological processes.

Spatial resolution of PET is inherently limited by distance of travel of the positron within the substance of the brain before annihilation. The range of travel before annihilation depends on the energy with which the positron is emitted from the nucleus of the radioactive isotope. In the case of the isotope ^{11}C, 75% of the emitted positrons will be annihilated within 2.1 mm (in water). For ^{18}F, which emits a less energetic positron, the corresponding distance is 1.2 mm. In addition, spatial resolution is limited by the fact that motion of the centre of mass of the positron–electron pair produces a spread of order 0.5° about the expected angle of 180° between the paths of the two gamma rays. For current cameras, the spatial resolution is such that a line source would have a width at half maximum of approximately 5 mm, and thus approaches the inherent limit set by the range of positron travel and motion of the centre of mass of the positron–electron pair.

The positron-emitting isotopes employed in PET are relatively short-lived, with half-lives for radioactive decay ranging from 2.1 min for ^{15}O to 110 min for ^{18}F. ^{11}C, which is especially suitable for labelling neuroreceptor ligands, has a half-life of 20 min. With short half-life isotopes the radioactivity level falls rapidly after the study, minimizing unnecessary radiation exposure.

There are two principal ways in which PET has been used to study the effects of antipsychotic drugs. The first is the imaging of changes in brain activity induced by antipsychotic drugs. The second is measurement of neuroreceptor occupancy during antipsychotic treatment.

7.2.1.1 Techniques for measuring changes in brain activity

Changes in brain activity can be studied by measuring regional glucose metabolism (rCMRglu) or regional cerebral blood flow (rCBF). rCMRglu can be determined from the distribution of [^{18}F]deoxyglucose, which accumulates in cells at a rate that reflects the rate of glycolysis. rCBF can be determined from the distribution of either inhaled $C^{15}O_2$ or injected $H_2^{15}O$ for which equilibrium between blood and tissue levels is attained rapidly. Hitherto, most PET studies of the changes produced by antipsychotic drugs have measured rCMRglu. However, measurement of rCBF has some advantages. First, rCBF appears to be a more sensitive measure of rapid changes in brain activity than metabolism (Fox & Raichle, 1986). This is likely to be especially important in studies in which neuropharmacological activation is combined with neuro-psychological activation to establish the effects of pharmacological agents on particular mental processes. Furthermore, multiple images of rCBF can be obtained in a single session, which is necessary if the time-course of acute changes following administration of pharmacological agent is to be established. An image of rCBF can be obtained with radiation exposure of order 0.5 mSv (cf. annual exposure to background radiation is of order 3 mSv; an X-ray computerized tomography image of the brain entails exposure to approximately 2.5 mSv). If exposure of up to 5 mSv is considered acceptable, as many as ten images can be obtained. The acquisition time for each image is approximately 2 min. Provided the interval between images is at least 10 min there is negligible interference by residual radioactivity from the preceding image.

A potentially confounding issue in the interpretation of changes in rCBF following administration of a pharmacological agent is the possibility that observed changes reflect direct vasomotor effects of the drug rather than the response to altered neuronal activity. This is less likely to be a problem when the aim of the study is to establish the effect of the pharmacological agent on a particular mental process because a similar degree of directly induced vasoactivity would be expected during the mental activity of interest and during the control mental state.

7.2.1.2 PET techniques for measuring ligand binding

For studies of neuroreceptor ligand binding, the isotopes ^{11}C or ^{18}F are generally used, because it is feasible to insert these isotopes into neuroreceptor ligands, and the half-lives of these isotopes roughly match the time-scale for accumulation of specifically bound ligand.

As the concentrations of neuroreceptors typically lie in the range 1-20 nM, it is important to be able to measure concentrations of ligands of 1 nM or less. The factors determining sensitivity can be appreciated by considering the following simplified calculation of the concentration of a neuroreceptor ligand that might be measured in practice. As the magnitude of statistical fluctuations in counting radioactive disintegrations is approximately the square root of the number of events counted, it is necessary to detect at least 10^3 disintegrations from the volume of interest if statistical errors are to be acceptably small. Allowing for loss due to absorption of gamma rays in the brain, and for the fact that a ring of detectors can only intercept gamma rays travelling approximately parallel to the plane of the ring, approximately 1 in 200 disintegrations might be detected. In labelling a ligand with a radioactive tracer such as ^{11}C it is feasible to achieve a specific activity of order 100 Ci/mmol ($= 3.7 \times 10^{12}$ Bq/mmol). This specific activity corresponds to labelling of approximately 1 in every 10^6 molecules of ligand with ^{11}C. Typically, disintegrations are counted for a period of 300 s. On the basis of the preceding figures, the amount of ligand required to give 10^3 counts in 300 s would be 0.2 pmol. If the volume of interest was 1 ml, this would correspond to a ligand concentration of 0.2 nM.

Many issues must be addressed in the preparation of a ligand that is suitable for measuring the characteristics of neuroreceptors using PET. First, it is necessary to achieve a sufficiently high proportion of labelled molecules of the ligand in a sample that is safe to administer to human subjects. Secondly, it is essential to ensure that the specificity of binding is such that it is possible to distinguish binding to the receptors of interest from non-specific binding.

Thirdly, it is necessary to make sure that metabolism over the time-scale of the study is minimal, or that it can be taken into account quantitatively. Metabolites that do not enter brain tissue make a minimal direct contribution to the image because the ratio of intravascular to extravascular radioactivity is small. However, even when metabolites do not cross the blood–brain barrier, a high rate of metabolism promotes rapid clearance of the radioligand from the brain and hence adds complexity to the task of modelling the time-course of accumulation of radioactivity. If clearance is too rapid, it is impossible to obtain conditions near to equilibrium. Metabolites that cross the blood–brain barrier present a problem if there are regional differences in non-specific binding. Metabolites that bind specifically to the receptors of interest present virtually insuperable problems.

In general, the relationships between the rate of passage across the blood–brain barrier, association to receptors, dissociation from receptors, and clearance via metabolism and excretion must be such that there is a period of time within the life of the radioligand when the process of specific binding to receptors plays a dominant role in determining the accumulation of radioactivity in the brain region of interest. In the initial phase, rate of tissue perfusion (rCBF) is the dominant factor determining the rate of accumulation of radioligand. If the ligand crosses the blood–brain barrier rapidly, this phase lasts only a few minutes. Provided clearance by metabolism and/or excretion is not too rapid, the subsequent time-course is determined largely by ligand binding. The observed pattern of temporal variation depends on the ratio of the rate constants for association and dissociation. If the rate of association greatly exceeds that of dissociation, the binding can be treated as irreversible. The ratio of specifically bound ligand to non-specific bound and free ligand increases approximately linearly with time. If the rates are of comparable magnitude, equilibrium will be achieved rapidly, and the ratio of specifically bound ligand to non-specifically bound and free ligand will tend to remain constant.

In summary, a suitable ligand is one that crosses the blood–brain barrier rapidly, exhibits little non-specific binding and is metabolized very slowly. In the period following the initial perfusion-dominated phase, it is best to ensure that either the rate of association is very much greater than the rate of dissociation so that binding can be treated as irreversible, or that the two rates are of comparable magnitude so that equilibrium is reached quickly. In view of the potentially confounding influence of processes such as tissue perfusion, transport across the blood–brain barrier, metabolism and excretion, and the possibility of significant occupation of receptors by endogenous neurotransmitters, measurement of receptor characteristics *in vivo* is inherently more complex than the corresponding measurements *in vitro*. However, measurements *in vivo* have the advantage that they examine receptors in their normal physiological environment.

Quantitative estimates of receptor characteristics must be based on a mathematical model that describes the accumulation of the radioligand in the brain region of interest. There is no model that can provide an adequate quantitative description of ligand binding in all circumstances. The models most widely used assume that the radioactivity is distributed in three compartments: (1) intravascular; (2) extravascular but not specifically bound; (3) bound to specific receptors of interest. The extravascular ligand that is not specifically bound (compartment 2) might be either free or non-specifically bound to unsaturable sites. Provided there is very rapid equilibrium between the free and non-specifically bound states of the ligand, the free ligand in the second compartment can be expressed as a constant fraction of the total amount of ligand in that compartment. The major differences between the various models arise from the assumptions about the relative rate of association and dissociation during the period of study.

7.2.1.3 The explicit dynamic model

Mintun *et al.* (1984) determined the numerical solution of the set of differential equations describing the rate of flow of ligand between the compartments. The method involves explicit calculation of the amount of ligand in each of three compartments, making no assumptions about relative rates of association and dissociation. It requires knowledge of regional blood flow and volume, and hence depends on explicit measurement of these quantities. The calculation yields the value binding potential, B_{max}/K_d, where B_{max} is the density of receptors in the region of interest and K_d is the dissociation constant, which is inversely proportional to the strength of binding. Mintun and colleagues point out that when tracer concentrations are below the pharmacologically effective range, it is intrinsically impossible to calculate B_{max} and K_d separately. Although the explicit method has the advantage of making relatively few assumptions, it is seldom applied because of the need to measure regional blood flow and volume.

7.2.1.4 The ratio method assuming irreversible binding

Wong *et al.* (1984) developed a model for the binding of the ligand N-methylspiperone to D_2 receptors in the striatum assuming that the specific binding is effectively irreversible during the time-course of the study. When the assumptions of the model are satisfied, the ratio of concentration of tracer in striatum to that in cerebellum increases linearly with time. The slope is proportional to the rate constant for binding. Wong and colleagues have demonstrated that for N-methylspiperone the predicted linearity is observed after the initial period in which blood flow is the dominating influence on the distribution of tracer. The method is less satisfactory in subjects with high B_{max} in whom binding is very rapid, because much of the binding occurs during the time when blood flow has a significant influence on distribution of tracer.

Although it is intrinsically impossible to calculate B_{max} and K_d separately when tracer concentrations are below the pharmacologically active range, Wong and colleagues argue that it is possible to obtain a valid estimate of B_{max} by performing two separate scans, one when the only added ligand is the radiolabelled N-methyl-spiperone, and the other in the presence of a dose of unlabelled haloperidol which blocks a substantial proportion of receptors. It is necessary to make assumptions about the blood–brain partition coefficient and the rate constants for haloperidol which introduce uncertainty into the validity of this method for comparing absolute values of receptor density in schizophrenic patients with those in normal individuals.

Fortunately, most of the uncertainties that prevail when the N-methylspiperone method is used to compare schizophrenic patients with controls do not apply to the use of this method to determine the relative occupancy of D_2 sites by antipsychotic medication by performing repeated measurements in the absence and in the presence of medication in a single individual. None the less, this method for estimating relative occupancy by repeated measurements in an individual case does assume that the strength of binding is not altered by the presence of the bound antipsychotic drug. While this is probably a valid assumption, it should be noted that in the case of binding of substrates to enzymes, there can be cooperative binding between binding sites such that the binding of one molecule of substrate produces a conformational change that enhances the binding of subsequent molecules of substrate. The occurrence of similar interactions between neuroreceptor-binding sites remains a possibility.

7.2.1.5 The equilibrium model

Farde *et al.* (1986) have demonstrated that the time-course of accumulation of [^{11}C]raclopride in the putamen implies that equilibrium between bound and unbound ligand occurs within the time-scale of a PET study. They determined the concentration of specifically bound ligand by subtracting concentration of radioactivity in the cerebellum (where there are very few D_2 receptors) from that in the putamen. They assumed that the concentration of free radioligand in the brain was approximately equal to the cerebellar concentration. (This assumption was justified by studies showing that there is very little non-specific binding of raclopride to brain tissue, together with evidence that there is minimal metabolism of raclopride over a period of 45 min.) They found that the concentration of specifically bound ligand in the putamen initially rose steeply, but after about 25 min it reached a maximum, and thereafter declined very slowly at a rate proportional to the slow decline of cerebellar activity. This observation implies pseudoequilibrium between bound and unbound ligand during this period of slow decline. Thus they were able to measure the concentration of bound ligand corresponding to a particular concentration of free ligand under conditions near to equilibrium.

By administering a range of doses of raclopride spanning the pharmacologically active range (with decreasing specific activity as raclopride dose increased so as to ensure that the dose of radioactivity remained at tracer level), they demonstrated that specifically bound ligand was related to concentration of free ligand by a hyperbolic curve indicating saturation of binding at high concentration of free ligand. By generating the hyperbolic curve which provided the best fit to the data, they estimated values of B_{max} and K_d in four healthy men. Furthermore, for each subject the Hill coefficient was near to unity, implying binding to a single species of receptor.

The proportion of D_2 receptors occupied by antipsychotic drug during treatment can be estimated by using the [^{11}C]raclopride technique to measure the reduction in number of receptors available. The Karolinska group (Farde *et al.*, 1986, 1988) determined the proportion of receptors occupied by comparing the observed amount of specific binding observed at a specific concentration of free ligand with the amount expected in the absence of any competing ligand, assuming values for B_{max} and K_d derived from saturation binding studies of control individuals. They found greater than 70% occupancy of D_2 receptors at therapeutic doses for neuroleptics representative of all major classes of typical neuroleptics.

The validity of such calculations of receptor occupancy depends on the validity of using values of B_{max} and K_d derived from studies of control individuals. In the study reported in 1986, the controls were healthy male subjects; in the 1988 study, the controls were drug-naive schizophrenic patients. In light of the probability that B_{max}

is elevated in patients who have had substantial prior exposure to neuroleptics it would clearly be better to determine B_{max} and K_d for each patient by a saturation binding study while unmedicated, and then use these values in the estimation of receptor occupancy during treatment. However, such a strategy would demand withdrawal of medication and also performance of multiple scans of each patient.

Farde et al. (1987) have also investigated the characteristics of the D_1 ligand, [^{11}C]SCH 23390. This ligand appears to reach equilibrium during the time-course of a PET study. However, the high rate of metabolism of SCH 23390 raises some doubt about the suitability of this ligand for accurate quantitative measurements in vivo. After 42 min, 85% of the radioactivity in blood is found in metabolites. Fortunately, the metabolites do not appear to cross the blood–brain barrier to a significant extent, so the distribution of radioactivity in brain would be expected to provide at least a good qualitative indication of specific D_1 ligand binding. Farde et al. (1987) demonstraed high levels of binding in basal ganglia and neocortex.

7.2.2 Single photon emission tomography (SPET)

SPET uses tracers labelled with isotopes which decay with the emission of a single photon. Because collimators (which necessarily absorb part of the emitted radiation) must be employed to define the direction of travel of detected photons, SPET is intrinsically less efficient than PET. Long-lived isotopes are generally used so it is not necessary to have a cyclotron nearby, and the technique is therefore more widely available.

SPET, like PET, can be used to measure the physiological response of the brain to pharmacological doses of antipsychotics, or to map the distribution of trace amounts of labelled antipsychotic drugs in the brain. Modelling of the processes governing distribution of SPET tracers is less advanced than is the case with PET tracers, so absolute quantitative measurements are not performed.

The SPET tracer most suitable for measuring rCBF is hexamethyl propyleneamine oxime (HMPAO) labelled with ^{99m}technetium (^{99m}Tc). The majority of this lipophilic tracer becomes fixed on first passage through the brain, so the distribution of radioactivity largely reflects blood flow in a brief period immediately following administration of the tracer. ^{99m}Tc has a half-life for radioactive decay of 6 h. Repeated independent measurements within the one day are not possible, though in principle the effects of administration of a pharmacological agent might be measured by employing the split dose technique. An initial dose of tracer is given under baseline conditions, the subject is scanned, the pharmacological agent of interest is administered, and a second dose of the tracer given at the time when the maximal effect of the pharmacological agent on brain function is expected. Finally a second scan is performed, and the difference between the two scans provides a measure of the effects of the pharmacological agent. The radiation exposure for a [^{99m}Tc]HMPAO study is typically 5 mSv. This relatively high radiation exposure places a severe limitation on the use of SPET for repeated rCBF measurements.

Iodobenzamine, a 6-methoxybenzamide compound, labelled with ^{123}I ($[^{123}I]IBZM$) is a suitable tracer for measurement of dopamine D_2 receptors using SPET. Like raclopride, it has a high specific affinity for D_2 receptors. The time-course of tissue radioactivity suggests that equilibrium between bound and unbound ligand is achieved within 20–40 min after administration of the tracer.

7.3 Effects of antipsychotic drugs on brain activity

The object of neuropharmacological challenge studies is the measurement of the effect of administration of a pharmacological agent on brain function. In their simplest form, these studies entail the measurement of brain activity before and after administration of the pharmacological agent of interest. In view of the fact that antipsychotic effects of dopamine blocking drugs develop over a period of several weeks' treatment, the main question of clinical interest with regard to these drugs is the effect of sustained administration over a prolonged period. The most consistent finding has been of increased metabolism in the basal ganglia after treatment. This was reported in the earliest studies (DeLisi *et al.*, 1985; Wolkin *et al.*, 1985) and has been confirmed in subsequent studies (for example, Szechtman *et al.*, 1988; Wik *et al.*, 1989; Bartlett *et al.*, 1991). There appear to be differences in detail between the effects of different antipsychotics. For example, Bartlett *et al.* (1991) found that haloperidol produced a relative increase in basal ganglion metabolism in the setting of a decrease in global cerebral metabolism, while thiothixene produced an absolute increase in basal ganglia metabolism accompanied by a parallel increase in global metabolism. In the absence of adequate information about the temporal relationship between changes in basal ganglia metabolism and therapeutic effects, it is difficult to determine the relevance of these changes to the antipsychotic effect of the drugs.

Various studies have examined the acute effects of dopamine agonists. Using PET to measure regional glucose metabolism, Cleghorn *et al.* (1991) found that apomorphine (0.75 mg/70 kg) produced a decrease in metabolism in the corpus striatum in neuroleptic-naive schizophrenic patients, but not in normal subjects. Since a small dose of a dopamine agonist can exacerbate psychotic symptoms in schizophrenic patients, the observed decrease in striatal metabolism induced by apomorphine in patients is consistent with the hypothesis that the increase in basal ganglia metabolism produced by antipsychotic drugs is relevant to their therapeutic effect.

In view of the progress in the use of PET to delineate the nature of the mental processes implicated in the production of schizophrenic symptoms (Liddle *et al.*, 1992), it is likely to be informative to examine the effects of pharmacological agents on the pattern of brain activity associated with specific mental processes that are implicated in the pathophysiology of the illness. This is especially likely to be so in the case of dopamine-blocking drugs because much evidence suggests that the role of dopamine is the modulation of mental activity. The appropriate strategy would employ combined neuropharmacological and neuropsychological challenge to determine the effects of drugs on the changes in brain activity associated with a specific mental task.

The combination of neuropharmacological and neuropsychological challenge is illustrated by the study of Daniels *et al.* (1990) in which they used SPET (with the tracer ^{133}Xe) to measure the effect of the indirect dopamine agonist amphetamine on the activation of prefrontal cortex associated with performance of the Wisconsin card-sorting test. This task demands the flexibility in problem solving that is characteristic of the role of the prefrontal cortex. Schizophrenic patients tend to perform this task poorly. Weinberger *et al.* (1986) had previously demonstrated that, in comparison with normal subjects, schizophrenic patients exhibit a lesser degree of activation of the dorsolateral prefrontal cortex during the task. Daniels and colleagues found that administration of amphetamine enhanced the patients' ability to activate the dorsolateral prefrontal cortex during the task. This finding implies that the abnormality of brain function associated with impaired Wisconsin card-sorting performance in schizophrenia can be reversed by administration of an indirect dopaminergic agonist.

Although this preliminary study should be interpreted with caution, it illustrates the feasibility of combining neuropharmacological and neuropsychological activation. Techniques employing either $H_2^{15}O$ or $C^{15}O_2$ to measure rCBF are in principle the most suitable for such studies. So far, applications of ^{15}O tracer techniques to delineate the effects of combined neuropharmacological challenge and neuropsychological activation have been confined to normal subjects (Friston *et al.*, 1991).

7.4 Occupation of neuroreceptors by antipsychotic drugs

7.4.1 Receptor occupancy and antipsychotic plasma levels

The PET group at New York University School of Medicine (Wolkin, 1990) have used [^{18}F]N-methylspiperone to measure receptor occupancy during treatment with haloperidol in 26 schizophrenic patients. They demonstrated a curvilinear relationship between receptor occupancy and plasma haloperidol level such that occupancy initially rose rapidly with increasing plasma level, achieving approximately 80% occupancy at 15 ng/ml, but beyond a plasma level of approximately 20 ng/ml marked increase in plasma level produced only a very slight increase in occupancy. This observation is consistent with the clinical evidence that there is little therapeutic benefit in increasing the dose of haloperidol beyond that required to produce a plasma level of 20 ng/ml.

While these results suggest some relationship between basal ganglia D_2 blockade *in vivo* and antipsychotic potency, they do not prove that the mechanism of the antipsychotic effects involves blockade of these receptors. The data obtained by Farde *et al.* (1988) for receptor occupancy during treatment with clozapine suggests that a very high degree of D_2 blockade is not essential for antipsychotic effects. They found 65% D_2 occupancy at a clozapine dose of 300 mg b.d. However, their calculation of receptor occupancy was based on values for B_{max} and K_d derived from drug-naive control patients, and would underestimate occupancy if prior treatment had induced an excess of receptors in the treated patient. Pilowsky et al. (1992) have produced more convincing evidence that clozapine can achieve antipsychotic effects at moderate levels of D_2 blockade. Using SPET with the ligand [^{123}I]IBZM, they found that a change from conventional antipsychotic treatment to clozapine resulted in increased therapeutic effect accompanied by decreased D_2 receptor occupancy in the basal ganglia.

7.4.2   The time-course of D_2 occupancy and antipsychotic effects

The antipsychotic effect of typical neuroleptic drugs develops over a period of several weeks. PET studies have provided direct confirmation that substantial levels of D_2 occupancy in the basal ganglia are achieved within hours of the administration of a single dose. For example, Nordstrom *et al.* (1991) performed repeated scans using [^{11}C]raclopride to determine the time-course of D_2 receptor occupancy in the putamen after single doses of haloperidol in normal subjects. They found occupancy greater than 70% at 3 h after a 4 mg dose, and occupancy greater than 80% at 3 h after a dose of 7.5 mg. Thus the delayed onset of therapeutic effect cannot be attributed to delayed access of neuroleptics to D_2 receptors *in vivo*.

Smith *et al.* (1988) used [^{18}F]N-methylspiperone to demonstrate that the occupancy of D_2 receptors falls rapidly to negligibly low levels within 7 days of discontinuation of haloperidol treatment. In contrast, clinical observations of the time of relapse after discontinuation of treatment suggest that therapeutic effects are maintained for a period of several weeks or even months. Thus, the therapeutic effects of antipsychotic drugs develop much more slowly than the achievement of D_2 blockade at the commencement of treatment, and can persist long after receptor occupancy has fallen to negligible levels on withdrawal of medication.

7.4.3   Receptor occupancy in treatment-resistant cases

Wolkin *et al.* (1989) have performed a thorough study of D_2 receptor blockade in treatment-resistant cases. Following a period of neuroleptic washout, symptoms were rated and D_2 receptor occupancy in the striatum was assessed using PET with [^{18}F]N-methylspiperone, in ten schizophrenic patients. Treatment with haloperidol was commenced and dose titrated according to treatment response up to a maximum plasma level of at least 10 ng/ml. PET scan and symptom ratings were repeated 4–6 weeks after commencement of treatment, and after at least 1 week on a fixed dose. Taking a decrease of less than 20% in total score on the Brief Psychiatric Rating Scale as the criterion for non-response to treatment, five patients were classified as non-responders and five as responders. The percentage decrease in the striatal D_2 receptor availability after haloperidol treatment was approximately 85% in each group. Furthermore, across the entire range of plasma levels, the degree of blockade in non-responders was at least as great as that in responders at similar plasma levels. Thus, in this patient group, poor response to treatment could not be attributed to failure to achieve blockade of striatal D_2 receptors.

7.5 Conclusions regarding antipsychotic drug action

While the findings from PET studies of the effects of antipsychotic drugs on brain function must be regarded as provisional, there is a degree of consistency in the findings that antipsychotic agents increase metabolic activity in the basal ganglia in schizophrenic patients. Furthermore, PET studies using radiolabelled D_2 ligands confirm that typical antipsychotics block D_2 receptors in the basal ganglia, and that a high degree of receptor occupancy is achieved at plasma levels which correspond to therapeutic doses of medication. However, a high degree of striatal D_2 receptor blockade is neither necessary nor sufficient for antipsychotic effects. Some patients exhibit persistent psychotic symptoms despite virtually complete striatal D_2 blockade. Conversely, therapeutic doses of atypical antipsychotics such as clozapine produce only a moderate degree of D_2 receptor blockade. The time-course of the antipsychotic effect is quite different from the time-course of D_2 blockade. Therefore, the achievement of the antipsychotic effect appears to involve some alteration in brain function apart from simple blockade of D_2 receptors.

Brain-imaging studies have demonstrated their potential for delineating the mechanism of antipsychotic drug action. However, the brain is a complex organ, and at this stage, the window opened by imaging techniques has revealed but a glimpse of the interaction between antipsychotic drugs and brain function.

References

Bartlett, E.J., Wolkin, A., Brodie, J.D. *et al.* (1991) *Psychiat. Res. Neuroimaging* **40**, 115–124.
Belliveau, J.W., Kennedy, D.N., McKinstry, R.C. *et al.* (1991) *Science* **254**, 716–719.
Cleghorn, J.M., Szechtman, H., Garnett, E. *et al.* (1991) *Psychiat. Res. Neuroimaging* **40**, 135–153.
Daniels, D.G., Weinberger, D.R., Breslin, N. *et al.* (1990) *Schizophrenia Res.* **3**, 28.

DeLisi, L.E., Holcomb, H.H., Cohen, R.M. *et al.* (1985) *J. Cereb. Blood Flow Metab.* 5, 201–206.

Farde, L., Hall, H., Ehrin, E. & Sedvall, G. (1986) *Science* 321, 258–261.

Farde, L., Halldin, C., Stone-Elander, S. & Sedvall, G. (1987) *Psychopharmacology* 92, 278–284.

Farde, L., Wiesel, F.-A., Halldon, C. & Sedvall, G. (1988) *Arch. Gen. Psychiat.* 45, 71–76.

Farde, L., Wiesel, F.-A., Stone-Elander, S. *et al.* (1990) *Arch. Gen. Psychiat.* 47, 213–219.

Fox, P.T. & Raichle, M.E. (1986) *Proc. Natl. Acad. Sci., USA* 83, 1140–1145.

Friston, K.J., Grasby, P.M., Frith, C.D. *et al.* (1991) In *Exploring Brain Functional Anatomy with Positron Tomography* (eds Chadwick, D.J. & Whelan, J.), pp. 76–87, New York, Wiley.

Gjedde, A. & Wong, D.F. (1991) *J. Cereb. Blood Flow Metab.* 11 (Suppl. 2), S824.

Liddle, P.F., Friston, K.J., Frith, C.D. *et al.* (1982) *Br. J. Psychiat.* 160, 179–186.

Mintun, M.A., Raichle, M.E., Kilbourn, M.R. *et al.* (1984) *Ann. Neurol.* 15, 217–227.

Nordstrom, A.-L., Farde, L., Halldin, C. & Sedvall, G. (1991) *Biol. Psychiat.* 29, 246S.

Pilowsky, L.S., Costa, D.C., Ell, P.J. *et al.* (1992) *Lancet* 340, 199–202.

Smith, F., Wolf, A.P. & Brodie, J.D. (1988) *Biol. Psychiat.* 23, 653–663.

Szechtman, H., Nahmias, C., Garnett, S. *et al.* (1988) *Arch. Gen. Psychiat.* 45, 523–532.

Weinberger, D.R., Berman, K.F. & Zec, R.F. (1986) *Arch. Gen. Psychiat.* 43, 114–124.

Wik, G., Wiesel, F.-A., Sjogren, I. *et al.* (1989) *Psychopharmacology* 97, 309–318.

Wolkin, A. (1990) In *The Neuroleptic Non-Responsive Patient: Characterization and Treatment* (eds Angrist, B. & Schulz, S.C.), pp. 35–49, Washington, DC, American Psychiatric Press.

Wolkin, A., Jaeger, J., Brodie, J.D. *et al.* (1985) *Am. J. Psychiat.* 142, 564–571.

Wolkin, A., Barouche, F. & Wolf, A.P. (1989) *Am. J. Psychiat.* 146, 905–908.

Wong, D.F., Wagner, H.N., Dannals, R.F. *et al.* (1984) *Science* 226, 1393–1396.

Wong, D.F., Wagner, H.N., Tune, L.E. *et al.* (1986) *Science* 234, 1558–1563.

CHAPTER 8

PHARMACOKINETICS OF ANTIPSYCHOTIC DRUGS

Stephen H. Curry

Drug Metabolism and Pharmacokinetics, Fisons Pharmaceuticals, Divisional Research and Development, Rochester, New York, USA

Table of Contents

8.1 Introduction

The earliest studies on the metabolism of phenothiazine neuroleptics were conducted soon after the initial use of chlorpromazine in the treatment of schizophrenia nearly 40 years ago. In one of the longest sagas of drug metabolism investigation, over 100 research groups have been involved in the writing of over 100 papers, some of them concerned with over 100 metabolites. The topic has been reviewed a number of times, but it is once again timely to take stock of the situation and to review current needs.

ANTIPSYCHOTIC DRUGS AND THEIR SIDE-EFFECTS
ISBN 0-12-079035-1

This particular review is primarily designed to place recent work in perspective in relation to statements accessible in earlier reviews (see, for example, Cooper, 1978, 1985; Curry, 1976b, 1981, 1985, 1988; Rivera-Calimlin, 1982; Greenblatt, 1985; Ko et al., 1985; Dahl, 1986; Baldessarini et al., 1988).

The key stages in the investigation of the metabolism and pharmacokinetics of neuroleptic drugs have been: (1) the development of urine-testing reagents following the realization that psychiatric patients are relatively non-compliant when it comes to taking prescribed medication (Forrest et al., 1961; Bolt et al., 1966; Forrest & Green, 1972); (2) identification of some of the many metabolites of neuroleptic drugs (Papadopoulas et al., 1980; Young, 1986); (3) the development of gas-chromatographic methods for the specific and sensitive assay of chlorpromazine and some of its metabolites in plasma, followed very rapidly by the discovery of presystemic elimination (the first-pass effect) as a major influence in interpatient variation in chlorpromazine plasma concentrations (Curry et al., 1982; Curry, 1968, 1976a); (4) the observation of a 'U-shaped' relation between neuroleptic effect and concentrations in plasma (Curry et al., 1970a,b; Rivera-Calimlin et al., 1973, 1978; Kucharski et al., 1984); (5) the realization that depot phenothiazines administered by intramuscular injection overcome first-pass effect problems in addition to those caused by poor compliance (Adamson et al., 1973); (6) the development of a radioreceptor assay applicable to routine monitoring (Creese & Snyder, 1977; Cohen, 1980, 1984; Kelly, 1984; Krska et al., 1986); and (7) the application of relatively modern pharmacokinetic techniques to detailed study of concentrations in plasma (Curry et al., 1970a,b; Curry & Hu, 1990; Marder et al., 1989).

Throughout this work, emphasis has been on: (1) use of high-quality assay (analytical) methods; (2) detection of the more important metabolites; (3) persistence of residues in the body long after dosing stops (elimination half-life); (4) whether enough of a clinical/pharmacokinetic relationship exists to justify routine clinical monitoring; (5) detection of, and correction for, poor patient compliance; (6) the contribution, if any, of active metabolites to pharmacological effect (Mackay et al., 1974; Kleinman et al., 1980; Dahl, 1982; Hawes et al., 1986); and (7) prolactin and other indicators of pharmacological exposure (McCreadie et al., 1984). These areas of interest to some extent conveniently provide a framework for the majority of the remaining sections of this review. In addition, there are sections on the first-pass effect and other related biochemical phenomena, and equivalence of oral and intramuscular dosage forms.

8.2 Analytical methods

The earliest attempts at assay of neuroleptic, especially phenothiazine, drugs involved extension of spectrophotometric and colorimetric methods, originally devised for standardization of dosage forms, to biological fluids. This was successful with *in vitro* studies, and with urine, but not with blood or its fractions. For example, an extremely valuable set of urine colour tests was established, for use in determining patient compliance, which was rapidly appreciated as a major problem in the then new field of pharmacotherapy of schizophrenia. Additionally, much was achieved with various forms of separation chromatography, on columns and paper, and with thin-layer chromatography plates in regard to identification of metabolites. However, these techniques were, at best, semiquantitative, and it was not until gas–liquid chromatography (GLC) was applied to the problem that a truly quantitative, instrumentalized chromatographic technique became available. By means of selective solvent extraction, and separation of chlorpromazine from its metabolites on GLC columns, plus detection and quantitation with electron capture instrumentation, it was possible for the first time to measure unequivocally a neuroleptic drug specifically and with sufficient sensitivity to confidently determine the concentration in plasma in a treated patient. Developments since this discovery have involved GLC with nitrogen detectors, and GLC linked to mass spectrometers, plus high-pressure liquid chromatography (HPLC), as well as reversion to biological methods, such as radioimmunoassay and radioreceptor assays. There is, nowadays, no reason why any particular drug or metabolite should not be specifically and sensitively assayed in plasma even though technical difficulties can be immense, and this has been achieved in most of the work published since 1970. It would be impossible in this review to review all of the published reports and to give an opinion on the validity of the assays used. Suffice it to say that in most of the work sufficient selectivity, sensitivity and responsivity has been achieved, and it is the biological data generated which have led to confusion in interpretion. However, radioreceptor assays deserve special attention.

8.2.1 Radioreceptor assays

It was the phenomenal technical difficulties involved in chemical assay of neuroleptic drugs that led to the development of the radioreceptor assay as a simple alternative. This method depends on the perception that there is a correlation between clinically effective neuroleptic dose and binding of the neuroleptic drug to biological material rich in the D_2 type of dopamine receptors. Binding is studied by displacing a radiolabelled ligand (for example, [^{3}H]spiroperidol) from a suspension of material extracted from the caudate nucleus of the rat. The neuroleptic displaces the ligand in proportion to its neuroleptic potency and its concentration. In this way, by mixing patient plasma, ligand and biological material, the distribution of the radiolabelled material gives a 'count' of the total neuroleptic activity in the patient plasma, regardless of its source.

Radioreceptor assays have their own modes of standardization. In most cases, the assays it calibrated on the basis of neuroleptic units (NU), where 1 NU is equivalent to 1 ng/ml of haloperidol. Since haloperidol has three times the potency in the system of chlorpromazine, 1 NU is equivalent to 3.0 ng/ml of chlorpromazine. Other drugs are intended to be similarly detected in relation to their potency, as are drug metabolites. However, in regard to the metabolites, this is a hope based on ignorance, since no adequate evaluation of their clinical potency in schizophrenic patients has been, or could be, conducted. Also, drugs at the high and low ends of the potency scale do not adequately conform. For example, since thioridazine is notably less potent than either chlorpromazine or haloperidol, 1 NU when thioridazine is the principal or only drug present represents many more nanograms per millilitre. By the same (or converse) token, 1 NU when fluphenazine is the principal or only drug present represents less than 0.3 ng/ml. Unfortunately, the radioreceptor assay underestimates thioridazine concentrations, and overestimates fluphenazine concentrations, even after the supposed in-built correction for potency is applied. The potency estimates involved are actually from *in vitro* binding studies, which do not correlate as well as originally hoped with *in vivo* phenomena. It has been very plausibly suggested, and the idea has been partially tested, that the relationships involved are confounded by differences among the drugs in brain/blood distribution, which is highest for fluphenazine, lowest for thioridazine (and mesoridazine) and intermediate for chlorpromazine and haloperidol (Sunderland & Cohen, 1987; Young *et al.*, 1989). Of course, this distribution, like almost all phenothiazine distribution phenomena, including, apparently, dopamine receptor binding, correlates very well with lipid solubility (partition coefficient). This was reinforced most recently by Morel *et al.* (1987) and Whelpton (1989).

8.3 Neuroleptic drug metabolites

Neuroleptic drugs, as typified by chlorpromazine, are extensively metabolized. Chlorpromazine itself is metabolized by sulphoxidation, demethylation, hydroxylation, deamination and dechlorination (to promazine). These metabolic reactions occur in combination. All of the reactions confer polarity, such that there is a modest decrease in lipophilicity and an increase in hydrophilicity with each reaction. When two or more reactions occur in combination, the decrease in lipophilicity is greater. The greatest hydrophilicity of all is induced by glucuronidation, which occurs when a hydroxylated metabolite becomes conjugated with glucuronic acid. It has been shown that only the first products of each metabolic reaction, for example, 7-hydroxychlorpromazine, demonomethyl and didesmethylchlorpromazine, chlorpromazine sulphoxide, and chlorpromazine N-oxide, bind importantly to dopamine receptors. Binding to D_1 receptors is perfectly correlated with lipophilicity. Binding to D_2 receptors correlates with lipophilicity except that 7-hydroxychlorpromazine binds more strongly than would be predicted, and certain other hydroxylated derivatives of chlorpromazine bind more strongly than does chlorpromazine itself. This is one reason why attention has focused on 7-hydroxychlorpromazine as the mediator of the effect of chlorpromazine, since dopamine theories of schizophrenia remain the major focus of mechanistic studies (Snyder *et al.*, 1974; Iverson, 1975; Creese *et al.*, 1976; Seeman *et al.*, 1976; Farde *et al.*, 1988; Hayes, 1989; Sibley, 1991).

Textbooks of pharmacology refer to the many active metabolites of chlorpromazine which contribute to its effect. This is not a fair representation of the truth. Only two metabolites of chlorpromazine have received any human evaluation of their effect, neither in an objective trial. In an open study, chlorpromazine sulphoxide was shown to have approximately one-seventh of the potency of chlorpromazine as a non-specific sedative. In another open study, a group of stablilized schizophrenics were shown not to relapse when switched from chlorpromazine to 7-hydroxychlorpromazine, and it was concluded that the two compounds are of approximately equal potency (Kleinman *et al.*, 1980). Chlorpromazine sulphoxide binds very little to dopamine receptors; 7-hydroxychlorpromazine binds strongly. It has been shown that antipsychotic effects can occur with chlorpromazine present in plasma, with none of its metabolites possessing dopamine receptor binding ability present. Thus the metabolic reaction is not essential for an antipsychotic effect. There can be little doubt that the active metabolites, numbering only three or four, contribute to the effect when present, but their presence is not essential. This, of course, plays havoc with monitoring schemes, since it greatly complicates the decision concerning what should be measured and how the measurements should be made.

Metabolism mostly represents a one-way conversion of relatively non-polar substrates to polar elimination products. There is virtually no interconversion. However, considerable interest has recently been focused on the interconvertibility of reduced and oxidized forms of haloperidol (Hawes *et al.*, 1986). As mentioned earlier, the active metabolites include demonomethylchlorpromazine, which has been examined in some detail in regard to age, race and sex effects on its concentrations (Young, 1986). Figure 1 summarizes current knowledge of the metabolic routes involved.

8.4   Presystemic elimination (first-pass effect)

This is the phenomenon of metabolism of orally administered drugs in the wall of the gastrointestinal tract, and/or in the portal circulation and liver, before the dose reaches the general (non-portal) circulation. It was first observed, within the present context, with chlorpromazine. It can cause relatively high metabolite to parent drug concentration ratios in plasma, in comparison with those arising after parenteral doses, and, depending on the pharmacological properties of the metabolites, activation or inactivation of the drug. It causes a relatively low pharmacokinetic area under the curve to occur for parent drug with oral doses. With chlorpromazine,

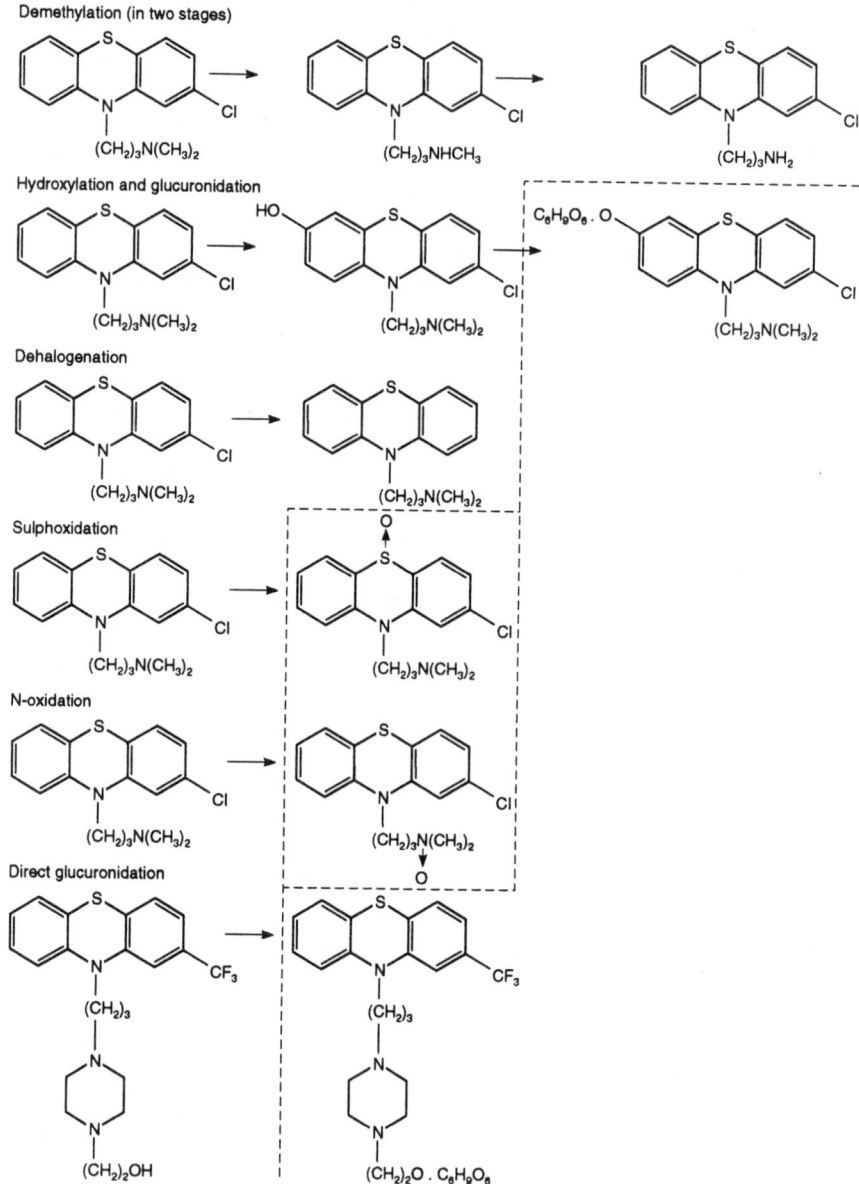

Figure 1 Metabolic routes for neuroleptic drugs.

presystemic elimination losses vary from 0 to 100%, depending on poorly understood factors. It is presumed that virtually all neuroleptic drugs are subject to a first-pass effect, but data on this are incomplete. The metabolites produced during presystemic elimination are excreted in urine and bile in much the same way as are the metabolites arising from parenteral dosing, so that a patient can be compliant, have very low concentrations of parent drug in plasma, and have 'normal' metabolite concentrations in urine. The first-pass effect is the major cause of inequivalence of oral and parenteral medication.

8.5 Enzyme induction

When enzyme induction occurs, the ability of the enzymes of the liver to convert drugs to metabolites increases, generally speaking because of an increase in the availability of the enzymes. With constant dosage, parent drug concentrations fall, and metabolite concentrations rise, so that metabolite to parent drug concentration ratios increase. Enzyme induction occurs in response to the presence of the drug being studied, or in response to the presence of an interfering drug. Phenobarbitone is the prototype inducer. Chlorpromazine is a self-inducer. Enzyme induction can lead to parent drug concentrations being lower at steady state than otherwise expected, or it can lead to concentrations falling as time progresses, with, in this case, metabolite concentrations maintained, increased, or themselves reduced because their further metabolism is enhanced.

8.6 Binding to plasma protein

Binding of drugs to plasma protein is a common problem. All neuroleptics bind reversibly to plasma protein. The bound percentage of the plasma content varies from 0% (some metabolites) to 99% (chlorpromazine). It is affected by the structure of the drug and by drug concentration. Bound molecules, at the time they are bound, are inert, in that they do not penetrate tissues, cross the glomerulus, or diffuse through the renal tubular epithelium. However, the dynamic nature of the binding must be appreciated. While the equilibrium constant is often very high, the rates on and off the binding site are also very high. If new molecules are added to the system re-equilibration is almost instantaneous. Thus the notion that binding delays tissue penetration or metabolism or renal excretion is considered by some investigators to be fallacious. However, the idea that binding affects the proportion of the dose involved at any particular time in the equilibrium between receptors and the biophase (the fluid surrounding the receptors– intracellular fluid, extracellular fluid and/or plasma water) is quite sound. Thus binding can be a factor in the intensity of response per unit of dose.

Virtually no attempts have been made to study free (unbound) neuroleptic concentrations (in plasma water) in the clinical setting, as has been done with phenytoin. It is possible that stronger clinical–chemical correlations would be observed if unbound levels were measured, but the assay problems involved seem to be virtually insuperable at present (Tang *et el.*, 1984; Garver, 1989).

8.7 pH-dependent phenomena

Most neuroleptics are weak organic bases (they are amines, with pK_a values in the region 8–11). As such, they cross membranes more readily in their non-ionized form, and when distributed between an aqueous medium and a lipid medium will transfer preferentially into the aqueous medium more readily if it is acidic. Thus conditions in the stomach do not favour absorption. Conditions in the intestine, although still 2 or 3 pH units away from the pK_a of the compound, are more favourable towards absorption (in fact, the vast surface area of the intestine, and the relatively long transit time in the intestine, ensure that the intestine and not the stomach is the major site of absorption). Also, relatively acidic urine will cause net transfer of neuroleptic drugs from blood into urine across the renal tubular membrane. However, since less than 1% of a neuroleptic dose is excreted as unchanged drug in urine even in favourable pH conditions, this is a relatively unimportant phenomenon.

8.8 Elimination half-life

The elimination half-life measures the kinetics of loss of drug from the body as a whole once all distribution equilibria have been achieved. With highly lipid-soluble drugs, such as neuroleptics, it is usually measured as the half-life of plasma level decay at the very low levels which prevail in the time period 24–72 h after a single dose, or in approximately the same time period after the last dose of a series of multiple doses. In the first 24 h after a single dose, by any route of administration, and at virtually all times during long-term treatment, the most recent dose is in the process of reaching distribution equilibrium between tissues into which the drug penetrates slowly, and plasma water. The elimination half-life represents metabolism and excretion of the final fraction of the single dose, or the body residue after the period of multiple dosing, but it is controlled by the relatively slow efflux which occurs from tissue stores. The elimination half-life can be immense, perhaps up to 60 days for chlorpromazine. It has little relevance to the desired effect of the drug, even though it represents mechanisms which keep significant amounts in the body for long periods with what is, after all, a very long-acting drug. However, it probably has considerable significance, in ways poorly understood at present, for toxicity.

Of considerable interest is the recent observation that the half-life of neuroleptic activity as measured by means of the radioreceptor assay is as much as 15–17 days after administration of haloperidol to rats (Cohen *et al.*, 1988). Generally speaking, rats eliminate drugs more rapidly than do humans, so from this data we might predict a very long half-life in humans. Also, a neuroleptic assay will include active metabolites with most drugs (although to a relatively minor extent with haloperidol). It should be noted that Irene Forrest and co-workers, over 30 years ago, reported that drug-derived material was detectable in urine for as long as 2 years following cessation of chlorpromazine treatment. Thus, without doubt, neuroleptic drugs persist in one form or another for a very long time, and this probably has significance for the relapse times after stopping dosing. However, since the route from the brain is via plasma, it is probably erroneous to think that neuroleptic drugs and their metabolites are ever present in tissues but absent from plasma. What actually happens is that they become analytically undetectable in plasma while still present in tissues (and detectable in urine). This was recently shown clearly with promazine (Curry & Hu, 1990).

8.9   U-shaped clinical–chemical relationships

In the very earliest work in this field of study, the observation was made that in a group of 11 patients, 3 were underdosed, with effectively zero plasma chlorpromazine concentrations in spite of dosing compliance, resulting from a virtual 100% first-pass effect (Curry *et al.*, 1970b). In the same work, two patients were overdosed, with plasma chlorpromazine concentrations above 500 ng/ml. These two patients benefited from reduction of dose and plasma level. The other six patients, with chlorpromazine concentrations in an intermediate range, were successfully treated. Underdosed patients were shown to be responsive to intramuscular dosing, especially with depot neuroleptics such as fluphenazine decanoate. Since the overdosed patients were shown to be responsive to reductions in oral dosage and consequent plasma levels it was concluded that they were exhibiting unwanted effects of chlorpromazine which, at the time, were difficult to distinguish from the disease being treated.

Thus a U-shaped clinical–chemical relationship was established. This observation has since been confirmed by several research groups, using a variety of drugs, and both specific (e.g. GLC and HPLC) and non-specific (radioimmunoassay and radioreceptor assay) techniques (Table 1). It has not been observed by a smaller group of investigators (Table 2), who may have restricted their studies to one limb of the U-shaped relationship. Figure 2 shows four representative figures from studies suporting the belief in a U-shaped relationship.

Table 1 Studies published in the period 1984–90 supporting the concept of a U-shaped relationship between neuroleptic plasma levels and clinical treatment outcome.

Drug	Patient group	Clinical method[a]	Plasma level method	Therapeutic range	Comments	Reference
Various	22 acute psychotics	BPRS	Radioreceptor assay	11–126 NU/ml	—	Kucharski et al. (1984)
Thiothixene	19 DSM-III inpatient schizophrenics	NHSI (% improvement)	GLC	2–15 ng/ml	Only one patient > 15 ng/ml	Mavroidis et al. (1984)
Fluphenazine	19 DSM-III inpatient schizophrenics	NHSI	GLC	0.13–0.7 ng/ml	—	Mavroidis et al. (1984a,b)
Haloperidol	17 DSM-III schizophrenics in acute exacerbation	NHSI	GLC	5–11 ng/ml 1–2.3 ng/ml	Plasma RBC	Garver et al. (1984)
Haloperidol	33 relapsing schizophrenics	BPRS	GLC	6.5–16.5 ng/ml 2.2–6.8 ng/ml	Plasma RBC	Smith et al. (1985)
Perphenazine	228 acute paranoid psychotic inpatients showing acute symptoms	Ad hoc (see text of paper)	GLC	2–6 nmol/l	Low doses required with increasing age	Hansen & Larsen (1985)
Trifluoperazine	36 acutely diagnosed psychotic inpatients	BPRS/GAS	GLC	1–2.3 ng/ml	Many more patients at low end of range than at the top end	Janicak et al. (1989)

Note: Older studies in this field have included: Curry & Marshall (1968), Sakalis *et al.* (1972, 1977), Van Putten (1974), Bergling *et al.* (1975), Gottschalk *et al.* (1975), Davis *et al.* (1978), May & Van Putten (1978), Wode-Heldgodt *et al.* (1978), Gelder & Kolakowska (1979), Cohen *et al.* (1980), Rubin *et al.* (1980), Chang *et al.* (1985), Curry *et al.* (1981), Dysken *et al.* (1981), Hansen *et al.* (1981), Magliozzi *et al.* (1981), Vaisanen *et al.* (1981), Van Putten *et al.* (1981, 1983), Morselli *et al.* (1982) and Mavroidis *et al.* (1983).

[a]BPRS, Brief Psychiatric Rating Scale; NHSI, New Haven Schizophrenic Index; GAS, Global Assessment Scale.

Table 2 Some recent studies in which the concept of a U-shaped relationship examined in Table 1 has been questioned.

Drug	Patient group	Clinical method[a]	Plasma level method	Overall results	Comments	Reference
Fluphenazine	24 schizophrenics (DSM-III)	Subjective rating	Radioreceptor assay	Non-responsive patients on high doses had high levels	May have reflected induction of side-effects	Brown & Silver (1988)
Zuclopenthixol	27 schizophrenics	CGI, CPRS and UKU	HPLC	*Inverse* correlation between effects and serum concentrations	Reflected over-dosing and induction of side-effects	Jorgensen *et al.* (1985)
Haloperidol	30 schizophrenics	Subjective rating	HPLC	5 ng/ml and up satisfactory; no upper plasma level limit found	Therapeutic 'plateau' suggested, no justification for high doses	Kirch *et al.* (1988)
Thiothixene	42 treatment-resistant schizophrenics	Subjective rating	HPLC	Patients showing moderate improvement had mean level of 26 ng/ml	Within range of other reports	Hollister *et al.* (1987)

[a]CGI, Clinical Global Impressions; CPRS, Comprehensive Psychopathological Rating Scale; UKU, See Lingjaerde *et al.* (1987).

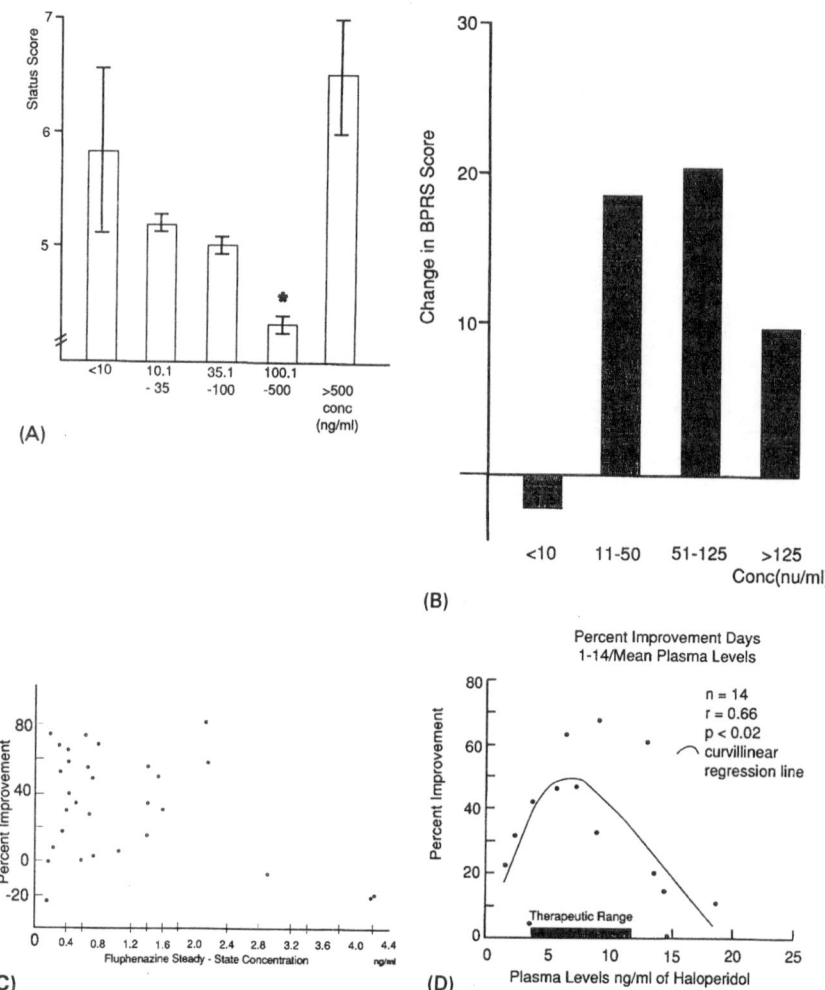

Figure 2 A composite diagram of figures from four publications illustrating the U-shaped relationship between neuroleptic drug response and plasma concentrations of the drugs concerned. (A) and (B) from Curry (1985); (C) from Dysken *et al*. (1981); (D) from Mavroidis *et al*. (1983). (All figures reproduced with permission of the copyright holders.)

8.10 Changeover from oral medication to depot neuroleptics

In spite of the immense body of relevant literature, it is still virtually impossible to make any hard-and-fast recommendation in this regard. We know all too little about comparative routes and rates of metabolism, parent drug and metabolite concentrations, time of dosage requirements, metabolite contributions to pharmacological action, etc. Generally speaking, it can be presumed that the depot neuroleptics have a greater bioavailability of pharmacologically active molecules than is the case with the oral dosage forms. Thus the daily depot dose is likely to be less than the daily oral dose of the same drug. Changing from one drug to another is, at present, a matter of trial and error. However, three groups of investigators have attempted objective study of this problem (Vasavan Nair et al., 1986; Nayak et al., 1987; Marder et al., 1989). Dosage equivalence when changing from oral to depot haloperidol dictates a 30–50% drop in daily dosage, and this is a consequence of the 30–40% first-pass effect applicable to oral but not intramuscular haloperidol (Nayak et al., 1987; Vasavan Nair et al., 1986). Changeover from oral fluphenazine to intramuscular fluphenazine decanoate is less precise, probably because the oral dose first-pass effect varies from, perhaps, 50% to 99% or more. In this case, a patient may be taking 10–25 mg per day of oral fluphenazine, but may need only 1 mg /day of the intramuscular dosage form. Extreme caution over an extended period of time is needed.

8.11 Prolactin

Prolactin proved to be something of a diversion in attempts to find pharmacological markers of neuroleptic drug effect. Prolactin release is under dopaminergic control, and since it is believed that the antipsychotic effect of neuroleptic drugs is exerted through dopaminergic pathways, it seemed reasonable to anticipate that there would be a correlation between the two variables. Indeed, prolactin levels are raised by neuroleptic drugs, but not with the same time-course, in that the times of maximal prolactin concentrations and peak drug concentrations do not coincide. No useful correlation between the effect of prolactin and the antipsychotic effect has been demonstrated (McCreadie et al., 1984).

8.12 Therapeutic monitoring

At issue is whether therapeutic monitoring should be practised, and if so, how it should be conducted. Of course, nobody would say that use of neuroleptics should be indiscriminate, with no patient checks, but there is a question of whether monitoring of events, such as plasma level changes, other than the desired effect is needed. The objectives of monitoring would include: (1) checks of patient compliance; (2) titration of plasma levels to a predetermined desirable range; (3) checks during gradual dose reduction to the minimum compatible with effective treatment; (4) detection of unwanted biochemical effects revealed through the study of biochemistry outside the context of pharmacokinetics; and (5) solution of medico-legal problems.

While modern techniques of patient care, patient education, and the availability of depot dosage forms have undoubtedly led to increased compliance, there is still an occasional, perhaps frequent need, for a chemical test to confirm compliance in a non-responding patient. While a positive chemical test of plasma will confirm compliance, a negative test can result equally well from a 100% first-pass effect in a compliant patient, as from non-compliance. It is psychologically disastrous to label a compliant patient non-compliant, so care must be exercised in interpreting a negative test of plasma. When there is a 100% first-pass effect in a compliant patient, the products of the first-pass effect are to be found in urine, so a non-specific urine colour test can actually be more valuable than a plasma test.

The desirable therapeutic range is from 30 to 350 ng/ml of chlorpromazine or its equivalent of other drugs. This translates to 10–100 ng/ml of haloperidol, or 10–100 neuroleptic units if the radioreceptor assay is applied. This is a broad therapeutic range, in total contrast with the narrow therapeutic ranges of such drugs as theophylline, digoxin, phenytoin and lithium, which cannot be used effectively without plasma level monitoring. Also, within the 30–350 ng/ml range for chlorpromazine, there can be fluctuations above and below the upper and lower limits as the result of the normal fluctuation between peak and trough plasma levels consequent on pulsed dosing, without any acute events occurring. Accordingly, therapeutic monitoring is not recommended for routine application. It should be saved for study of treatment-resistant patients – for the solution of problems.

There has been some discussion regarding whether or not the patients in whom a plasma level/clinical outcome relationship is observed belong to a subgroup. Almost 20 years ago, in the earliest literature concerned with chlorpromazine plasma levels, it was observed that non-responders could be in the low or high plasma level ranges of the U-shaped relationship. In the one group, responses improved when neuroleptic plasma levels were increased. In the other group, responses improved when plasma levels were decreased. However, both groups could include patients who showed no useful response at any level. This concept was recently reinforced in a communication in which the authors suggested that 'neuroleptic plasma levels may predict response in patients who meet a criterion for improvement' (Levinson et al., 1988). Any monitoring scheme must include a mechanism for excluding true non-responders.

It has been of great interest to watch a dramatic change in prescribing practice over the last 20 years during which therapeutic monitoring of neuroleptics has been possible. In the 1960s, a well-respected prescribing practice was to increase neuroleptic dosage for as long as was needed to induce reversible side-effects of the Parkinson's disease type, and then reduce dosage a little so that the side-effects disappeared, or to prescribe anticholinergic drugs with neuroleptic dosage maintained. Thus, the patients received the maximum tolerable neuroleptic doses. It was believed that this optimized the chances of therapeutic success. As time progressed, it was realized that tardive dyskinesia, the highly undesirable long-term, difficult to reverse, neurological side-effect of neuroleptic drug treatment was most likely to occur in patients who received relatively high doses for relatively long periods of time. Thus, the risk of tardive dyskinesia was reduced by prescribing, not the maximum tolerable dose, but the minimum dose compatible with a useful effect (Kane, 1983, 1986; Faraone *et al.*, 1986; McEvoy *et al.*, 1986). This has resulted in patients in whom a useful effect has occurred being given ever smaller doses, plus non-drug therapy, and successful treatment. This supports the idea that neuroleptic drugs do not specifically suppress schizophrenia, although nobody can deny the fact that they suppress some symptoms of schizophrenia, but that they reverse a vicious circle of psychopathology. In this a relatively high dose (and plasma level) is needed for initial reversal of the pathological process, but as treatment continues, progress can be maintained by reducing doses and reducing plasma levels – in some cases to zero. This theory places plasma level perspective in relation to the natural course of schizophrenia (Davis & Andriukaitis, 1986). It seems self-evident that, in achieving dose reduction, plasma level monitoring is desirable, perhaps necessary, so that if pathology reappears, there is a reference point available for future treatment.

How should monitoring be conducted; when is it necessary? Ideally, monitoring would involve a comprehensive screen of measurable effects, blood chemistry, and drug and metabolite concentrations. In practice, the decision is between specific chemical assay of the parent drug and (perhaps) one or two known, important metabolites, and the radioreceptor assay. While some investigators prefer whole blood (Simpson *et al.*, 1973; Garver *et al.*, 1977, 1984; Smith *et al.*, 1985) most would recommend sampling plasma or serum. The method applied will be dependent on availability of resources. In some institutions, largely those with medical school links, specific assay is sometimes available, and it is used effectively and efficiently by knowledgeable personnel. Specific chemical assay services can also be purchased through various contract laboratories. In a very much larger number of institutions, the best that can be hoped for is availability of a radioreceptor assay measurement. Unfortunately, even this is limited in its availability. The currently available assays involve a ^{3}H ligand, measured using liquid scintillation spectrometry. Few psychiatric hospital laboratories have much need for liquid scintillation spectrometry. They do conduct radioimmunoassays, using gamma counters, and there is a genuine need for a radioreceptor assay using a gamma emitting isotope in its ligand. The use of the radioreceptor assay seems to have declined in recent years, probably as much for this reason as for any other.

8.13 Conclusion

Investigation on a vast scale over a considerable period of time has led to the existence of a large body of information concerning pharmacokinetic aspects of neuroleptic drug therapy. Pharmacokinetic monitoring of therapy is warranted when difficult treatment problems persist but it involves specialized laboratory techniques and personnel skills not widely available. It is hoped that future drugs applicable to the treatment of schizophrenia will be less prone to produce unwanted effects and will give more predictable relief from the symptoms of the disease, reducing the need for the monitoring schemes which are apparently so difficult to provide.

References

Adamson, L., Curry, S.H., Bridges, P.K. et al. (1973) Dis. Nerv. Syst. 34, 181-191.

Baldessarini, R.J., Cohen, B.M. & Teicher, M.H. (1988) Arch. Gen. Psychiat. 45, 79-91.

Bergling, R., Mjorndal, T., Oreland, L. et al. (1975) Clin. Pharmacol. 15, 178-186.

Bolt, A.G., Forrest, I.S. & Serra, M.T. (1966) J. Pharmacol. Sci. 55, 1205-1208.

Brodie, B.B. (1967) J. Am. Med. Assoc. 202, 600-609.

Brown, W.A. & Silver, M.A. (1988) J. Clin. Psychopharmacol. 5, 143-147.

Chang, S.S., Javaid, J.I., Dysken, M.W. et al. (1985) Psychopharmacology 87, 55-58.

Cohen, B.M. (1980) Psychiat. Res. 1, 173-178.

Cohen, B.M. (1984) In Guidelines for the Use of Psychotropic Drugs (eds Stancer, H., Garfinkel, P.E. & Rakoff, V.M.), New York, Spectrum Publications.

Cohen, B.M., Lipinski, J.F., Pope, H.G. et al. (1980) Psychopharmacology 70, 191-193.

Cohen, B.M., Babb, S., Campbell, A. & Baldessarini, R.J. (1988) Arch. Gen. Psychiat. 45, 879-880.

Cooper, T.B. (1978) Clin. Pharmacokinet. 3, 14-38.

Cooper, T.B. (1985) J. Clin. Psychopharmacol. 5, A11-A16.

Creese, I. & Snyder, S.H. (1977) Nature 270, 180-182.

Creese, I., Burt, D.R. & Snyder, S.H. (1976) Science 192, 481-483.

Curry, S.H. (1968) Analyt. Chem. 40, 1251-1255.

Curry, S.H. (1976a) Psychopharmacol. Commun. 2, 1-15.

Curry, S.H. (1976b) Br. J. Clin. Pharmacol. 3, 20-28.

Curry, S.H. (1981) In Plasma Levels of Psychotropic Drugs and Clinical Response (eds Burrows, G.D. & Norman, T.), New York, Marcel Dekker.

Curry, S.H. (1985) J. Clin. Psychopharmacol. 5, 263-271.

Curry, S.H. (1988) In Pharmacology and Drug Treatment of Schizophrenia (eds Bradley, P. & Hirsch, S.), Oxford, Oxford University Press.

Curry, S.H. & Brodie, B.B. (1967) Fedn Proc. 26, 761.

Curry, S.H. & Hu, Y.-P. (1990) Psychopharmacol. Bull. 26, 95-98.

Curry, S.H. & Marshall, J.H.L. (1968) Life Sci. 7, 9-17.

Curry, S.H., Davis, J.M., Janowsky, D.S. & Marshall, J.H.L. (1970a) Arch. Gen. Psychiat. 22, 207-215.

Curry, S.H., Marshall, J.H.L., Davis, J.M. & Janowsky, D.S. (1970b) Arch. Gen. Psychiat. 22, 289-296.

Curry, S.H., Stewart, R.B., Springer, P.K. & Pope, J.E. (1981) Lancet i, 395-396.

Curry, S.H., Brown, E.A., Hu, OY-P. & Perrin, J.H. (1982) J. Chromatogr. 231, 361-376.

Dahl, S.G. (1982) Ther. Drug. Monit. 4, 33-40.

Dahl, S.G. (1986) Clin. Pharmacokinetics 11, 36-61.

Davis, J.M. & Andriukaitis, S. (1986) J. Clin. Psychopharmacol. 6, 2S-10S.

Davis, J.M., Erickson, S. & Dekirmenjian, H. (1978) In Psychopharmacology: a Generation of Progress (eds Lipton, M.A., DiMascio, A. & Killiam, K.F.), pp. 905-916, New York, Raven Press.

Dysken, M.W., Javaid, J.I., Chang, S. *et al.* (1981) *Psychopharmacology* **73**, 205–210.

Faraone, S.V., Curran, J.P., Laughren, T. *et al.* (1986) *Psychiat. Res.* **19**, 311–322.

Farde, L., Wiesel, F.-A., Halldin, C. & Sedvall, G. (1988) *Arch. Gen. Psychiat.* **45**, 71–76.

Forrest, F.M., Forrest, I.S. & Mason, A.S. (1961) *Am. J. Psychiat.* **118**, 300–307.

Forrest, I.S. & Green, D.E. (1972) *J. Forensic. Sci.* **17**, 592–617.

Garver, D.L. (1989) *J. Clin. Psychopharmacol.* **9**, 277–281.

Garver, D.L., Dekirmenjian, H., Davis, J.M. *et al.* (1977) *Am. J. Psychiat.* **134**, 304–307.

Garver, D., Hirschowitz, J., Glicksteen, G.A. *et al.* (1984) *J. Clin. Psychopharmacol.* **4**, 133–137.

Gelder, M. & Kolakowska, T. (1979) *Compr. Psychiat.* **20**, 397–408.

Gottschalk, L.A., Biener, R., Noble, E.P. *et al.* (1975) *Compr. Psychiat.* **16**, 323–337.

Greenblatt, D.J. (1985) *J. Clin. Pharmacol.* **25**, 239–240.

Hansen, L.B. & Larsen, N.-E. (1985) *Psychopharmacology* **87**, 16–19.

Hansen, L.B., Larsen, N.-E. & Vestergard, P. (1981) *Psychopharmacology* **74**, 306–309.

Hawes, E.M., Hubbard, J.W., Martin, M. *et al.* (1986) *Ther. Drug Monit.* **8**, 37–41.

Hayes, P.E. (1989) *Wellcome Trends in Hospital Pharmacy* **11**, 8–10.

Hollister, L.E., Lombrozo, L. & Huang, C.C. (1987) *Int. Clin. Psychopharmacol.* **2**, 77–82.

Iverson, L.L. (1975) *Science* **188**, 1084–1089.

Janicak, P.G., Javaid, J.I., Sharma, R.P. *et al.* (1989) *J. Clin. Psychopharmacol.* **9**, 340–346.

Jorgensen, A., Aaes-Jorgensen, T., Gravem, A. *et al.* (1985) *Psychopharmacology* **87**, 364–367.

Kane, J.M. (1983) *Schizophrenia Bull.* **9**, 528–532.

Kane, J.M. (1986) *J. Clin. Psychopharmacol.* **6** (1), 205–235.

Kelly, R.C. (1984) *Diagn. Med.* **7**, 37–40.

Kirch, D.G., Bigelow, L.B., Karpi, E.R. *et al.* (1988) *Schizophrenia Bull.* **14**, 283–289.

Kleinman, J.E., Bigelow, L.B., Rogol, A. *et al.* (1980) In *Phenothiazines and Structurally Related Drugs: Basic and Clinical Studies* (eds Usdin, E., Eckert, J. & Forrest, I.S.), New York, Elsevier.

Ko, G.N., Korpi, E.R. & Linnoila, M. (1985) *J. Clin. Psychopharmacol.* **5**, 253–262.

Krska, J., Sampath, G., Shan, A. & Soni, S.D. (1986) *Br. J. Psychiat.* **148**, 187–193.

Kucharski, L.T., Alexander, P., Tune, L. & Coyle, J. (1984) *Psychopharmacology* **82**, 194–198.

Levinson, D.F., Simpson, G.M., Singh, H. *et al.* (1988) *Arch. Gen. Psychiat.* **45**, 878–879.

Lingjaerde, O., Ahlfors, U.G., Bech, P. *et al.* (1987) *Acta Psych. Scandanavica Supplementum* **334**, 1–100.

McCreadie, R.G., Mackie, M., Wiles, D.H. *et al.* (1984) *Br. J. Psychiat.* **144**, 625–629.

McEvoy, J.P., Stiller, R.L. & Farr, R. (1986) *J. Clin. Psychopharmacol.* **6**, 133–138.

Mackay, A.V.P., Healey, A.F. & Baker, J. (1974) *Br. J. Clin. Pharmacol.* **1**, 425–430.

Magliozzi, J.R., Hollister, L.E., Arnold, K.V. & Earle, G.M. (1981) *Am. J. Psychiat.* **138**, 365–367.

Marder, S.R., Hubbard, J.W., Van Putten, T. & Midha, K.K. (1989) *Psychopharmacology* **98**, 433–439.

Mavroidis, M.L., Kanter, D.R., Hirschowitz, J. & Garver, D.L. (1983) *Psychopharmacology* **81**, 354–356.

Mavroidis, M.L., Kanter, D.R., Hirschowitz, J. & Garver, D.L. (1984a) *J. Clin. Psychiat.* **45**, 370–373.

Mavroidis, M.L., Kanter, D.R., Hirschowitz, J. & Garver, D.L. (1984b) *J. Clin. Psychopharmacol.* **4**, 155–157.

May, P.R.A. & Van Putten, T. (1978) *Arch. Gen. Psychiat.* **38**, 202–207.

Morel, E., Lloyd, K.G. & Dal, S.G. (1987) *Psychopharmacology* **92**, 68–72.

Morselli, P.L., Bianchetti, G. & Dugas, M. (1982) *Ther. Drug Monit.* **4**, 51–58.

Nayak, R.K., Doose, D.R. & Vasavan Nair, N.P. (1987) *J. Clin. Pharmacol.* **27**, 144–150.

Papadopoulas, A.S., Chard, T.G., Crammer, J.L. & Lader, S. (1980) *Br. J. Psychiat.* **136**, 591–596.

Rivera-Calimlin, L. (1982) *Ther. Drug Monit.* **4**, 41–49.

Rivera-Calimlin, L., Castaneda, L. & Lasagna, L. (1973) *Clin. Pharmacol. Ther.* **14**, 978–986.

Rivera-Calimlin, L., Gift, T., Nasrallah, J. *et al.* (1978) *Commun. Psychopharmacol.* **2**, 113–121.

Rubin, T.T., Forsman, A., Heykarts, J. *et al.* (1980) *Arch. Gen. Psychiat.* **37**, 1069–1074.

Sakalis, G., Curry, S.H., Mould, G.P. & Lader, M.H. (1972) *Clin. Pharmacol. Ther.* **13**, 931–946.

Sakalis, G., Chan, T.L., Sathananthan, G. *et al.* (1977) *Commun. Psychopharmacol.* **1**, 157–166.

Seeman, P., Lee, T., Chan-Wong, M. & Wong, K. (1976) *Nature* **261**, 717–718.

Sibley, D.R. (1991) *Trends Pharmacol. Sci.* **12**, 7–9.

Simpson, G.M., Lament, R., Cooper, T.B. *et al.* (1973) *J. Clin. Pharmacol.* **13**, 288–297.

Smith, R.C., Dekirmenjian, H., Davis, J.M. *et al.* (1977) *Commun. Psychopharmacol.* **1**, 319–324.

Smith, R.C., Baumgartner, R., Shvartsburd, A. *et al.* (1985) *Psychopharmacology* **85**, 449–455.

Snyder, S.H., Banerjee, S.P., Yamamura, H.I. & Greenberg, D. (1974) *Science* **184**, 1243–1253.

Sunderland, T. & Cohen, B.M. (1987) *Psychiat. Res.* **20**, 299–305.

Tang, S.W., Glaister, J., Davidson, L. *et al.* (1984) *Psychiat. Res.* **13**, 285–293.

Tune, L.E., Creese, I., DePaulo, J.R. *et al.* (1980) *Am. J. Psychiat.* **137**, 187–190.

Vaisanen, K., Vuikari, M., Rimon, R. & Raisanen, P. (1981) *Acta Psychiat. Scand.* **63**, 262–265.

Van Putten, T. (1974) *Arch. Gen. Psychiat.* **31**, 67–72.

Van Putten, T., May, P.R.A. & Jenden, D. (1981) *Psychol. Med.* **11**, 729–734.

Van Putten, T., May, P.R.A., Marder, S.R. *et al.* (1983) *Psychopharmacology* **79**, 40–44.

Vasavan Nair, N.P., Surrani-Gadotte, B., Schwartz, G. *et al.* (1986) *J. Clin. Psychopharmacol.* **6**, 30S–307S.

Whelpton, R. (1989) *J. Pharm. Pharmacol.* **41**, 856–858.

Wode-Heldgodt, B., Borg, S., Fyro, B. & Sedvall, G. (1978) *Acta Psychiat. Scand.* **58**, 149–173.

Young, A.S., Faraone, S.V. & Brown, W.A. (1989) *J. Clin. Psychopharmacol.* **9**, 361–363.

Young, R.C. (1986) *Ther. Drug Monit.* **8**, 23–26.

PART II
CLINICAL ISSUES

CHAPTER 9

THE ASSESSMENT OF ANTIPSYCHOTIC MEDICATION IN CLINICAL TRIALS

Steven R. Hirsch

Department of Psychiatry, Charing Cross and Westminster Medical School, University of London, London, UK

Table of Contents

9.1 Introduction

No one study, however well defined, can give a comprehensive or definitive answer to the range of important questions which must be addressed in evaluating a medicinal treatment for psychosis. Regardless of the statistical power or the magnitude of the observed differences in a particular study, confidence in the results can only be truly acquired by repeated replication in different hands and with different patients.

The issue of evaluation could not be more timely in the forthcoming decade because physiological, pharmacological, and animal behavioural studies have raised our

ANTIPSYCHOTIC DRUGS AND THEIR SIDE-EFFECTS
ISBN 0-12-079035-1

hopes that new compounds with non-pharmacological effects have been discovered and will, we hope, prove to be more effective in the treatment of psychosis than treatments available hitherto, and with less of the traditional neurological side-effects and risks of long-term tardive dyskinesia.

An outline of the traditional phases of clinical pharmacological studies in relation to requirements for registration provide a framework for this chapter, but the key and clinically most difficult issue is establishing the antipsychotic efficacy of a drug; this will be given the most attention, including a discussion of particular designs to overcome the inevitable clinical problems. Our discussion will be informed by the conclusions of a consensus meeting on the methodology of clinical trials in Europe dedicated to the methodology of antipsychotic drug evaluation which took place in Zurich in October 1990 (Angst *et al.*, 1991).

9.2   Phase I studies

Phase I studies take place after *in vitro* and animal pharmacological and toxicological studies have suggested that a compound is likely to have a desired clinical effect without causing intolerable or unwanted effects. Such studies traditionally take place, first of all, in normal human volunteers for a given single dose, and then with repeated doses of the drug under study, first in very low dosage which is then gradually increased until some adverse effects are noted. Pharmacokinetic studies are usually carried out to determine plasma levels and the elimination half-life from serum, and to confirm the routes of excretion and the safety of the medication. Normal human, clinical pharmacological studies are conducted to determine the pattern of action of the medication with particular attention to speed of onset and sedation or other side-effects. In some instances, patient volunteers are used instead of normal volunteers. The primary focus at this phase is safety.

9.3   Phase II studies

At this stage, medication is given to patients exhibiting symptoms to determine whether there are therapeutic effects without unacceptable side-effects and to confirm judgements based on animal studies, and in normal volunteers about side-effects and the tolerable and effective range of dose. While some hold the view that even at this stage only placebo-controlled trials can efficiently deal with accurate information, a broadly accepted view is that open, uncontrolled studies carried out by experienced psychiatrists with small numbers of patients is the preferred way to proceed. Although they cannot give proof of efficacy they provide information which is useful in planning double-blind studies. Open clinical studies are carried out to evaluate the safety of new drugs when initially introduced in patients and to identify the more common adverse effects. It may help to identify target symptoms of syndromes and discover new actions. They may be useful in helping the clinician to judge the time-course of the major actions on symptoms and estimate the therapeutic dose range and doses at which undesirable side-effects begin to appear. Thus, open clinical trials generate hypotheses but these must then be tested in well-controlled, double-blind studies.

Open studies in the early phases of phase II investigation introduce the clinician and supporting staff to new substances in a manner which is more easily accepted than a formal clinical trial. If the drug proves to be trouble free with some promising benefits, the stage is then set for double-blind, placebo-controlled studies.

Open studies allowing for flexible doses, increasing in a stepwise fashion, can help to determine an effective therapeutic dose and give an indication as to what dose is excessive or causes unwanted side-effects. This information can then be used to set the dosage level when more systematic placebo-controlled studies are carried on in the next stage of investigation.

Later stage phase II studies are carried out in patients to determine whether the drug is effective for the treatment of psychosis, and this is inextricably linked with the need to register the drug for clinical use. The Federal Drug Administration in the United States and the Committee on Safety of Medicines in Great Britain, as well as many other national drug commissioning authorities, require at least one well-organized, placebo-controlled study to establish that a particular drug is pharmacologically active. Demonstrating that a drug is as effective as standard drugs currently in use for the treatment of the condition is not sufficient because in any particular sample of patients the observed clinical effects could be due to spontaneous remission during treatment, either with the standard drug or the experimental drug. Equally, a particular group of patients may comprise poor responders to standard, therapeutically effective treatment as well as the drug under test. In both instances, the two treatments will have equal outcomes which could lead to the misleading conclusion that the new treatment is as effective as the standard treatment, when it may not be. In any group of patients, the most efficient test that a drug is effective is to demonstrate a significant difference between the response to placebo and the active substance.

As discussed later in this paper, placebo-controlled studies are the most efficient way to determine that a drug is clinically effective because the number required to demonstrate a significant clinical effect is much smaller than with any other design. Therefore, there is a strong argument for commencing placebo-controlled studies as soon as the likely clinical parameters of an effective dose, and the dose which begins to cause side-effects, are established. The placebo-controlled studies are therefore commenced in the second phase of phase II studies.

9.4 Phase III studies

Phase III is the stage at which extended clinical studies are carried out with a larger number of patients with the aim of establishing the drug's profile of action in comparison with standard established medication. Despite the large number of new substances which have been introduced into the market since the discovery of chlorpromazine in the mid-1950s, none had proven superior to chlorpromazine in their antipsychotic action (Hirsch, 1986), until a number of groups showed that clozapine is more effective than chlorpromazine in certain clinical groups. Many new substances which have been introduced into the market or are being tested today have been developed mainly to reduce the risk of unwanted side-effects, particularly extrapyramidal symptoms and, in some cases, tardive dyskinesia. Speed of onset has also been an area of clinical interest. While placebo-controlled studies are the most efficient type of study, clinicians find it is much easier to compare a new drug to a standard existing drug once its efficacy has been established in a placebo-controlled context. For the purpose of determining profile of action in respect to clinically desired effects and unwanted side-effects, comparisons of a new drug with an existing drug is satisfactory. This is also a more practical way to look at drug metabolism, interaction with other drugs, and the benefits of drugs when used for maintenance, long-term treatment to prevent re-occurrence of side-effects.

9.5 Phase IV studies

Phase IV refers to post-marketing studies carried out after the drug has been introduced into the market. Drug surveillance in large numbers in order to determine the incidence of side-effects and identify special, unpredicted effects can be done at this stage in order to generate new hypotheses. It also provides a better way of determining how a drug acts in so-called 'real life' conditions in a wide range of patients. Drug surveillance studies in phase IV have become more common in recent years.

9.6 Fixed- versus flexible-dose studies

Fixed-dose studies lack the reality of the normal clinical situation but are advantageous in certain specific goals such as determining dose–treatment relationships. Variability is reduced, and a standardized clinical experiment is provided which allows for a more accurate determination of efficacy at a certain dose level. In practice, the advantages are often overestimated because the individual variation between patients to a single dose is usually greater than the patients' response to the variation of the dose. Thus, in a standardized fixed-dose trial there is a danger that some patients will inevitably be underdosed and others will be given too high a dose, thereby paradoxically increasing the variability of response. A generally accepted clinical perspective is that an open trial is probably the better way to determine the optimal dose in the early phases of drug trials.

Allowing a clinician to flexibly increase the dose according to what he/she regards to be an appropriate clinical response is a more naturalistic way of proceeding as it mimics the normal clinical situation. Dose-response rates are more difficult to evaluate, particularly from case records, because patients who do not respond will have had their dose pushed to a maximum and some 20% of patients fail to respond at any dose. Thus, with currently available treatments at the higher dose range there is a tendency to collect patients with a poor response because poor responders inevitably end up being treated with higher doses. The marked variations in the standard clinical doses between clinicians in various countries suggest that the average dose is a clinically inspired variable, reflecting a local tendency to treat patients at a relative higher or lower mean dose. One possible way of overcoming this difficulty is to use a slowly progressive, stepwise escalation of dose, increasing the dose weekly from a predetermined level believed to be at or just below the effective antipsychotic dose. Another approach is to allow for a preliminary phase to determine the apparent optimal dose in a given patient, and then after 4 weeks to switch to a fixed-dose strategy.

9.7 Patient selection

The importance of patient selection in determining the outcome of clinical trials is often underestimated. A fuller discussion of this issue can be found elsewhere (Hirsch & MacRae, 1986). Open studies in the early stages are likely to include mild to moderately ill patients, as are placebo-controlled studies, because of the tendency to avoid difficult patients with problematic behaviours. Studies of outpatients with chronic disorders are unlikely to include patients who are treatment-resistant, and studies in acutely admitted patients are likely to include more than a representative number of patients who will remit spontaneously as well as milder patients who are able to give informed consent. Drug-withdrawal studies tend to include patients who respond to medication and have been well-stabilized without relapsing in the past, unless patients are entered at the time they are first given maintenance medication when they are admitted with an acute episode. Multi-centred trials do not overcome this problem, but do increase variability due to selection of patients because the different centres may include different types of patients. As long as the researcher realizes these sources of bias and designs the clinical trial to take account of the inherent tendency towards bias arising from the patient selection processes, these factors can be put to good use in helping to design a more relevant trial.

9.8   Statistical aspects

Statistical evaluation of results is based on either establishing equivalence between a new treatment and a standardized treatment, or establishing a difference. Placebo-controlled trials are the most efficient way to do this because the difference between the experimental and control group is maximized. If there is an apparent difference between two groups, statistical tests are used to exclude type 1 errors, that is, the likelihood that the observed difference has not occurred by chance. Placebo-controlled trials of standard neuroleptics can expect 15–25% of the placebo group to markedly improve spontaneously and 60–75% of the group on active medication, say a 40% difference. If a new drug is as good as a standard neuroleptic, one would only require 17 patients to be treated with the new drug and 17 on placebo to find a difference which is statistically significant at the 0.05 level. Furthermore, the difference between the response to placebo and the response to the experimental drug gives a direct measure of the specific pharmacological effect of the new treatment over and above non-specific effects observed on the placebo.

If, on the other hand, one is comparing a new drug to a standard neuroleptic, and the new drug is about as effective as a standard neuroleptic, the hypothesis being tested is that the new drug is as good or better than standard medication. This requires a statistical test of equivalence, or what is referred to as the statistical 'power' of the procedure using estimates of confidence intervals. In establishing the power of a particular treatment, that is, the likelihood that a type II error has been avoided, one would calculate the probability that the observed similarity between the two treatments has not occurred by chance and that a true difference has not been missed because the number of patients tested was not sufficient to show a difference when there was one. Thus, one is trying to reduce the risk of concluding that there is no difference between treatments when a genuine difference exists. In order to exclude the possibility that an observed difference of 20% or less between two treatments has not occurred merely as a matter of chance, with a power at the 95% level, one would need 154 patients in each group, assuming that the improvement rate for one of the two treatments would be 70%. If the improvement rate of one of the two treatments was 60%, one would require 161 patients. If the improvement rate of one of the two treatments was 60% and one wanted to show that a 10% difference between the two treatments is significant, that is, not miss a difference of 10% if it were present, and at the same time one wanted to be sure that if the difference was less than 10% this had not occurred by chance at the 95% confidence level, then one would need 589 patients in each treatment group!

When comparing a drug to a standard treatment, there are other problems that should be considered. Even if the two treatments are, in fact, identical one cannot be sure that this did not occur merely because the passage of time and the natural course of the disorder affected both groups equally. With an active drug for a comparator (control), an observed difference between two treatments may be due to use of clinically unequivalent doses of the two drugs. Many studies which find that one drug is more efficacious than another, or has fewer side-effects, have found such effects because the doses of the two drugs being compared are not clinically equivalent.

9.9 Rating instruments

Clinical trials in psychiatry require a structured or semi-structured standardized method for rating symptoms in order to reduce the variability due to different raters and to reduce bias by providing well-defined, operational criteria for the assessment of individual rating items. Generally, the choice of instruments involves a trade-off between instruments which are sensitive and likely to detect small changes, and instruments which are highly specific with well-defined ratings which tend to rely on easily detectable phenomena. In practice, the global ratings which allow the clinician to use his or her judgement are more likely to pick up small changes because they draw on a wider range of phenomena, as compared to scales which depend on well-defined criteria which give the clinician less latitude in making individual ratings. An example of the former is the Brief Psychiatric Rating Scale (BPRS), and examples of the latter are the Present State Examination (PSE) and the Comprehensive Psychopathological Rating Scale (CPRS).

9.10 Clinical designs for specific purposes

A methodological approach to a study is chosen according to the aims of the study and the hypothesis being tested. Studies have various purposes, including determination of short-term efficacy and long-term efficacy, dosage levels, frequency of side-effects, and the ability to determine the effect on particular target symptoms, such as positive symptoms of schizophrenia, hallucinations and delusions, or negative symptoms such as social withdrawal and poverty of movement.

Open studies used in phase I and phase II, and the choice of placebo-controlled studies versus the use of a standard well-established drug as a comparator for controls, have been discussed above. The ideal clinical design includes both a placebo to rule out spontaneous non-specific causes of change and a measure of the pharmacological efficacy, but will also include a standard drug as a third arm of treatment in order to show that the particular sample of patients will respond to the medication which is especially important if the experimental drug is no better than placebo. An active drug comparator also gives an indication of the difference between the new drug and the active standard drug, which helps to evaluate its special role in the clinician's armamentarium.

A different approach is to take patients who are already established on a given medication and have shown some clinical benefit, either in the acute phase or in the chronic phase, and substitute the new drug to see if the patient either improves further or deteriorates. Again, it is preferable to have a placebo as a third arm to ensure that the patients being studied are pharmacologically responsive to treatment and to see if the drug under test is partially or wholly inactive as compared to the placebo and standard treatment.

In practice, clinicians, nursing staff and patients as well as their families are usually reluctant to agree for patients to go into clinical trials, particularly when the patients are very disturbed. A modified clinical design to overcome this problem has been proposed by Hirsch & Barnes (1990). Patients are given a standard neuroleptic for a week to bring the most florid stage of acute disturbance under control and acclimatize the patient to an acute inpatient setting. After one week, the patients are randomized to continue on the standard drug or switched to placebo for the following 3–6 weeks. Again, a three-arm study would be better, randomizing patients to placebo, standard and experimental treatments. Patients who continue on a standard neuroleptic would be expected to continue to improve while patients on placebo should deteriorate back towards the baseline. The difference between placebo, standard and experimentally treated groups can then be tested at the end of the study period. One would normally commence the trial from the moment treatment is instituted with the standardized treatment, switching after one week; but an alternative is to treat patients openly with the standardized treatment and then ask for consent at the end of one week to switch to the two- or three-armed type of study. Another alternative is to treat the patients openly with the experimental drug for 2–4 weeks and then switch to a placebo control versus standard or experimental medication to continue for a short or long time period, according to the aims of the study. This latter design will select for patients who are both prepared to receive the experimental drug from the outset and have shown some reasonable response, establishing whether they are pharmacological responders or not by the placebo control in the second phase.

Studies of patients who are well established on a standard treatment or an experimental treatment inevitably involve selection bias, tending to include patients who respond well under the experimental condition and excluding patients who fail to respond. It follows that if there is any inherent pharmacological benefit to the medication being tested, beneficial effects should be demonstrable in a placebo-control design because of the inherent tendency of patients with schizophrenia to relapse while not on medication. Such studies are ethically justifiable in the light of the limited benefit of current medication which has high rates of side-effects, and by the fact that patients are closely observed and quickly taken out of the trial if they are not shown to benefit or at the first sign of deterioration. One must remember that nearly all patients will eventually relapse even if treated continually with current neuroleptic medication (see Curson et al., 1985).

9.11   Other measures of pharmacological efficacy

In addition to clinical studies, information about pharmacological effects in humans is beginning to emerge using positron emission tomography (PET) and single photon emission tomography (SPET) (see Chapter 7) as well as EEG and EEG brain-mapping. PET can be used with radioactively tagged carbon-11 isotopes of the active drug to show where the neuroleptic is taken up in the brain by brain receptors. Farde *et al.* (1988) in Sweden and Smith *et al.* (1988) have shown that neuroleptics with D_2 receptor-blocking properties are taken up in the basal ganglion while Lundberg *et al.* (1989) have shown that clozapine, which is a weak D_2 receptor blocker but a strong D_1 and 5-HT$_2$ receptor blocker, is taken up in the forebrain. Liddle *et al.* (1992) have shown that patients with specific clinical groupings of symptoms have specific areas of brain hypofunction and hyperfunction during resting state. The syndromes are the psychomotor poverty syndrome, with psychomotor slowness and poverty of affect and movement; disorganization syndrome with formal thought disorder and incongruity of affect; and reality distortion syndrome, with hallucinations and delusions. If this is so, one can, in the future, expect changes in cerebral blood flow to be demonstrable using PET, if new antipsychotic medications can effectively treat specific symptom groupings.

9.12   Conclusion

Clinical studies of the efficacy of treatment in schizophrenia are time-consuming and require tremendous commitment by clinicians, nurses and clinical research teams. However, it is only with this type of commitment which involves vigorous research with patients who will give their consent to treatment, and carefully observed studies which minimize the danger to patients and maximize the accuracy of scientific observation, that we can progress to develop a new focus of medication.

References

Angst, J., Bech, P., Bobon, D. *et al.* (1991) *Pharmacopsychiatry* **24**, 149–152.
Curson, D.A., Barnes, T.R., Bamber, R.W. *et al.* (1985) *Br. J. Psychiat.* **146**, 464–480.
Farde, L., Wiesel, F.-A., Halldin, C. & Sedvall, G. (1988) *Arch. Gen. Psychiat.* **45**, 71–76.
Hirsch, S.R. (1986) In *Psychopharmacology and Treatment of Schizophrenia* (eds Bradley, P.B. & Hirsch, S.R.), pp. 286–340, Oxford, Oxford University Press.
Hirsch, S.R. & Barnes, T.R.E. (1990) In *Methodology of the Evaluation of Psychotropic Drugs (Psychopharmacology Series 8)* (eds Benkert, O., Main, W. & Rickels, K.), pp. 26–36, Berlin, Springer-Verlag.

Hirsch, S.R. & MacRae, K.D. (1986) In *The Psychopharmacology and Treatment of Schizophrenia* (eds Bradley, P.B. & Hirsch, S.R.), pp. 212–233, Oxford, Oxford University Press.

Liddle, P.F., Friston, K.J., Frith, C.D. *et al.* (1992) *Br. J. Psychiat.* **160**, 179–186.

Lundberg, T., Lindstrom, L.H., Hartvig, P. *et al.* (1989) *Psychopharmacology* **99**, 8–12.

Smith, B., Wolf, A.P. & Brodie, J.D. (1988) *Biol. Psychiat.* **23**, 653–663.

CHAPTER 10

INDICATIONS FOR ANTIPSYCHOTIC DRUGS

Robin G. McCreadie

Department of Clinical Research, Crichton Royal Hospital, Dumfries, UK

Table of Contents

The principal indications for antipsychotic drugs are the management of schizophrenia both in the acute phase and as maintenance therapy, mania, delusional depression and behavioural disturbance in dementia. What follows is not a comprehensive review of the many hundreds of papers published on the indications for antipsychotics over the past 40 years. Rather, what is highlighted are key papers which have significantly increased our understanding of the antipsychotic drugs and their clinical uses.

10.1 Schizophrenia

Before 1952 the management of the acutely disturbed schizophrenic was largely custodial care, and unproved treatments such as insulin coma and leucotomy. The first antipsychotic, chlorpromazine, was introduced in psychiatric practice in France early in 1952. A French surgeon, Laborit, found that chlorpromazine had a tranquillizing effect without lowering the level of consciousness. Psychiatrists at his hospital, the Val De Grace, were the first to use the drug in psychiatric patients, and shortly thereafter Delay and colleagues also used the drug in their hospital, and reported on its therapeutic effect (Delay et al., 1952).

Chlorpromazine was clearly a major advance in therapeutics – the controlled trials came many years later. Other phenothiazines, butyrophenones and thioxanthenes followed, and later came diphenylbutylpiperidines and substituted benzamides. Currently the Monthly Index of Medical Specialties (MIMS) in the United Kingdom lists over 20 antipsychotic drugs. Such a large number suggests that either the illness schizophrenia has many symptoms which can be 'picked off' by different drugs or that no one drug is much better than any other.

10.1.1   Acute schizophrenia

By the late 1950s there were at least ten phenothiazines being used in the treatment of schizophrenia, although some psychiatrists remained sceptical about their value. In 1961, in the United States, the NIMH Psychopharmacology Service Center began a co-ordinated, double-blind study involving over 400 acutely ill schizophrenic patients treated at nine collaborating hospitals (NIMH, 1964). Chlorpromazine, fluphenazine and thioridazine were compared with placebo. Within 6 weeks, 95% of drug-treated patients showed some degree of improvement, demonstrated through global, symptom and behaviour assessments; 75% showed marked or moderate improvement. At the end of 6 weeks, 46% of patients were rated as having no symptoms or borderline illness. Placebo patients, while not improving as much as drug patients, did show some improvement: more than 20% were much improved by the end of 6 weeks. This, however, was the proportion of placebo patients who could be maintained for 6 weeks – almost a third of placebo patients who started the study were dropped before 6 weeks as treatment failures. No significant differences in clinical efficacy were found among the three active phenothiazines; specifically there was no evidence that chlorpromazine was more effective in patients requiring sedation or fluphenazine more effective in withdrawn patients.

The NIMH study examined only drugs of the phenothiazine group. Drugs belonging to other groups, the butyrophenones (e.g. haloperidol), thioxanthenes (e.g. flupenthixol), diphenylbutylpiperidines (e.g. pimozide) and substituted benzamides (e.g. sulpiride) have been less extensively investigated. However, studies which have shown the active drug to be more effective than placebo include nine on haloperidol and two on pimozide (Davis, 1985).

An elegant study of the thioxanthene flupenthixol in the late 1970s not only showed that it was effective in acute schizophrenia, but increased our understanding of the mode of action of antipsychotics (Johnstone et al., 1978). Flupenthixol has α and β isomers. The α isomer blocks the dopamine receptor, the β isomer does not. Forty-five patients with acute schizophrenia received either the α isomer or the β isomer or placebo. The drug effect, which appeared only in the third and fourth week of the trial, was greatest with α flupenthixol; the β isomer was no more effective than placebo. This clinical study supports the view that antipsychotics act through their effect on the dopamine system.

Studies quoted so far have shown that antipsychotics are effective in acute schizophrenia. Which symptoms respond to treatment? A further analysis of the NIMH study (Goldberg *et al.*, 1965) found that the clinical effects of drug treatment went far beyond those suggested by the term 'tranquillizer'. In addition to a change in excitement and anxiety, there was a reduction in symptoms such as apathy and motor retardation. Symptoms in which there was an improvement on drug treatment, but not on placebo, included irritability, hebephrenic symptoms (for example, grimacing and silly giggling) and indifference to the environment. This study suggested, therefore, that a wide range of symptoms respond to antipsychotic medication.

More recently, the concept of positive and negative symptoms (though long described, its origin is obscure; Berrios, 1985) has become fashionable once again (Crow, 1980). Positive symptoms include hallucinations, incoherence, delusions and incongruity of affect. There is less agreement as to what constitutes negative symptoms, though most psychiatrists would accept blunting of mood, poverty of thought and underactivity. The study by Johnstone *et al.* (1978) on α- and β-flupenthixol examined individual symptoms and found improvement was largely confined to positive symptoms. Both non-specific symptoms, such as anxiety and depression, and negative schizophrenic symptoms showed little tendency to improve and no differential response to drug therapy. The authors suggested, therefore, that the scope of the antipsychotic effect may be more limited than that suggested by the NIMH study. However, they point out that negative symptoms rated in a clinical interview may not be the same as negative features assessed by behavioural ratings. Such features as withdrawal may be secondary to delusional ideas. There is probably as yet no convincing evidence that antipsychotic drugs significantly improve negative symptoms.

Is any one antipsychotic drug better than any other in the treatment of acute schizophrenia? The answer would appear to be no. If the answer were yes, then clinical psychiatrists throughout the world would have spotted it many years ago. Even the new generation of antipsychotics, such as remoxipride, show no difference in efficacy when compared with standard drugs such as haloperidol. For example, Lewander *et al.* (1990) analysed nine double-blind studies which compared remoxipride with haloperidol. Studies lasted 4–6 weeks, and improvement was assessed by the Brief Psychiatric Rating Scale and the Clinical Global Impression Scale. The results showed that remoxipride had a therapeutic effect comparable to that of haloperidol on psychotic symptoms. The benefits of the newer antipsychotics lie more in fewer side-effects, especially less sedation and extrapyramidal side-effects. However, it is every clinician's experience that some individual patients may respond poorly to one antipsychotic, but not to another. The reasons for this are unclear. Between-individual differences in pharmacokinetic and pharmacodynamic factors are no doubt important.

Although no one drug is better than any other in dealing with core schizophrenic symptoms, the sedative action of some antipsychotics may be useful when dealing with an acutely disturbed patient. High-potency compounds such as haloperidol may be preferable, as patients may require high doses. The less potent drugs may cause disabling side-effects such as hypotension.

10.1.2 Maintenance therapy in schizophrenia

Once the acute episode has subsided, schizophrenics should remain on lower doses of antipsychotic medication as maintenance therapy (see Chapter 12). The need for maintenance therapy after an acute episode was demonstrated in the 1970s by a study from the MRC Social Psychiatry Unit in London (Leff & Wing, 1971). Thirty-five patients out of an original 116 entered the trial. Thirty-two had a Catego diagnosis of florid schizophrenia. When they had recovered from an acute schizophrenic illness and had been discharged from hospital they received in a double-blind study either trifluoperazine, chlorpromazine or placebo. Over 1 year, 35% of the drug patients relapsed, compared with 80% of placebo patients. The paper also studied in detail the 81 patients who did not enter the study. They included those considered well enough not to need maintenance therapy (an opinion subsequently shown to be substantially correct), and those thought to be too precarious to risk taking off drugs – most of the latter relapsed without indeed being taken off drugs. The authors concluded that maintenance therapy was likely to be effective in patients with an 'intermediate prognosis'.

In a double-blind study from the United States (Hogarty & Ulrich, 1977), 374 schizophrenic outpatients were randomly assigned to chlorpromazine or placebo therapy following a 2-month period of drug stabilization after discharge. An analysis of the actual experiences of drug- and placebo-treated patients over the subsequent 3-year period showed that over the entire 3 years the monthly risk of relapse on drug (2.9%) was much less than that on placebo (9.6%). The risk of relapse among successfully maintained patients did decline, but did not disappear with the passage of time. For example, at month 1 the risk of relapse on drug was 4%. By month 24 the risk was 1.5%.

Davis (1975) reviewed 24 controlled studies on the use of maintenance antipsychotic drugs. Out of 1068 patients who received placebo, 698 (65%) relapsed, in contrast to 639 out of 2127 who received maintenance antipsychotics (30%). This review confirmed the effectiveness of maintenance therapy in schizophrenia.

If patients do benefit from maintenance therapy, how long should such therapy continue? The answer may be, indefinitely. For example, a second study from the MRC Social Psychiatry Unit (Hirsch et al., 1973) examined patients, a third of whom had been on intramuscular drugs for more than 2 years. Eighty-one chronic schizophrenic outpatients, who had been maintained on fluphenazine decanoate injections for 8 or more weeks, either continued on this drug or were switched under double-blind conditions to placebo injections. After 9 months, 8% of patients on active medication had relapsed, compared with 66% on placebo. Relapse was accompanied by a resurgence of specifically schizophrenic symptoms, and by an increase in abnormalities described by relatives.

A further discontinuation study (Cheung, 1981) examined patients who had been successfully maintained for even longer on neuroleptics. Thirty patients had had no relapses for 36–60 months, and had been continuously maintained on neuroleptic medication. Fifteen continued in a double-blind study with neuroleptics, and 15 received benzodiazepines. Over 18 months, two patients on neuroleptics, but eight on benzodiazepines relapsed, a statistically significant difference. The author emphasizes again, as did Leff & Wing (1971), that the schizophrenic patients in this study represented a group of intermediate prognosis.

Drugs used as maintenance therapy are either oral or long-acting intramuscular preparations. The latter are especially popular in the United Kingdom, and were introduced largely to improve patient compliance (see Chapter 13). There is no evidence that one oral antipsychotic is any better than any other in preventing relapse, nor one intramuscular drug better than another. However, comparisons between oral and intramuscular preparations are few. One study (Falloon *et al.*, 1978) compared oral pimozide with intramuscular fluphenazine decanoate. Forty-four patients returned to the community following hospital treatment of an acute schizophrenic episode. They received, in a double-blind study for 1 year, either oral pimozide or injectable fluphenazine decanoate every 2 weeks. The principal criteria of outcome were a schizophrenic relapse, depressive symptomatology, adverse effects, and the regularity of medication. Oral pimozide was at least as effective as intramuscular fluphenazine, with 24% relapsing compared with 40%. The frequency of extra-pyramidal symptoms tended to decrease on pimozide and increase with fluphenazine.

This study suggests that oral antipsychotics are as useful as long-acting intramuscular drugs. This may be so in a research setting. In everyday clinical practice, however, it is unlikely that patients on oral medication would be so closely supervised.

In view of the propensity of antipsychotics to produce side-effects, especially tardive dyskinesia, a recent attempt has been made, not to prescribe patients continuous antipsychotic medication as maintenance therapy, but only to prescribe such drugs when relapse appears imminent (Jolley *et al.*, 1990). In this study, 54 outpatients who met DSM-III criteria for schizophrenia, and were in remission, received either active or placebo depot fluphenazine decanoate. Both groups received brief courses of oral haloperidol when prodromal symptoms or relapse occurred. Of 19 relapses recorded over 2 years, 10 were preceded by non-psychotic prodromal signs. Survival rates for both relapse and hospitalization were worse with intermittent treatment than continuous treatment over the 2-year period; 92% of controls and only 54% of patients given intermittent treatment survived the 2-year period without hospitalization.

Prolonged or frequent relapses as well as episodes of prodromal symptoms were more frequent with intermittent treatment. The authors concluded that continuous depot neuroleptic prophylaxis was superior to brief intermittent therapy.

10.1.3 Drug-resistant schizophrenic patients

In a small number of patients, estimated at 10–20% of the schizophrenic population, florid psychotic symptoms will not respond to typical neuroleptic drug therapy. What then should be done? In the 1970s there was a vogue for very high dose treatment for chronic drug-resistant patients. However, controlled studies did not support this approach. For example, in a double-blind study of 6 months duration (McClelland *et al.*, 1976) a very high dose of fluphenazine decanoate (250 mg weekly) was compared with a standard dose (12.5 mg weekly) in 50 chronic schizophrenic patients. Assessment was by the Brief Psychiatric Rating Scale and the Wing Ward Behaviour Scale. Both treatment groups improved, but there was no significant difference between them. Extrapyramidal side-effects were not significantly higher in the very high-dose group. In another study (McCreadie & MacDonald, 1977), a double-blind chlorpromazine-controlled trial, high-dosage haloperidol (100 mg daily) did improve the mental state of some patients over 3 months. However, the majority of patients on haloperidol showed a deterioration in ward behaviour, possibly related to drowsiness. They also developed abnormal liver function tests.

High-dose therapy, therefore, is probably not helpful. Recently, however, there has been increased interest in the use of clozapine in drug-resistant patients. Clozapine, a dibenzodiazepine, is an 'atypical neuroleptic' in that its binding to D_1 and D_2 receptors is relatively weak, and more equivalent than that of most typical neuroleptics (see Chapters 2 and 11). It is a potent muscarinic acetylcholine receptor antagonist, and also has serotonin, adrenergic and histaminergic blocking activity. The side-effects of granulocytopenia, however, has limited its everyday use. In a multicentre, clinical trial Kane *et al.* (1988) assessed its efficacy in patients resistant to standard neuroleptics. DSM-III schizophrenics who had failed to respond to at least three different neuroleptics entered a single-blind, prospective trial of haloperidol (mean dose 61 mg) for 6 weeks. Patients whose condition remained unimproved ($N = 268$) then received in a double-blind study either clozapine (up to 900 mg daily) or chlorpromazine (up to 1800 mg daily) for 6 weeks. Assessment included the Brief Psychiatric Rating Scale, the Clinical Global Impression Scale and the Nurses Observation Scale for Inpatient Evaluation. Thirty per cent of the clozapine-treated patients responded compared with 4% of the chlorpromazine-treated patients. The improvement included negative as well as positive symptom areas. The authors concluded that this response to clozapine demonstrated that the subgroup of severely ill schizophrenic patients previously considered by many to be beyond the reach of conventional therapy does remain capable of experiencing substantial medication response. They also pointed out that this is the first time that any specific antipsychotic drug has been shown to be superior to another in a well-defined group of treatment-resistant patients. The study suggested that with capable monitoring clozapine should be considered in patients with drug-resistant schizophrenic illnesses.

10.2 Mania

Antipsychotic drugs have been extensively studied in schizophrenia. Their use in mania, although widespread, has received little scientific attention by way of controlled studies. However, one large, well-designed, double-blind study was published in 1972 (Prien et al., 1972). In an 18-hospital collaborative study, 255 newly admitted manic patients were randomly assigned to chlorpromazine or lithium carbonate for a 3-week period. Treatments were compared in terms of early termination, symptom change and toxicity. Chlorpromazine was clearly superior to lithium in treating the highly active patient. Chlorpromazine acted more quickly, produced significantly fewer dropouts, and had a lower incidence of severe side-effects. The difference between chlorpromazine and lithium was less pronounced among mildly active patients, but lithium appeared to be the better treatment. It left the patient feeling less sluggish and fatigued, and produced fewer side-effects. Further smaller studies have confirmed the two principal findings of this study, namely, that antipsychotics are more effective in the seriously disturbed manic than lithium, and that they act more quickly. No studies have clearly suggested that any one antipsychotic is more effective than any other; one found that although chlorpromazine was effective globally it produced fewer changes in manic ideation and behaviour than haloperidol (Shopsin et al., 1975).

10.3 Delusional depression

For many clinicians electroconvulsive therapy is the treatment of choice in patients with delusional depression. However, a number of studies have suggested that a combination of an antipsychotic and an antidepressant may also be useful. One of the best-designed studies was that by Spiker and colleagues (1985). It examined three groups of patients who fulfilled the Research Diagnostic Criteria for major depressive disorder, psychotic subtype with the presence of a delusion. In a double-blind, randomized design 17 patients received the antipsychotic perphenazine, 19 the antidepressant amitriptyline and 22 amitriptyline plus perphenazine. Medication was given for 5 weeks and progress assessed through the use of the Hamilton Rating Scale for Depression, the Brief Psychiatric Rating Scale, and the Raskin Global Rating Scale. A responder was defined as a patient who was no longer delusional nor

163

depressed. Seventy-eight per cent of the patients assigned to amitriptyline plus perphenazine were responders, compared with only 14% of those treated with amitriptyline alone, and 19% of those treated with perphenazine alone. Clearly the combination of amitriptyline and perphenazine was superior.

10.4 Functional psychosis

It has long been clinicians' experience that the distinction between schizophrenia and affective illness can be difficult to make; such a distinction indeed is probably unnecessary in the drug treatment of the acute episode. It is the nature of the symptoms rather than the underlying diagnosis that determines which drugs are used; namely, antidepressants for depressive symptoms, antipsychotics for psychotic symptoms and lithium or antipsychotics for manic symptoms. This longstanding approach by clinicians to the management of functional psychosis was examined in detail in a double-blind study by Johnstone *et al.* (1988). The efficacy of the neuroleptic pimozide, lithium and a combination of the two was compared with that of placebo in a 4-week trial in 120 functionally psychotic patients, each of whom was assessed for psychotic symptoms by the Krawiecka Scale, manic symptoms by the Bech–Rafaelson Scale, and depressive symptoms by the Montgomery–Asberg Scale. The sample was subdivided into those with predominantly elevated mood, those with predominantly depressed mood, and those with no consistent mood change. Pimozide reduced psychotic symptoms in all groups of patients. It had no significant effect on depressed mood. The patients were then reclassified in terms of DSM-III criteria, and the results recalculated for these classifications. This method of reclassification made no difference to the results.

This study confirms the principal indications for antipsychotics – namely psychotic symptoms in whatever illness they appear.

10.5 Dementia

Although antipsychotic drugs have been used for over 30 years in the management of demented elderly patients, their usefulness has yet to be made clear. In one double-blind study (Ather *et al.*, 1986), 74 patients aged 65 years or over with a diagnosis of dementia (including Alzheimer and arteriosclerotic forms) and requiring treatment for longstanding agitation, confusion and restlessness received either thioridazine or chlormethiazole. Active treatment was for 4 weeks, and treatment efficacy was examined through the use of the Crichton Geriatric Behaviour Rating Scale, and the Behaviour Rating Scale of the Clifton Assessment Procedures for the Elderly. Thioridazine and chlormethiazole were found to be equally effective in controlling behavioural disturbance associated with dementia. However, confusion and nocturnal awakening were controlled more effectively with chlormethiazole. A greater incidence of adverse effects was associated with thioridazine treatment.

In a recent review of antipsychotics in the behavioural treatment of dementia (Sunderland & Silver, 1987), the authors identified 20 double-blind or placebo-controlled studies published between 1954 and 1986. The studies involved 1207 patients with a mean age of 74 years. The diagnosis ranged from 'mentally disturbed elderly' to organic brain syndrome. Thus, the patient group is a heterogeneous one with numerous underlying aetiologies for the cognitive impairments. Sixty per cent of the double-blind studies showed beneficial effects with antipsychotics. The symptoms of excitement, agitation, hallucinations and hostility were found to be the most responsive to antipsychotics. However, there was also a high placebo response with behavioural symptoms and a relatively small percentage showed marked clinical improvement. The authors concluded that when used acutely at low doses for specific purposes, for example, treatment of agitation, the drugs can be both safe and effective. Although extrapyramidal and anticholinergic side-effects were no greater than in other psychiatric populations, little if any attention has been paid to the possible deleterious effects of antipsychotics on cognition.

10.6 Miscellaneous indications

Tourette's disorder   In Tourette's disorder with multiple muscle and vocal tics, some patients' movements diminish significantly with an antipsychotic drug. Haloperidol appears to be the drug of choice, although there does not seem to be any large double-blind controlled study demonstrating its effectiveness over other antipsychotics. Most reports are of a few patients only (for example, Shapiro & Shapiro, 1968).

Mental handicap   The mentally handicapped person with a psychotic illness should, of course, be given an antipsychotic. However, antipsychotic drugs in large doses are not infrequently used to manage the individual with severe aggressive or self-injurious behaviour. There is little evidence that antipsychotics are of any benefit in the treatment of groups of such patients (Craft, 1958). It is probable that they do no more than sedate and depress all behaviours. Behaviour modification programmes should be tried first with severe aggressive or self-injurious behaviour. If such programmes fail, antipsychotic drugs may then be tried.

Depression   In depression, it has been claimed that the antipsychotic flupenthixol may be effective in low doses. In a double-blind study (Young et al., 1976) 60 depressed outpatients received either amitriptyline (75–225 mg/day) or flupenthixol

(1.5–4.5 mg/day) for 6 weeks. There were no significant differences between the two drugs, but the trends favoured flupenthixol, especially in the alleviation of anxiety. The authors pointed out that the patients were not severely depressed and that the improvement on both drugs might have been due partly to anxiolytic drug effects. This view is supported in a small, placebo-controlled, crossover study of neurotic outpatients, where anxiety symptoms were helped more than depressive symptoms by flupenthixol (Predescu *et al.*, 1973). Clearly, larger placebo-controlled studies of both moderately and severely depressed patients are needed to determine the usefulness of flupenthixol in the treatment of depression.

Anorexia nervosa In anorexia nervosa, chlorpromazine has been widely prescribed on account of its appetite-stimulating properties. It has been examined in open studies as the only physical treatment (Crisp, 1966) or in combination with modified insulin treatment (Dally & Sargant, 1966). Both studies supported the use of chlorpromazine, at least in the short term, as a way of inducing weight gain. There have been no controlled double-blind studies. The use of chlorpromazine has diminished in recent years with greater emphasis now on behavioural and psychotherapeutic techniques. It is also important to remember that chlorpromazine itself may induce amenorrhoea.

Monosymptomatic hypochondriacal delusional states In monosymptomatic hypochondriacal delusional states, the oral antipsychotic pimozide is said to be of value. However, the reported studies contain few patients and are rarely double-blind. An open study of 26 patients simply reported that 19 had an 'excellent response' (Munro, 1980). In a small, double-blind, placebo-controlled crossover study, 11 patients with delusions of infestation were treated with pimozide for 6 weeks; 10 improved, with significant relief of itch and delusions (Hamann & Avnstorp, 1982). There is no reason to suppose that pimozide should be more effective than any other antipsychotic; there have been no double-blind studies comparing pimozide with other antipsychotics.

References

Ather, S.A., Shaw, S.H. & Stoker, M.J. (1986) *Acta Psychiat. Scand.* **73** (Suppl. 329), 81–91.
Berrios, G.E. (1985) *Arch. Gen. Psychiat.* **42**, 95–97.
Cheung, H.K. (1981) *Br. J. Psychiat.* **138**, 490–494.
Craft, M.J. (1958) *J. Ment. Defic. Res.* **1**, 91–95.
Crisp, A.H. (1966) *Br. J. Psychiat.* **112**, 505–512.
Crow, T.J. (1980) *Br. Med. J.* **280**, 66–68.
Dally, P. & Sargant, W. (1966) *Br. Med. J.* **ii**, 793–795.
Davis, J.M. (1975) *Am. J. Psychiat.* **132**, 1237–1245.
Davis, J.M. (1985) In *Comprehensive Textbook of Psychiatry* (eds Kaplan, H.I. & Sadick,

B.J.), pp. 1481-1513, Baltimore, Williams & Wilkins.

Delay, J., Deniker, P. & Harl, J.M. (1952) *Ann. Med. Psychol.* **110**, 112-117.

Falloon, I., Watt, D.C. & Shepherd, M. (1978) *Psychol. Med.* **8**, 59-70.

Goldberg, S.C., Klerman, G.L. & Cole, J.C. (1965) *Br. J. Psychiat.* **111**, 120-133.

Hamann, K. & Avnstorp, C. (1982) *Acta Dermatovener (Stockholm)* **62**, 55-58.

Hirsch, S.R., Gaind, R., Rohde, P.D. *et al.* (1973) *Br. Med. J.* **1**, 633-637.

Hogarty, G.E. & Ulrich, R.F. (1977) *Arch. Gen. Psychiat.* **34**, 297-301.

Johnstone, E., Crow, T.J., Frith, C.D. *et al.* (1978) *Lancet* **i**, 848-851.

Johnstone, E.C., Crow, T.J., Frith, C.D. & Owens, D.G.C. (1988) *Lancet* **ii**, 119-125.

Jolley, A.G., Hirsch, S.R., Morrison, E. *et al.* (1990) *Br. Med. J.* **301**, 837-842.

Kane, J., Honigfeld, G., Singer, J. & Meltzer, H. (1988) *Arch. Gen. Psychiat.* **45**, 789-796.

Leff, J.P. & Wing, J.K. (1971) *Br. Med. J.* **3**, 599-604.

Lewander, T., Westerbergh, S.E. & Morrison, D. (1990) *Acta Psychiat. Scand.* **82** (Suppl. 358), 92-98.

McClelland, H.A., Farquharson, R.G., Leyburn, P. *et al.* (1976) *Arch. Gen. Psychiat.* **33**, 1435-1439.

McCreadie, R.G. & McDonald, I.M. (1977) *Br. J. Psychiat.* **131**, 310-316.

Munro, A. (1980) *Br. J. Hosp. Med.* **24**, 34-38.

NIMH Psychopharmacology Service Centre Collaborative Study Group (1964) *Arch. Gen. Psychiat.* **10**, 246-261.

Predescu, V., Ciurezu, T., Timtofte, G. & Roman, I. (1973) *Acta Psychiat. Scand.* **49**, 15-27.

Prien, R.F., Caffey, E.M. & Klett, C.J. (1972) *Arch. Gen. Psychiat.* **26**, 146-153.

Shapiro, A.K. & Shapiro, E. (1968) *Br. J. Psychiat.* **122**, 345-350.

Shopsin, B., Gershon, S., Thomson, H. & Collins, F. (1975) *Arch. Gen. Psychiat.* **32**, 34-42.

Spiker, D.G., Weiss, J.C., Dealy, R.S. *et al.* (1985) *Am. J. Psychiat.* **142**, 430-436.

Sunderland, T. & Silver, M.A. (1987) *Int. J. Geriat. Psychiat.* **3**, 79-88.

Young, J.P.R., Hughes, W.C. & Lader, M.H. (1976) *Br. Med. J.* **i**, 1116-1118.

ACUTE TREATMENT

John M. Kane

Department of Psychiatry, Hillside Hospital, Division of Long Island Jewish Medical Center, Glen Oaks, New York, USA

Table of Contents

11.1 Introduction

The acute treatment period usually refers to that phase of the illness which includes obvious psychotic signs and symptoms with behavioral dysfunction as well as impairment in psychosocial and/or vocational functioning. Although the mode of onset of an acute episode varies enormously, as a rule an acute exacerbation consists of an increase in positive symptoms such as delusions, hallucinations and thought disorder. In many instances an exacerbation of so-called negative symptoms, such as withdrawal, anhedonia, and lack of motivation may also occur. It is important to recognize that even within an episode of schizophrenia the form and content of symptoms may change over time. In addition, clinicians have to confront the fact that some important manifestations of a schizophrenic illness are subjective (for example, hallucinations and delusions) and that the extent to which the patient is willing or able to report these phenomena reliably or consistently may vary. As a result it is sometimes difficult to establish a true baseline for the evaluation of a specific treatment effect. In some cases, in fact, patients may appear to be worsening as they improve since they are becoming more open and trusting and therefore more accurately reporting unusual thoughts or perceptual experiences.

ANTIPSYCHOTIC DRUGS AND THEIR SIDE-EFFECTS
ISBN 0-12-079035-1

Table 1 Typical dosages of frequently used antipsychotics: approximate relative potency of antipsychotic agents.[a]

Generic	Relative potency	Usual range of total daily dose[b]	
		Acute (mg/day)	Maintenance (mg/day)
Phenothiazines			
Chlorpromazine	100	200–1000	50–400
Thioridazine	100	200–800	50–400
Mesoridazine	50	100–400	25–200
Acetophenazine	20	60–100	40–80
Prochlorperazine	15	60–200	20–60
Perphenazine	10	12–64	8–24
Trifluoperazine	5	10–60	4–30
Triflupromazine	25	30–150	20–100
Fluphenazine	2	5–60	1–15
Thioxanthenes			
Thiothixene	5	10–120	6–30
Chlorprothixene	100	50–600	50–400
Butyrophenones			
Haloperidol	2	5–50	1–15
Dibenzoxazepines			
Loxapine	10	20–160	10–60
Dihydroindolones			
Molindone	10	40–225	15–100
Dibenzodiazepines			
Clozapine	50	300–900	200–400
Long-acting injectable preparations			
Fluphenazine decanoate			6–100[c]
Haloperidol decanoate			50–200[d]

[a]These are approximate estimates of relative potency. It should be noted that relative potency may not be the same in the higher dosage ranges as it is in the lower.

[b]Dosage may vary with individual responses to the antipsychotic agent employed.

[c]Prolixin decanoate may be given at intervals of up to 3–4 weeks. Dosage requirements vary widely.

[d]Haloperidol decanoate should be given every 4 weeks. Dosage requirements vary widely.

The context in which an acute episode or exacerbation occurs is also important in planning both the acute and subsequent continuation or maintenance treatment plan. Many patients relapse because they have discontinued their antipsychotic medication. It is important to establish the reasons for this and to initiate necessary psychoeducation and consider planning for the use of guaranteed medication to facilitate compliance. All too frequently the focus is on treating the acute episode and not paying adequate attention to factors leading up to it so that future episodes can be prevented. Other factors might include environmental stress, substance abuse or inadequate dosage of maintenance medication.

Antipsychotic medications remain the mainstay of the acute treatment for schizophrenia. Recent research has helped to clarify a variety of clinical concerns in the use of these drugs; however, some questions remain. This review is an attempt to summarize the current status of acute antipsychotic drug treatment for schizophrenia, to highlight recent advances and to discuss areas of controversy.

11.2 Indications

The most clear-cut indication for antipsychotic drug treatment remains schizophrenia. Psychotic signs and symptoms such as delusions, hallucinations, thought disorder and suspiciousness can be seen in a variety of disorders and are not specific to schizophrenia. It is critical, therefore, to establish a differential diagnosis and rule out other causes of psychotic states which might require other treatments. Although numerous investigators over the past 25 years have attempted to identify useful predictors of acute antipsychotic drug response, these efforts have not succeeded to the point of identifying individuals with schizophrenia for whom an acute trial of medication would not be recommended unless there were some absolute medical contraindications. The overwhelming majority of patients with schizophrenia benefit to some extent from antipsychotic medication and most benefit considerably.

Clinical issues which require consideration during an acute treatment trial include: choice of drug; dosage; duration; and what strategies should be employed if the patient is not responding adequately.

11.3 Choice of drug

Typical dosages of frequently used antipsychotics and their approximate relative potencies are listed in Table 1. With the possible exception of clozapine, which will be discussed subsequently, there are no consistent data to suggest differences in clinical efficacy among currently marketed antipsychotic drugs. It is possible that such differences do exist, but that clinical trials with the required methodology to establish potential differences have not been carried out. Almost all of the data available are based on comparisons of mean changes in response measures from random-assignment, parallel group clinical trials. However, even though similar response rates (for example, 70–80%) may be observed within each treatment group, the possibility that a given individual might respond better to one drug than another cannot be ruled out. Surprisingly, there are remarkably few data which address this question despite its obvious clinical importance. Many clinicians report anecdotal experiences in which a patient who has failed to respond to drug A improves when switched to drug B. The problem, however, remains in interpreting this phenomenon when the passage of additional time (on any medication) may have been the critical factor in producing further response. This is particularly critical when changes are made within the first 4–6 weeks, since considerable variability is seen in the time-course of response during acute treatment. Patients may continue to show substantial improvement after the first weeks, but in many cases at least 50% of the improvement is likely to be seen within that time-frame.

The fact that antipsychotic drugs demonstrate considerable differences in relative affinities for various brain receptors does lend some support to the possibility that these compounds may differ in their clinical effects (Richelson, 1985). At the same time, however, correlations have been demonstrated between milligram clinical potency and dopamine D_2 receptor affinity for a large series of antipsychotic drugs (Seeman et al., 1976; Creese et al., 1977). It has been well established that neuroleptic drugs differ in their propensity to produce various adverse effects, as a result of varying receptor affinities (Richelson, 1984), and such differences may be important when choosing a particular medication for individuals with known sensitivity to particular adverse effects or for whom the occurrence of a particular adverse effect would be an obvious problem (see Table 2). Despite our assumptions regarding equivalent efficacy, one of the most important factors in choosing a specific medication for a given individual is the patient's previous therapeutic response; therefore, unless there is a good rationale for doing otherwise, it makes sense to utilize the same medication to which the patient has responded well in the past.

Many clinicians continue to prefer highly sedating, low-potency antipsychotics (for example, chlorpromazine, thioridazine, mesoridazine) in the treatment of patients who are aggressive or highly agitated. The literature, however, does not support any advantage for one class of drug as opposed to another in this context, with high- and low-potency drugs being equally efficacious (Bailine et al., 1987). In addition, there is no evidence that high-potency drugs (for example, haloperidol, fluphenazine, trifluoperazine) produce more improvement than low-potency drugs in emotionally withdrawn or psychomotorically retarded patients (Goldberg et al., 1972).

There is one additional factor which might influence the choice of medication for acute treatment, and that is whether or not a long-acting injectable medication will ultimately be prescribed for maintenance treatment. Some clinicians prefer to give a

Table 2 Affinities of antipsychotics for human brain receptors.

	D$_2$	Muscarinic acetylcholine	Histamine H$_1$	α-Adrenergic
Highest	*cis*-Thiothixene	Clozapine	Mesoridazine	Mesoridazine
	Fluphenazine	Thioridazine	Promazine	Chlorpromazine
	Perphenazine	Mesoridazine	Clozapine	Thioridazine
	Trifluoperazine	Chlorpromazine	Loxapine	Promazine
	Trifluopromazine	Promazine	*cis*-Thiothixene	Haloperidol
	Haloperidol	Loxapine	Perphenazine	Clozapine
	Prochlorperazine	Prochlorperazine	Chlorpromazine	Fluphenazine
	Chlorprothixene	Trifluoperazine	Thioridazine	Perphenazine
	Mesoridazine	Perphenazine	Prochlorperazine	*cis*-Thiothixene
	Chlorpromazine	Fluphenazine	Fluphenazine	Prochlorperazine
	Thioridazine	*cis*-Thiothixene	Trifluoperazine	Trifluoperazine
	Loxapine	Haloperidol	Haloperidol	Loxapine
	Molindone	Molindone	Molindone	Molindone
	Promazine			
Lowest	Clozapine			

Table adapted from Richelson (1984) with permission. Copyright © 1984, Physicians Postgraduate Press.

trial of the same drug in oral form before prescribing the decanoate and in some patients this transition may be more acceptable. In our view, in many settings (particularly in the US) long-acting injectable drugs are underutilized and more thought should be given to setting the stage for their use during the acute treatment phase. This is not to say that we recommend the use of long-acting drugs during the acute treatment phase; oral, liquid or short-acting parenteral preparations provide much more flexibility in terms of dosage titration and management of potential adverse effects. However, clinicians involved in the acute treatment phase should consider the long-term treatment plan and play a role in helping to initiate it. It is much easier in many cases to discuss maintenance treatment with the patient prior to his or her leaving the hospital and even to give a low 'test dose' of a long-acting injectable preparation rather than leaving this to the next clinician who takes over the treatment in the community. A subsequent change in medication or route of delivery is easier for the patient to accept if it has been expected from early on.

11.4 Dosage

Given the potential short- and long-term adverse effects associated with antipsychotic drugs, the utilization of minimum effective dosage is an important goal. The relationship between drug dosage and clinical response is a complex one because of the overall heterogeneity of response to antipsychotic drugs and the various other factors besides dosage which can influence outcome. Some patients may improve regardless of dose (in effect placebo responders), but rather in response to hospitalization, reduction of stress, spontaneous improvement, etc. while other patients may be poor responders to medication regardless of the dose or duration of treatment. In addition, patients vary enormously in their time-course of response.

In general, there are important methodologic issues in establishing minimum effective dosage requirements or optimum dose ranges for acute treatment. Random-assignment, fixed-dose comparisons are really necessary to clarify dose–response relationships. The reason being that if doses are adjusted on the basis of clinical response, then those patients who tend toward the unresponsive end of the spectrum or patients who respond more slowly than others will end up receiving the highest doses. It is not easy for an individual clinician to attribute cause and effect when altering medication dose in a specific patient. If, for example, a patient fails to respond adequately to an initial dose given for 3–4 weeks and the clinician decides to significantly raise the dose or even switch to another medication, it may not be valid to attribute subsequent improvement to the change when it may have occurred solely because of the passage of additional time. Without controlled trials it is difficult to draw conclusions regarding the value of such alternative treatment strategies.

In those studies which have compared high doses (that is, 2000 mg/day chlorpromazine equivalents or higher) to standard-dose treatment there is no evidence of statistically significant advantages for the high-dosage treatment (for example, Erickson *et al.*, 1978; Donlon *et al.*, 1980; Neborsky *et al.*, 1981; see Baldessarini *et al.*, 1988; Davis *et al.*, 1989, for reviews of such studies). There may be an occasional patient experiencing low drug bioavailability or increased rates of metabolism with a particular drug who would benefit from an unusually high dose, but clearly such patients are in the minority and all patients should first have a trial of moderate doses before being exposed to high doses. (The role of blood levels in this context is discussed in Chapter 8.) In general, the literature supports 400–700 mg/day chlorpromazine or equivalent as adequate for the majority of patients (Klein & Davis, 1968; Baldessarini *et al.*, 1988).

Since high-potency neuroleptics are generally well tolerated apart from parkinsonian side-effects (which can be managed or prevented with antiparkinson medication) at very high doses, there had been a tendency among some clinicians to use higher doses of such compounds. In many settings there has been increasing pressure to discharge patients from hospital more and more quickly and clinicians have attempted to hasten response by more rapid escalation and/or the use of higher doses. There is no evidence, however, that such strategies produce significantly more rapid response and they are associated with higher rates of adverse effects.

Baldessarini *et al.* (1988) reviewed 19 studies comparing different antipsychotic drug dosages in the treatment of acute psychoses of various types. The weight of these studies provides no support for utilizing high-dose, or 'rapid neuroleptization' strategies. Dosages about 500–600 mg of chlorpromazine or 10–15 mg of haloperidol or fluphenzaine within the first 24 h after admission or during the first few days of treatment did not produce any consistent clinical advantages.

An example of such a trial is that of Erickson *et al.* (1978), who randomly assigned 42 acutely decompensated schizophrenic patients to receive, on a double-blind basis, either a 5-day loading dose of 60 mg intramuscular haloperidol as compared to 15 mg orally per day. After the first 5 days, the high-intramuscular-dose group received 15 mg per day orally as did the control group. There were no advantages for the high-loading dose group on any of the clinical therapeutic measures, but they did experience more dystonic reactions.

Intramuscularly administered medication does have a somewhat faster effect in that a peak blood level is reached within 30 min, whereas following the first oral dose a peak blood level may not be reached for 90 min. This difference may be important for highly agitated or violent patients, but ultimately the same blood level will be achieved with oral or liquid medication so that the prolonged use of the intramuscular route of administration is not necessary.

It is necessary to remind ourselves that although we may see some very rapid effects of antipsychotic drugs (within hours or days) it can take 4–6 weeks to see only 50% of the ultimate degree of response and the ultimate level of improvement may not be seen for many weeks. For example, in a study of newly admitted, first-episode schizophrenic patients, Lieberman *et al.* (1991) found that the mean interval between starting medication and achieving maximum improvement (in effect the absence of clinically significant psychopathology) to be 35 weeks with a median of 11 weeks. (The issue of when and if to change medications or increase dosage if patients are not responding adequately after several weeks will be discussed subsequently.)

11.5   Antipsychotic drug dosage equivalencies

Given the number of antipsychotic medications available and the need which can arise to change drugs or to translate dosage findings with one drug to the utilization of another, the issue of equivalencies becomes important.

Table 1 suggests dose equivalences of various antipsychotic drugs using chlorpromazine as the standard agent against which others are compared. Unfortunately, the data on which these equivalencies are based are limited. In general, these estimates are derived from double-blind, clinical trials comparing one antipsychotic to another with clinicians adjusting dose as they see fit. When the data are analyzed at the end of the trial, comparisons can be made of the dosages employed and a conversion ratio suggested. Alternatively, some clinical trials are designed with predetermined dosage ratios set by the investigator or sponsor based on some estimate of what they believe the conversion ratio to be. In addition, data from open trials or placebo-controlled trials can be pooled to attempt to identify a clinically effective dosage range. For reasons which were discussed previously, these data sources may not necessarily permit the identification of minimum effective dosages or dosage ranges and in order to do that fixed-dose comparisons of different dosage levels are really necessary. There are other potential problems with customary conversion ratios, such as the fact that the ratio which may be appropriate at the lower end of the dosage spectrum may not apply at higher dosage levels.

It has been documented that clinicians frequently use dissimilar dosing practices with high-potency as compared to low-potency antipsychotics. In one survey (Baldessarini *et al.*, 1984), the mean chlorpromazine equivalent dose of the two most potent antipsychotics (haloperidol and fluphenazine) was 3.54 times as high as the mean doses prescribed of chlorpromazine or thioridazine.

Several recent studies have employed different fixed doses of high-potency neuroleptics and concluded that for haloperidol and fluphenazine doses in the range of 10–20 mg are equally effective and better tolerated than higher doses (Levinson *et al.*, 1990; Van Putten *et al.*, 1990; Rifkin *et al.*, 1991).

11.6   Strategies for treating non-responsive patients

Despite the tremendous clinical benefit generally associated with antipsychotic drug treatment, a substantial minority of schizophrenic patients derive little if any benefit. Although the management of these patients poses an enormous challenge to clinicians, this is a population that has not been well-studied in terms of alternative treatment strategies. This is the context in which many clinicians will employ high-dose treatment, switch to different agents or add adjunctive pharmacotherapy with lithium, carbamazepine, benzodiazepines or even a trial of electroconvulsive therapy. Though there are numerous anecdotal reports suggesting the value of these strategies in particular patients, there are remarkably few systematic, well-controlled trials which support the use of any particular approach. Even the most obvious and basic question of whether or not it makes sense to switch from one class of neuroleptics to another has not been adequately studied.

Table 3 summarizes the results of four double-blind trials comparing standard-dose and 'mega'-dose treatment in patients who had failed to respond adequately to antipsychotic drug treatment. There were no statistically significant advantages for the high-dose treatment in any of these studies; however, it is of interest to note that a substantial proportion of patients participating in these trials were rated as improved. This raises a question as to whether or not the length of the previous trial had been adequate, or to what extent non-somatic treatment factors may have contributed to this further improvement.

Although we do not recommend routine use of blood levels, when patients fail to respond to an adequate trial of an antipsychotic drug, this is an instance when a blood level might be indicated to identify patients with unusually low (or unusually high)

Table 3   Therapeutic response in neuroleptic-resistant schizophrenia.

Investigator	Drug(s)	Dosage (daily)	Overall improvement combined groups	
Itil et al. (1970)	Fluphenazine Fluphenazine	30 mg 300 mg	9/17	53%
McCreadie & McDonald (1977)	Haloperidol Chlorpromazine	100 mg 600 mg	7/20	35%
Quitkin et al. (1975)	Fluphenazine Fluphenazine	30 mg 1200 mg	13/31	42%
Bjorndal et al. (1980)	Haloperidol Haloperidol	15 mg (mean) 103 mg (mean)	10/23	43%

blood levels. However, there have been very few controlled studies exploring the value of manipulating blood levels into a putative therapeutic range. Volavka *et al.* (1990) have reported preliminary results from such an investigation, but did not find significant effects from manipulating blood levels of haloperidol (into or out of) a specific blood level range.

After 4–6 weeks of antipsychotic drug treatment with minimal or no response it does seem reasonable to initiate a 'therapeutic' trial of some alternative medication. In our experience from an ongoing controlled trial, switching from fluphenazine to haloperidol after 4 weeks has not produced substantial improvement during the subsequent 4 weeks (Kane *et al.*, 1991, unpublished data). These preliminary findings are somewhat discouraging, but more data need to be collected before firm conclusions can be drawn. It may also remain true that a few individual patients might benefit from such a strategy even though group means do not change substantially over time.

When clinicians do entertain such therapeutic trials in unresponsive patients, it is critical to establish target signs and symptoms and to assess their response over time. In our experience in reviewing large numbers of medical records of unresponsive patients, it is very common to see various non-standard treatments or treatment combinations continued for long periods of time without any clear documentation as to any beneficial effect.

As a general rule we recommend two or three different classes of antipsychotic drugs given in adequate doses (at least 400–700 mg/day chlorpromazine equivalents) for 4 weeks before the initiation of alternative approaches such as adjunctive lithium or a trial of clozapine (one of these trials should employ dosage of at least 1000 mg/day chlorpromazine equivalents). Although 4 weeks can be a very long time to wait with a patient who is difficult to manage, the time-course of response varies enormously among patients with schizophrenia. Although some investigators have suggested that early response to treatment (for example, within the first 24–48 h) may be predictive of ultimate response after 4–6 weeks (May *et al.*, 1976, 1980), the sensitivity and specificity of this approach has not been adequately established to justify switching treatments and even if they were, it is not at all clear what treatment would then be most appropriate.

11.7 Clozapine

Although clozapine first underwent clinical trials in Europe and briefly in the US in the 1970s, its worldwide distribution has been limited by a higher incidence of agranulocytosis than that associated with other antipsychotic medications. Clozapine was not marketed in the US or the UK until a large-scale clinical trial was conducted establishing its superiority in carefully selected, treatment refractory patients (Kane *et al.*, 1988).

For this study, 268 individuals who had failed to respond to at least three periods of treatment with antipsychotic drugs from at least two different chemical classes given in dosages equivalent to or greater than 1000 mg/day (chlorpromazine equivalents) for a period of 6 weeks and who also failed to respond to a prospective, single-blind, 6-week trial of haloperidol (up to 60 mg/day or higher plus benztropine mesylate 6 mg/day) were eligible to participate in a 6-week random assignment, double-blind trial comparing clozapine and chlorpromazine (plus benztropine mesylate). When a priori criteria were employed, 30% of the clozapine-treated patients were categorized as responders as compared to only 4% of the chlorpromazine-treated patients. Clozapine produced significantly greater improvement on the Brief Psychiatric Rating Scale, Clinical Global Impressions Scale and Nurses Observation Scale for Inpatient Evaluation.

The average daily dose of chlorpromazine in the trial was 1200 mg and that of clozapine was 600 mg. This study provided strong support for the usefulness of clozapine in some patients who had failed to respond to standard neuroleptic treatment and supported the observations of numerous clinicians throughout Europe and the US as to clozapine's novel properties.

The proportion of patients who did experience clinically meaningful response in this trial was similar to that found in several European studies (Povlsen et al., 1985; Lindstrom, 1987; Naber et al., 1989). At the present time we do not have any well-validated predictors which could help in identifying those patients most likely to respond to clozapine, so that a trial would be appropriate for any individuals who are refractory to standard antipsychotic agents, unless there are contraindications to the use of clozapine.

In addition, clozapine is relatively free of adverse neurologic side-effects such as drug-induced parkinsonism, tardive dyskinesia or tardive dystonia (Casey, 1989). Therefore, individuals who have such neurologic adverse effects may also be candidates for clozapine treatment.

The current estimate of the risk of agranulocytosis based on systemically collected data in the United States is 1.0% after 52 weeks of clozapine treatment (Lieberman 1991). This risk does vary over time, with the majority of cases occurring between 6 weeks and 6 months of clozapine treatment. Although the incidence of agranulocytosis does appear to decline substantially after 1 year of clozapine treatment, cases have been reported to occur later than that, and, therefore, at the present time weekly white blood cell counts (CBCs) are recommended for the duration of clozapine treatment. The agranulocytosis associated with clozapine is reversible if the drug is discontinued. However, even with careful monitoring this adverse effect can in some cases be fatal. Therefore, the use of clozapine should involve a thorough consideration of the overall benefit-to-risk ratio and a careful discussion with the patient and family in order to elicit appropriate informed consent. Other adverse effects associated with clozapine include sedation, tachycardia, hypersalivation, transient hyperthermia, hypotension and seizures (Safferman et al., 1991). The risk of seizures appears to be dose related, with the highest risk occurring among patients receiving 600 mg/day or more (Devinsky *et al.*, 1991).

11.8 Conclusions

Clearly, antipsychotic medication remains a critical element in the acute treatment of schizophrenia. Given heterogeneity in clinical presentation, pharmacodynamic factors and the drug responsiveness of the underlying illness, antipsychotic drugs cannot be prescribed in a rote fashion. A variety of clinical issues should be considered in choosing the drug, the dose, the duration of the trial and the overall goals of the acute treatment phase. It is important to view this treatment as one aspect of a larger treatment plan and to assure that the previous history and the long-term treatment needs are well considered in planning and evaluating the acute treatment.

Much remains to be learned about establishing the most appropriate strategies for poor responders, and clinicians should be open to new approaches based on emerging literature but with particular emphasis on well-controlled and generalizable clinical trials.

References

Bailine, S., Lesser, M.S., Krubit, G. *et al.* (1987) *Psychiat. Hosp.* **18**, 127–129.

Baldessarini, R.J., Katz, B. & Cotton, P. (1984) *Am. J. Psychiat.* **141**, 748–752.

Baldessarini, R.J., Cohen, B.M. & Teicher, M.H. (1988) *Arch. Gen. Psychiat.* **45**, 79–91.

Bjorndal, N., Bjerre, M., Gerlach, J. *et al.* (1980) *Psychopharmacology* **67**, 17–23.

Casey, D.E. (1989) *Psychopharmacology* **99**, S47–S53.

Creese, I., Burt, D.R. & Snyder, S.H. (1977) *Science* **192**, 596–598.

Davis, J.M., Barter, J.T. & Kane, J.M. (1989) In *Comprehensive Textbook of Psychiatry* (eds Kaplan, H.I. & Sadock, B.J.), 5th edition, pp. 1591–1626, Baltimore, Williams and Wilkins.

Devinsky, O., Honigfeld, G. & Patin, J. (1991) *Neurology* **41**, 369–371.

Donlon, P.T., Hokin, J.T. & Tupin, J.P. (1980) *Arch. Gen. Psychiat.* **37**, 691–695.

Erickson, S.E., Hurt, S.W. & Chang, S. (1978) *Psychopharmacol. Bull.* **14**, 15–16.

Goldberg, S.C., Frosch, W.A., Prossman, A.K. *et al.* (1972) *Arch. Gen. Psychiat.* **26**, 367–373.

Itil, I.M., Keskiner, A., Heinemann, L. *et al.* (1970) *Psychosomatics* **11**, 456–463.

Kane, J., Honigfeld, G., Singer, J. & Meltzer, H.Y. (1988) *Arch. Gen. Psychiat.* **45**, 789–796.

Klein, D.F. & Davis, J. (1968) *Diagnosis and Drug Treatment of Psychiatric Disorders*, Baltimore, Williams & Wilkins.

Levinson, D.S., Simpson, G.M., Singh, H. *et al.* (1990) *Arch. Gen. Psychiat.* **47**, 761–768.

Lieberman, J.A. (1991) Clozapine update: Agranulocytosis. Presentation at the annual NCDEU Meeting, Key Biscayne, Florida, 30 May.

Lieberman, J.A., Mayerhoff, D., Loebel, A. *et al.* (1991) *Schizophrenia Res.* **4**, 289–290.

Lindstrom, L.H. (1987) *Acta Psychiat. Scand.* **77**, 524–529.

May, P.R.A., Van Putten, T., Yale, C. *et al.* (1976) *J. Nerv. Mental Dis.* **162**, 177–183.

May, P.R.A., Van Putten, T. & Yale, C. (1980) *Am. J. Psychiat.* **137**, 1088–1089.

McCreadie, R.G. & McDonald, I.M. (1977) *Br. J. Psychiat.* **131**, 310–316.

Naber, D., Leppig, M., Grohmann, R. & Hippius, H. (1989) *Psychopharmacology* **99**, S73–S76.

Neborsky, R., Janowsky, D., Munson, E. & Depry, D. (1981) *Arch. Gen. Psychiat.* **38**, 195–199.

Povlsen, U.J., Noring, U., Fog, R. & Gerlach, J. (1985) *Acta Psychiat. Scand.* **71**, 176–185.

Quitkin, F., Rifkin, A. & Klein, D.F. (1975) *Arch. Gen. Psychiat.* **32**, 1276–1281.

Richelson, E. (1984) *J. Clin. Psychiat.* **45**, 331–336.

Richelson, E. (1985) *J. Clin. Psychiat.* **46**, 8–13.

Rifkin, A., Doddi, S., Karajgi, B. *et al.* (1991) *Arch. Gen. Psychiat.* **48**, 166–170.

Safferman, A., Lieberman, J., Kane, J. *et al.* (1991) *Schizophrenia Bull.* **17**, 247–261.

Seeman, P., Lee, T., Chau-Wong, M. & Wong, K. (1976) *Nature* **261**, 717–719.

Van Putten, T., Marder, S. & Mintz, J. (1990) *Arch. Gen. Psychiat.* **47**, 754–758.

Volavka, J., Cooper, T.B., Meisner, M. *et al.* (1990) *Psychopharmacol. Bull.* **26**, 13–17.

CHAPTER 12

MAINTENANCE ANTIPSYCHOTIC MEDICATION

John M. Davis, Philip G. Janicak, Abhin Singla and Rajiv P. Sharma

Illinois State Psychiatric Institute, University of Illinois, Chicago, Illinois, USA

Table of Contents

12.1 Introduction

Soon after antipsychotic drugs were discovered, it became apparent from a large number of open clinical studies and case histories that a substantial number of patients relapsed upon their withdrawal and that maintenance pharmacotherapy prevented this (Johnson, 1976a,b). The efficacy of antipsychotics in preventing relapse when used for prophylactic treatment is also supported by 35 random-assignments, double-blind studies which reported the number of patients who relapsed on placebo versus maintenance medication (Table 1, Davis, 1975; results initially summarized are updated here). Patients were randomly assigned to either placebo or antipsychotic medication (at least 6 weeks with oral therapy or 2 months with intramuscular depot treatment). Of the 3720 patients, 55% on placebo relapsed, compared to 21% on maintenance medication. On the basis of the Mantel–Haenszel (1959) meta-analytic method, the combined studies indicated a highly significant difference ($\chi^2 = 483$, d.f. $= 1, P < 10^{-107}$).

Table 1 Antipsychotic prevention of relapse.

Reference	Number of patients	Relapse on placebo (%)	Relapse on drug (%)	Difference in relapse rate (placebo–drug) (%)
Schauver *et al.* (1959)	80	18	5	13
Diamond & Marks (1960)	40	70	25	45
Blackburn & Allen (1961)	53	54	24	30
Gross & Reeves (1961)	109	58	14	44
Adelson & Epstein (1962)	281	90	49	41
Freeman & Alson (1962)	94	28	13	15
Troshinsky *et al.* (1962)	43	63	4	59
Whitaker & Hoy (1963)	39	65	8	57
Caffey *et al.* (1964)	259	45	5	40
Kinross-Wright & Charalampous (1965)	40	70	5	65
Garfield *et al.* (1966)	27	31	11	20
Melnyk *et al.* (1966)	40	50	0	50
Engelhardt *et al.* (1967)	294	30	15	15
Morton (1968)	40	70	25	45
Prien & Cole (1968)	762	42	16	26
Prien *et al.* (1969)	325	56	20	36
Baro *et al.* (1970)	26	100	0	100
Rassidakis *et al.* (1970)	84	58	34	24
Clark *et al.* (1971)	19	70	43	27
Leff & Wing (1971)	30	83	33	50
Hershon *et al.* (1972)	62	28	7	21
Hirsch *et al.* (1973)	74	66	8	58
Hogarty & Goldberg (1973)	374	67	31	36
Gross (1974)	61	65	34	31
Chien & Cole (1975)	31	87	12	75
Clark *et al.* (1975)	35	78	27	51
Schiele (1975)	80	60	3	57
Andrews *et al.* (1976)	31	35	7	28
Rifkin *et al.* (1977)	62	68	7	61
Levine *et al.* (p.o.) (1980)	33	59	33	26
Levine *et al.* (i.m.) (1980)	34	30	18	12
Wistedt (1981)	38	63	38	25
Cheung (1981)	28	62	13	49
Nishikawa *et al.* (1982)	55	100	85	15
Ruskin & Nyman (1991)	18	50	13	37

Summary statistics, $P < 10^{-107}$

This finding represents overwhelming statistical evidence that in schizophrenia, antipsychotics prevent relapse. Some of these studies included remitted patients studied in outpatient trials; others were still symptomatic with active psycho-pathology and being treated as either inpatients or outpatients. In fully remitted patients the antipsychotic medication could be characterized as having a clear prophylactic effect. In partially remitted patients, this effect could be characterized as continued maintenance treatment. In the latter case, symptomatology worsened substantially with drug discontinuation. To illustrate support for the effectiveness of long-term medication, we will summarize a few individual studies.

The rate of relapse of patients differs markedly from study to study (Table 1). This may be due to the differing durations of the studies, with patients studied for a longer period of time having a greater likelihood of relapse. In addition, the definition of relapse differs. Obviously, the relapse rate will be higher if one defines it as a modest re-emergence of psychotic symptoms than if one defines it as an emergence of psychotic symptoms sufficient to cause rehospitalization. If one uses the former criteria, the relapse rate may be 5–20% per month, whereas the more conservative criteria might be 1–10% per month. In each study the placebo group is compared to the drug group, and so the difference in relapse rates holds constant all the above-mentioned factors. In several of the studies listed in Table 1, an active placebo was used. Although these studies had a small sample of patients, the drug–placebo difference was still present even when an active placebo was used.

Hogarty & Goldberg (1973) studied 374 outpatients with schizophrenia. After discharge and a stabilization period on phenothiazines, they were randomly assigned to chlorpromazine or placebo. Half of each group received psychotherapy from an individual caseworker plus vocational rehabilitation counseling. After 1 year, relapse had occurred in 73% of the patients receiving the placebo-without-psychotherapy treatment, and 63% of the placebo-plus-psychotherapy patients. By contrast, only 33% of the chlorpromazine-only patients and 26% of the drug-plus-psychotherapy group suffered a relapse. Overall, only 31% of the drug-treated group relapsed, compared to 68% on placebo. The relapse rate with chlorpromazine dropped to 16% with the exclusion of those who abruptly stopped their medication. These patients showed few signs of schizophrenic symptoms at their monthly evaluations until the onset of their relapse, when they became abruptly more psychotic. Thus, almost half of these relapses occurred due to medication non-compliance. Psychotherapy groups had statistically insignificant fewer relapses than patients not receiving psychotherapy, but those who underwent treatment with drugs as well as psychotherapy functioned better than patients receiving drug alone. Psychotherapy may take more time to work, since its effect was more apparent after 2 years of treatment. It appears that these two treatments complement each other, as psychotherapy improves psychosocial functioning while drugs prevent relapses.

A VA collaborative project (Caffey et al., 1964) studied 171 patients who received a placebo and 88 patients on either chlorpromazine or thioridazine. Relapse occurred in

45% of the placebo group and only 5% of the drug treatment group. In this study, compliance was assured, for the study was inpatient and nurses administered the medication.

12.2 Time-course of relapse

An important issue in the maintenance treatment of schizophrenia is the rate of relapse upon discontinuation of therapy. In order to determine whether relapse occurred at a constant or varying rate all the datasets of patients studied over the course of long-term placebo therapy were analyzed. It was found that relapse tended to occur along an exponential function similar to that seen with the half-life of drugs in plasma (Figure 1). This would indicate that relapse occurs at a constant rate (Davis *et al.*, 1980). Beginning with a fixed number of patients in a study group, the number of patients relapsing at fixed time points will always be a constant percentage of the overall number of patients remaining in the study. With increased time, the actual number of

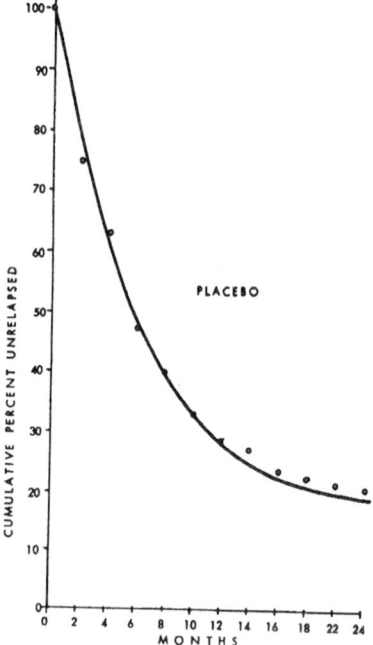

Figure 1 The time course of schizophrenic patients relapsing on placebo, plotted as percentage not yet relapsed versus time.

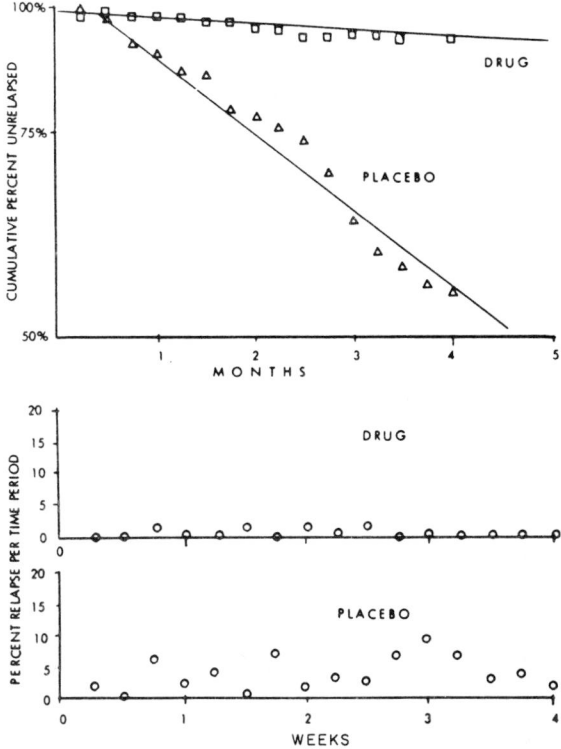

Figure 2 Relapse of schizophrenic subjects plotted as percentage not yet relapsed (natural log scale) versus time. A straight line indicates that the relapse rate is constant.

patients relapsing will decrease due to a diminishing patient pool. For example, if we begin with 100 study patients and a constant relapse rate of 10% per month, 10 patients will relapse at the end of the first month, leaving 90 patients in the trial. In the second month, 10% of 90, or 9 patients will relapse, leaving 81 patients. At the end of the third month, 8 patients will relapse, leaving 73 patients. Relapse will continue to occur at this constant rate of 10% per month, even though the absolute number of relapsing patients seems to be decreasing.

Data from several large collaborative studies were plotted, and the results fit the exponential model (for constant relapse rate) more accurately than the linear model. The VA hospital collaborative study (Caffey *et al.*, 1964) shows a constant relapse rate of 15.7% per month (Figure 2). The NIMH Hogarty & Goldberg (1973) study yielded a relapse rate of 10.7% for those on placebo (Figure 3). A collaborative NIMH study (Prien & Cole, 1968) yielded a constant relapse rate of 8% per month (Figure 4). Since these curves are exponential, the mathematical analyses resemble those considerations that would be applied to the half-life of drugs in plasma. The least-squares analyses of the empirical data provided an excellent fit, with r^2 approaching 0.95.

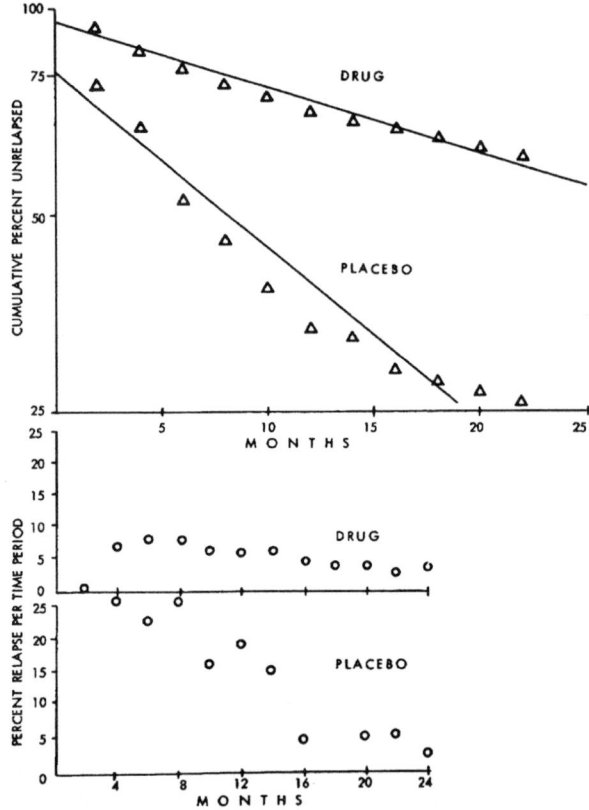

Figure 3 Relapse of schizophrenic subjects plotted as percentage not yet relapsed (natural log scale) versus time. A straight line indicates that the relapse rate is constant.

In a long trial, it should be noted, however, that all patients at risk for relapse will have relapsed. Those patients not at risk will not relapse, leaving a constant number of patients, essentially '5-year' survivors. If a patient does not relapse after a long period of time, one might assume he never will. In an attempt to clarify this point, Hogarty and co-workers (1976) followed their placebo group 2 or more years after the initial study. They found that almost all patients had relapsed or were lost to follow-up. Indeed, after 18 months, the empirical data hinted that the relapse rate was decreasing, but so few patients remained that the placebo group did not yield a sufficient number of unrelapsed patients for accurate study.

Another area of study is the relapse rate of patients who have been successfully maintained without relapse over the course of 2–3 years on maintenance medication. If relapse is prevented for some period of time, do patients lose their capacity to relapse or will the rate still be about 10% per month? In the drug-treated groups of Hogarty and

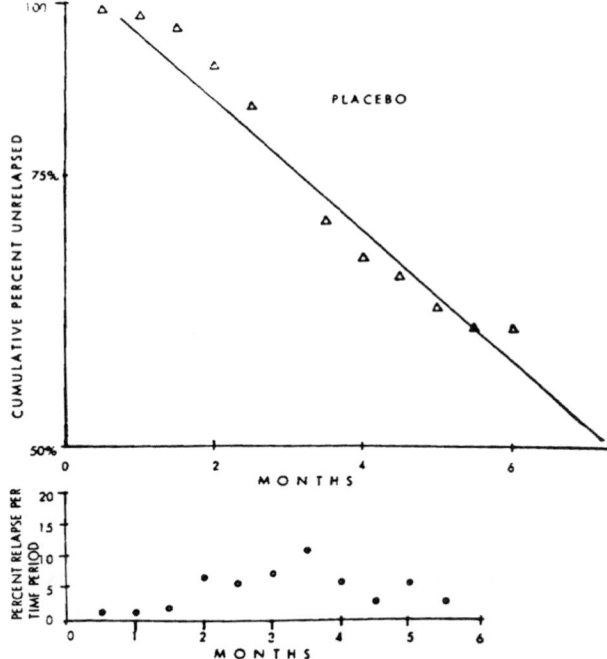

Figure 4 Relapse of schizophrenic subjects plotted as percentage not yet relapsed (natural log scale) versus time. A straight line indicates that the relapse rate is constant.

co-workers (Hogarty & Goldberg, 1973; Hogarty *et al.*, 1976; Hogarty & Ulrich, 1977) there were ample patients for this type of assessment. When the antipsychotics were withdrawn after 2–3 years of successful treatment, the initial relapse rates were similar to those rates in patients who had been taken off maintenance medications after only 2 months of therapy. They continued to relapse in an exponential manner, with a constant rate of 10% per month.

All too frequently the literature states that 50% of patients relapse with drugs, while 50% do not and therefore are not in need of medication. The follow-up period in most of the studies (in Table 1) was only 4–6 months, at which time a rate of 10% per month yields about a 50% relapse rate per year. Had the period been extended to 1 year, the rate would have increased to 75%. If the study period had been extended to 2 years, about 87% would have relapsed. It is not known whether the curve goes on to 100% relapses or not (Davies *et al.*, 1980). If the observation of constant relapse is correct, the great majority of patients will relapse when switched to placebo if followed up for long enough. We think this is a reasonable observation if it is borne in mind that this applies to the type of patient being studied in these investigations, that is, patients in maintenance medication clinics.

12.3 Indications for maintenance

The role of maintenance medication for a single episode of reactive psychosis has not been studied. It is reasonable to use short-term treatment for 6 months or so to ensure a solid recovery without necessarily resorting to long-term maintenance. The length of the therapy should be determined on the basis of the knowledge of the illness as well as the patient's life situation. Reactive schizophrenic patients can have one episode and never relapse, and in these cases, long-term maintenance medication may not be necessary. Whether maintenance therapy is needed for a patient after a first episode remains a clinical judgment (Davis *et al.*, 1989).

After a patient has had several episodes, there are good data from the above studies that indicate the usefulness of maintenance treatment. Patients with good prognostic signs (that is, those with the greatest drug/placebo difference) who have had many episodes but make a good recovery, benefit most from maintenance medication. Patients who have poor prognostic signs tend to benefit least from psychotherapy (that is, those that have the least drug/psychotherapy versus no treatment difference; Goldberg *et al.*, 1977). Psychotherapists urge patients to confront the problem. This may induce a stress with which a patient on the verge of decompensation may not be able to cope. This would indicate that patients who have persistent psychotic symptoms may not do as well in psychotherapy. To put it another way, in these more fragile patients, a therapist who has high expressed emotion may not be that helpful to the patient. Prien and his colleagues (1971) found that the continuously hospitalized, very chronic patients maintained on low-dose neuroleptics have a lower chance of relapse than those who needed more medication. Table 2 presents these data as relapse percentages in chronic schizophrenia per category of previous medication and chronicity (Prien *et al.*, 1969, 1971).

Due to the hazard of long-term side-effects, such as tardive dyskinesia, it is desirable to limit the use of neuroleptics. While many patients may require maintenance

Table 2 Percentage clinically deteriorated or relapsed by current medication dose and chronicity (length of hospitalization) in chronic schizophrenia.

Chronicity[a]	Dose (mg chlorpromazine equivalents)	*N*	% Relapsed
Very chronic	<300	45	22
Chronic	<300	54	53
Very chronic	>300	108	70
Chronic	>300	64	73

[a]Very chronic = 15 years or over. Chronic = less than 15 years.
From Prien & Cole (1968) and Prien *et al.* (1969, 1971).

neuropleptic treatment, it is clearly possible that there may be some patients who do not. Hence, if clinicians were able to predict which patients would not relapse, selected patients could be managed without medication. To test whether it is possible to identify patients who do not need medication and then switch them to placebo, Morgan & Cheadle (1974) conducted the following study. They selected 74 out of 475 patients as suitable candidates for management without the use of medication. Only 5 of these 74 remained relapse-free after several years without maintenance medication. Relapse in the other 69 occurred an average 4.5 months after removal of the drugs. This clearly indicates that even selected, good-risk chronic schizophrenic patients are at a high risk of relapse if not maintained on antipsychotics.

12.4 Targeted treatment

It is quite possible that prophylactic treatment does not really prevent episodes but rather treats them as they occur, that is, maintenance therapy automatically treats the episode so it does not become full-blown (Davis *et al.*, 1989). In that case, it might be possible for the clinician to follow a patient, and when a relapse begins (or there are early warning signals that relapse is about to occur), to medicate quickly to abort the relapse. Most patients who relapse do so abruptly, and we are not convinced that it would be possible to vigorously treat and abort a relapse once the process has started. Yet, it is certainly true that some relapses are preceded by a week or two of prodromal signs. This has led to four double-blind studies targeting treatment to an impending relapse as an alternate strategy to continuous maintenance medication.

In targeted treatment, pharmacotherapy is not used prophylactically but rather when prodromal symptoms of a relapse become manifest. Chronic schizophrenics, in the few days or week preceding a relapse, often have non-specific prodromal symptoms such as anxiety, depression, fear of going crazy, loss of interest, discouragement about the future, labile mood, reduced attention, preoccupation, fear of future adversity, fear of not fitting in, being overwhelmed by demands, loss of interest in dress, reduced energy, loss of control, boredom, racing thoughts, indecisiveness and nightmares. Targeted treatment utilizes these prodromal symptoms as an indication of when to initiate treatment in a patient maintained drug-free. Targeted treatment would benefit the patient by eliminating the need for continual neuroleptics, thus presumably reducing the risk of tardive dyskinesia.

Jolley *et al.* (1989, 1990) reported that of 25 patients in a continuous-medication control group, only 3 relapsed, with 2 requiring hospitalization. Of the 24 patients in a target treatment group, 12 relapsed and 8 required hospitalization. Herz *et al.* (1990) compared over 100 patients on continuous or targeted therapy. In the targeted group, there were more relapses, and survival analysis indicated a significantly better result with continuous medication. Herz and co-workers (1991) studied 101 patients, and found that 15 out of 50 targeted patients relapsed, with 12 requiring rehospitalization, while only 8 out of 51 in the maintenance treatment group relapsed, with 3 hospitalized. Carpenter *et al.* (1990) performed a similar comparison in a non-double-blind study. Fifty-three per cent of the 57 targeted therapy patients relapsed, with hospitalization, while 36% of the 59 continuous-therapy patients relapsed with rehospitalization. Survival analysis demonstrated again that the continuous therapy was clearly more effective than the targeted therapy in reducing the rate of relapse. Carpenter *et al.* (1990) noted that the relapse rate with continuous treatment was 1.6 versus 3.18 for the targeted therapy.

Gaebel and co-workers (1991) instituted a multicentre study in Germany. The patients were randomly assigned to early intervention, crisis intervention, or maintenance therapy. Of the 364 patients studied, 159 completed their 2-year trial. Twenty-three per cent of the maintenance-medication group relapsed, in contrast with 63% of the crisis intervention group and 45% of the early intervention group. Note that the early intervention group would have received substantially more neuroleptics than the crisis intervention group. The targeted treatment was a variant of low-dose therapy where patients were on neuroleptics much of the time, namely, the periods when they manifested prodromal symptoms. We can only approximate the German data to enter in our meta-analysis since it was only available in abstract form. We assume that one-third of the patients went into the continuous maintenance medication group and two-thirds into no-maintenance medication groups. With randomization, the number of patients in the two arms would be almost exactly equal. Use of the Mantel–Haenszel test in our meta-analysis is probably reasonable; hence, one could multiply the 23% of patients who did not relapse with maintenance medication by the assumed 121 patients in each arm of the trial. We could also average the 63% and the 45% of the two non-medication strategies and then multiply this mean (53.5%) times the 242 patients in these two arms of the trial. Entering these numbers in the meta-analysis would show that 25% of continuously medicated patients relapsed, in contrast to 50% in the targeted treatment groups (of one form or another, including crisis intervention). This is highly statistically significant, to $P < 0.000\,000\,000\,02$ level.

If we just focus on an overall analysis of the three published studies for which we have explicit data, we find that 23% of the continuous group and 38% of the targeted group required hospitalization. Using the Mantel–Haenszel test ($\chi^2 = 6.7$; d.f. = 1; $P = 0.01$), this difference is statistically significant. In these studies, the targeted drug patients were generally on drugs for shorter periods, sometimes only 50% of the time.

In summary there are four studies of targeted compared to continuous treatment, and all show that the results were poor with the targeted maintenance strategy.

A similar alternate strategy would be to maintain patients on a continuous lower dose (either intramuscular or oral) of medication, increasing the dose if prodromal signs of relapse occur. Studies have shown that the standard dose is more effective than low-dose neuroleptics, but again, many factors should be considered before deciding on a final approach. Jolley *et al.* (1990) found that 53% of the relapses were preceded by prodromal signs. This would seem to suggest that patients on continuous low-dose therapy should have an increase in maintenance medication to abort relapse should prodromal symptoms begin to appear.

12.5 Dosage of medication

There have been four dose–response studies of maintenance depot medication. Generally, most groups used a standard dose of 25 mg fluphenazine decanoate given intramuscularly every 2 weeks, although some used dosage ranges, with the standard compared to lower doses. The lowest dose used was that of Kane and co-workers (1983, 1984), who chose 1.25–5 mg. In their study, 3 patients in the standard dose group relapsed and 61 patients remained well. Of those in the low-dose group (1.25–5 mg), 26 patients relapsed and 36 remained well. It is clear that doses down in the range of a few milligrams of fluphenazine decanoate every 2 weeks are clearly below the critical threshold. Hogarty and co-workers (1988) used doses of 25 mg versus an average of 3.8 mg, and Marder *et al.* (1987) used doses of 25 mg in comparison to 5 mg. In Marder's study, patients who showed very early signs of relapse could have their dose slightly increased. We consider the 5–25 mg dose their fixed starting dose. Of those on the standard dose of 25 mg, 10 relapsed and 21 remained well. Of those on the lower dose, 22 relapsed and 13 remained well. When the patients had early signs of relapse, their dose was increased, and the dose–response relationship began to level out to no difference. Hogarty found a non-significant difference between his two doses. In his standard-dose group, 19 did not relapse, while 6 relapsed, whereas in the low-dose group, 21 did not relapse and 9 did. While this was a statistically non-significant difference, more relapses did occur in the lower dose group. Johnson *et al.* (1987) used a different drug, flupenthixol decanoate. Of those on the regular dose, 4 of 31 relapsed in 18 months, and of those who received half the usual dose, 12 of 28 relapsed in this time period. Johnson's low-dose group was in a range equivalent to that of the Hogarty and Marder low-dose groups.

If these three studies are considered collectively, we begin to see an increased relapse rate at these doses, and the breakpoint for the minimally effective dose would probably be just slightly higher. This would indicate that the clinician must balance several factors when choosing the proper therapy: (1) long-term risk of tardive dyskinesia, (2) the problem of dysphoric side-effects, (3) the likelihood of a severe relapse, (4) the likelihood of suicide, and (5) the disruption of a minor relapse. It may be preferable to avoid more serious side-effects at the cost of a few more relapses, if the relapses do not require hospitalization or produce serious impairment in social functioning. We would recommend treating most patients with the minimally effective dose and supplementing depot medication when early warning signals of relapse occur. When using depot medication, supplements should be made with oral doses because the pharmacokinetics of depot medication are such that it takes months to reach steady state. For oral medication, raising the dose brings about an altered steady state in several days.

12.6 Choice of medication

All antipsychotics are equally effective. The choice is made on the basis of side-effects and half-life. Pimozide is a specific dopamine antagonist that has some merit as a maintenance medication for schizophrenia due to its long oral half-life and low side-effect profile (Clark *et al.*, 1971, 1975). Due to non-compliance with the prescribed therapy, many schizophrenic patients suffer relapse. To reduce this risk, long-acting depot intramuscular fluphenazine enanthate and decanoate, as well as haloperidol decanoate, have been developed (del Guidice *et al.*, 1975). Table 3 compares the relapse rate of depot versus oral drug ($P = 0.000\,2$ Mantel–Haenszel test). The usefulness of depot medication is supported by studies by Johnson and co-workers (Johnson, 1979; Johnson *et al.*, 1983; Johnson & Wright, 1990), who use matched controls, Marriott & Hiep (1976), Tegeler & Lehmann (1981), and Freeman (1980), who use mirror image controls, that is, the relapse in patients on oral medication and later on depot medication.

There is a trade-off between the risk of tardive dyskinesia using adequate dose, long-term medication and the higher risk of relapse but lower risk of tardive dyskinesia with low-dose or intermittent treatment. We need to consider what happens if patients do have a relapse, which implies the occurrence of psychotic behavior that may interfere with vocational and social functioning and, at the extreme, may result in violence or suicide. In short, there is the cost of the psychotic episode to the patients, their families, and society.

Table 3 Difference between oral and depot formulation.

Reference	Total number of patients	Study duration	Percentage difference (oral–depot)
del Guidice *et al.* (1975)	82	1 year	48
Crawford & Forest (1974)	29	40 weeks	27
Schooler *et al.* (1979)	214	1 year	9
Rifkin *et al.* (1977)	51	1 year	2
Falloon *et al.* (1978)	41	1 year	–16
Hogarty *et al.* (1979)	105	2 years	25

12.7 Effect of antipsychotic drugs on the course of schizophrenia

A second consideration is whether a relapse or an untreated episode affects the natural course of a psychotic disorder. Does effectively treating schizophrenia improve the natural course of the illness? And, conversely, does ineffective treatment of an episode produce a worsening in the natural course of the illness? We reviewed two studies which provide data on the effects of treating or not treating an episode. May and collaborators (1976a,b) investigated the long-term outcome of 228 hospitalized schizophrenic patients randomly assigned to five treatment plans: ECT, a phenothiazine alone, psychotherapy alone, a phenothiazine in combination with psychotherapy, and no specific treatment (control group). Following successful treatment, patients were discharged into the community. Those patients with poor responses were generally in the groups not receiving drug or ECT. After a 6-month to 1-year period, 48 non-responding, hospitalized patients from all treatment groups received pharmacotherapy and psychotherapy. All but 2 of these patients responded to the combination and all 48 patients were eventually discharged. The principal difference among the groups at this point was that those initially randomly assigned to no drug or ECT treatment had their episode prolonged for 6 or more months until a drug was started. All 228 patients were then followed for 3–5 years after their index admission. When the total numbers of days of rehospitalization after the initial release were compared, there was a large difference among these treatment groups. Specifically, those who received only psychotherapy spent about twice as much time hospitalized as those who received pharmacotherapy and psychotherapy, despite the fact that post-study treatment was similar across both groups, that is, current treatment was then an uncontrolled variable (Figure 5). Those who received no drug/no psychotherapy also did substantially poorer than the drug/no psychotherapy group. It is of particular interest that the patients who initially received ECT did as well in terms of subsequent days hospitalized as those who received drug treatment.

An important aspect of May's study is that there was a significant drug-free period – 6–12 months. This is significant evidence that antipsychotics alter the natural course of schizophrenia. Thus, therapy with ECT or antipsychotics during the patient's initial episode resulted in a better outcome several years later. This would suggest that experiencing an episode is harmful, but the precise mechanism involved in producing this harm is unknown. Perhaps a psychotic episode induces some physical damage, making future episodes more likely; or perhaps the disruptive psychotic behavior plus the long hospital period have irreparable effects on social or family functioning. Both of these possibilities may be true. Whatever the reason, it appears that initiating therapy with antipsychotics or ECT at the onset of an acute episode may improve long-term outcome. Future research should be conducted in this area.

Greenblatt *et al.* (1965) compared four variations of drug and social therapies in

THREE YEARS FOLLOW-UP AFTER FIRST RELEASE

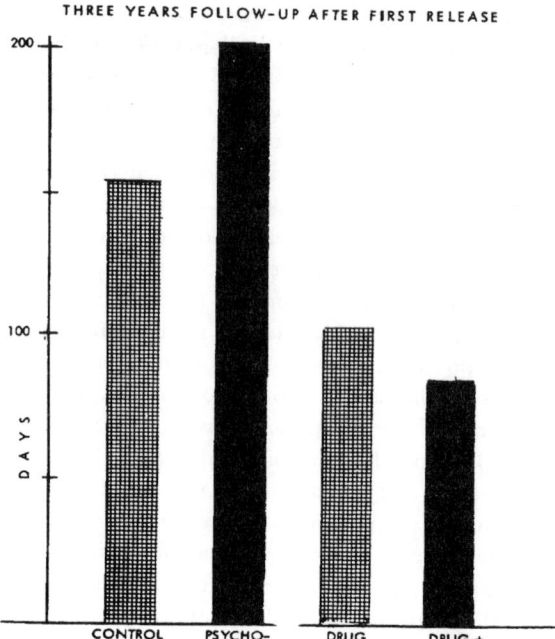

Figure 5

chronic schizophrenics continuously hospitalized for many years. These patients were randomly divided into drug and non-drug groups, and each group was further subdivided into intensive and minimal social therapy groups. Since these patients had been continuously hospitalized for many years and received medication, the outcome of the two no-drug groups is of interest in evaluating the effect of a long drug-free period on ultimate outcome. With respect to the short-term outcome, at the 6-month point the greatest improvement occurred in the two medication groups (drugs with psychotherapy and drugs alone). There was also a trend after 6 months for greater symptomatic improvement in the drug plus intensive social therapy group (33%), in comparison with the drug plus minimal social therapy group (23%). Those patients receiving intensive social therapy and no drugs fared poorly during the 6-month trial. This group then received 6 more months of psychosocial treatment plus drugs. For the long-term outcome, the intensive social therapy without drugs mitigated against improvement, and when finally placed on medication, this group was never able to catch up with those initially treated with drugs plus intensive social therapy.

One would have thought this group might have done the best since it had 1 year of intensive psychosocial treatment plus 6 months of drugs, but this was not the case. The

6 months drug-free seemed to produce a carry-over negative effect. While the sample size is small, this treatment was not statistically significantly helpful, and indeed, in terms of direction of the effect, seems harmful. By contrast, the psychosocial plus drug intervention direction of effect was helpful. In terms of ultimate outcome, intensive social therapy appeared to be important in discharging patients into the community since most of the patients discharged were in the intensive social therapy plus drug group.

12.8 Maintenance drug and psychosocial treatment

Schizophrenic patients from families with high expressed emotion (demanding, critical, high expectations) have a higher relapse rate than those from families with low expressed emotion (Leff *et al.*, 1982; Brown *et al.*, 1972; Vaughn & Leff, 1976; Vaughn *et al.*, 1984). This finding suggests that schizophrenic patients may be vulnerable to emotional confrontations. Several research groups have attempted to reduce high expressed emotion and, hence, reduce relapse rates through the use of family therapy. Families are taught techniques for coping with their schizophrenic member, and perhaps more importantly, they are educated about the disorder itself, including the need for medication compliance.

Table 4 shows the effect of psychosocial treatment on relapse rates in seven studies. All patients received maintenance antipsychotics, and the experimental variable manipulated was the presence or absence of some form of psychosocial treatment. Thus, these studies assessed whether psychoeducation/family therapy has an additional beneficial effect above and beyond that produced by drugs. Since the number of patients who relapsed in each treatment group was measured, we could combine data from these seven studies (Hogarty *et al.*, 1974, 1979, 1988, 1991; Goldstein *et al.*, 1978; Falloon *et al.*, 1982; Tarrier *et al.*, 1988; Leff *et al.*, 1990). We found a consistently better outcome (in terms of the likelihood of relapse) for patients with psychoeducation/family therapy intervention than with antipsychotics alone, a difference that was statistically significant ($\chi^2 = 16.5$; d.f. =; $P = 0.00005$). The psychosocial treatments used in these seven studies employed somewhat similar techniques; however, not all treatments were focused exclusively on lowering the family's expressed emotion toward the schizophrenic member. Nevertheless, the consistently better outcome in these studies for those receiving some type of psychoeducation/family therapy along with antipsychotic medication is a promising finding.

Results from medication and psychosocial interventions in post-discharge planning have been hopeful, and linking the inpatient setting with the outpatient environment appears to be crucial in preventing relapse.

Table 4 Outcome of patients treated with antipsychotic drugs with or without psychosocial treatment.

Reference	Evaluation interval	Drug alone		Drug and psychosocial therapy	
		Well	Relapsed	Well	Relapsed
Falloon *et al.* (1982)	9 months	9	9	16	2
Goldstein *et al.* (1978)	6 weeks	42	8	44	2
Hogarty *et al.* (1979)	2 years	25	27	30	23
Hogarty *et al.* (1991)	2 years	11	10	39	15
Tarrier *et al.* (1988)	9 months	8	8	29	3
Leff *et al.* (1990)	2 years	3	9	6	6
Hogarty *et al.* (1974)	2 years	73	22	80	15
Total		171	93	244	66
% Well/ relapsed		65	35	79	21

12.9 Postpsychotic depression

There is a significant difference between unremitted or partially remitted schizophrenics with pronounced negative symptoms and outpatient schizophrenics in remission who have a depressive episode. In the latter case, the patient is in relative remission from schizophrenia but presents with an acute episode of depression. Siris *et al.* (1987) selected candidates with a history of schizophrenic episodes who had recovered and experienced a major depression with resolution upon administration of tricyclic antidepressants. Thirty-three patients, all receiving both maintenance neuroleptics and maintenance tricyclic antidepressants, were studied in a double-blind study on continuing neuroleptics plus random administration of either a tricyclic or placebo. The imipramine group was found to have a statistically superior outcome (P = 0.020, two-tailed Fisher's test) on the global outcome of each of the subscales in depression. There was no difference in the measure of psychosis or side-effects in the two groups.

Siris *et al.* (1990) also conducted a follow-up study on the previous tricyclic treatment group. Patients were maintained on fluphenazine decanoate and benztropine, as well as adjunctive imipramine. For 6 months treatment was continued, and then patients were either tapered to a placebo or continued on the tricyclic regimen for one more year. The 6 who were tapered relapsed to a depressive state, while only 2 of the 8 patients remaining on imipramine relapsed. This is statistically significant, $P = 0.009$. Of note is that the relapsed patients again responded favorably once adjunctive imipramine was reinstituted.

Johnson (1981) studied 50 schizophrenic patients in remission who were randomly distributed to receive nortriptyline or placebo for a 5-week trial. At the end of the trial there were more subjects (7 or 28%) in the nortriptyline group free of depression at the end of the trial than in the placebo group (8%).

Prusoff *et al.* (1979) conducted a study with 40 schizophrenic outpatients with a depressive episode who had amitriptyline or placebo added to their maintenance perphenazine requirements. Of the 20 patients remaining in the study for 6 months, there was a slight degree in overall improvement in 92% of the patients receiving the antidepressant, but this effect was ascribed more to the overall improvement in most patients rather than a significant improvement in just a few. In general, the improvement in depression was modest and not statistically impressive, and there was also a suggestion of worsening in psychosis.

In summary, we feel episodes of superimposed depression should be treated but that antidepressants do not help negative symptoms in chronic schizophrenic patients.

12.10 Supersensitivity

Supersensitivity psychosis (SSP) has been described as the early emergence of psychosis upon the discontinuation of long-term neuroleptic treatment and hypothesized to be secondary to an upregulation of dopamine receptors. This occurs in a dopaminergic neural circuit relevant to psychoses, analogous to tardive dyskinesia, which has been hypothesized as a neuroleptic-induced supersensitivity consequent to striatal neuroleptic blockade (that is, dopaminergic receptor upregulation in the neural circuit relevant to movement). Hypothetically, there could be similar receptor supersensitivity in the postsynaptic dopaminergic pathway involved in schizophrenia. Withdrawal of neuroleptics may induce rebound psychosis, just as it may cause withdrawal tardive dyskinesia. Chouinard & Steinberg's (1984) criteria for the diagnosis are presented in Table 5, and patients who fit this criteria can be found in Hunt *et al.* (1988). Peet (1991), in a chart review study of 55 outpatients, found 7 who met the Chouinard & Steinberg (1984) criteria for SSP. Singh *et al.* (1990) tested 5 patients with a clinical history of supersensitive psychosis, and 5 with no such history. It was predicted that the SSP patients would relapse more rapidly upon

Table 5 Criteria for supersensitivity psychosis.

I. History of receiving neuroleptics or antipsychotics for at least 6 months

II. A. Patient has had a decrease or discontinuation of medication:
1. has shown appearance of psychotic symptoms within 6 weeks for oral medication, or
2. has shown appearance of psychotic symptoms within 3 months for i.m. medication, or
    B. Has had no decrease or discontinuation of medication during treatment
1. has shown greater frequency of relapse with time, and/or
2. tolerance to the antipsychotic effect of the neuroleptic.

III. At least two of the following criteria for definite and one for probable:
    A. Those who had a decrease of medication
1. psychotic symptoms upon decrease of medication were:
          (i) not previously seen, or
          (ii) are of greater severity
2. patient has shown greater frequency of relapse with time
3. tolerance to the antipsychotic effect
4. tardive dyskinesia is present (a standard examination must be used)
5. rapid improvement of psychotic symptoms when the effective neuroleptic dose is increased after a decrease or discontinuation of medication
6. patient has shown clear exacerbation of psychotic symptoms by stress
7. if patient is treated only with i.m. long-acting, has shown appearance of psychotic symptoms at the end of the injection interval, or
    B. Those who had no decrease of medication (only one required if II.B.1 + 11.B.2)
1. tardive dyskinesia is present (a standard examination is required)
2. patient has shown clear exacerbation of psychotic symptoms by by stress
3. if patient is treated only with i.m. long-acting, has shown appearance of psychotic symptoms at the end of the injection interval.

IV. Exclusion criteria:
1. Patients in the acute phase of the illness
2. Patients with continued psychotic illness which did not respond to neuroleptic treatment.

discontinuation of neuroleptics than the non-SSP patients. In the study, the neuroleptic medication was abruptly replaced by placebo without any tapering, and the emergence of psychosis or tardive dyskinesia was evaluated. The authors did not find evidence of relapse into psychosis in any patients in a 2-week period. As the relapse rate of untreated schizophrenics is 10–15% per month, we would expect some relapses during this period. Thus, one would have to show in the early phase after drug withdrawal that there is an increased relapse or at least the emergence or worsening of symptoms than would otherwise be expected. We must balance the prepared mind to be alert to this possibility until there is clear evidence either way, and for now, we would give this hypothesis the verdict of not proven.

12.11 Conclusion

Continuous maintenance antipsychotics, at least in the moderately low-dose range, afford the best chance for avoiding relapse in schizophrenic patients. The utilization of maintenance strategies must always be considered in the context of the long-term consequences to minimize more serious adverse effects (that is, tardive dyskinesia and supersensitivity psychosis). Further, psychosocial therapies can enhance the beneficial effects of medication, thus improving the overall quality of a patient's life.

References

Adelson, D. & Epstein, L.A. (1962) *J. Nerv. Mental Dis.* **134**, 543–554.

Andrews, P., Hall, J.N. & Snaith, R.P. (1976) *Br. J. Psychiat.* **128**, 451–455.

Baro, F., Brugmans, J., Dom, R. *et al.* (1970) *J. Clin. Pharmacol.* **10**, 330–341.

Blackburn, J. & Allen, J. (1961) *J. Nerv. Mental Dis.* **133**, 303–307.

Brown, G.W., Birley, J.L.T. & Wing, J.K. (1972) *Br. J. Psychiat.* **121**, 241–258.

Caffey, E.M., Diamond, L.S., Frank, T.V. *et al.* (1964) *J. Chronic Dis.* **17**, 347–358.

Carpenter, W.T., Hanlon, T.E., Heinrichs, D.W. *et al.* (1990) *Am. J. Psychiat.* **147**, 1138–1148.

Cheung, H.K. (1981) *Br. J. Psychiat.* **138**, 490–494.

Chien, C.P. & Cole, J.O. (1975) In *Drugs in Combination with Other Therapies* (ed. Greenblatt, M.), pp. 13–14, New York, Grune Stratton.

Chouinard, G. & Steinberg, S. (1984) In *Guidlines for Psychotropic Drugs* (eds Stancer, H.C., Garfinkel, P.E. & Rakoff, V.M.), pp. 205–227, New York, Spectrum Publications.

Clark, M.L., Huber, W., Serafetinides, E.A. & Colmore, J.P. (1971) *Clin. Trial J.* (Suppl.) **2**, 25–32.

Clark, M.L., Huber, W., Hill, D. *et al.* (1975) *Dis. Nerv. Syst.* **36**, 137–141.

Crawford, R. & Forrest, A. (1974) *Br. J. Psychiat.* **124**, 385–391.

Davis, J.M. (1975) *Am. J. Psychiat.* **132**, 1237–1245.

Davis, J.M., Dysken, M.W., Haberman, S.J. et al. (1980) Adv. Biochem. Pharmacol. 24, 471–481.

Davis, J.M., Marter, J.T. & Kane, J.M. (1989) In Comprehensive Textbook of Psychiatry (5th edition), Vol. 2 (eds Kaplan, H.I. & Saddock, B.J.), pp. 1591–1626, Baltimore, Williams & Wilkins.

del Guidice, J., Clark, W.G. & Gocka, E.F. (1975) Psychosomatics 16, 32–36.

Diamond, L.S. & Marks, J.B. (1960) J. Nerv. Mental Dis. 131, 247–251.

Engelhardt, D.M., Rosen, B., Freedman, D. et al. (1967) Arch. Gen. Psychiat. 16, 98–99.

Falloon, I., Watt, D.C. & Shepherd, M. (1978) Psychol. Med. 8, 59–70.

Falloon, I.R.H., Boyd, J.L., McGill, C.W. et al. (1982) New Engl. J. Med. 306, 1437–1440.

Freeman, H. (1980) In Long-term Effects of Neuroleptics (Adv. Biochem. Psychopharmacol.) (eds Cattabeni, F. et al.), pp. 559–564, New York, Raven Press.

Freeman, L.S. & Alson, E. (1962) Dis. Nerv. Syst. 23, 522–525.

Gaebel, W., Kopcke, W., Linden, M. et al. (1991) Schizophrenia Res. 4, 288.

Garfield, S., Gershon, S., Sletten, L. et al. (1966) Dis. Nerv. Syst. 27, 321–325.

Goldberg, S.C., Schooler, N.R., Hogarty, G.E. & Roper, M. (1977) Arch. Gen. Psychiat. 34, 171–184.

Goldstein, M.J., Rodnick, E.H., Evans, J.R. et al. (1978) Arch. Gen. Psychiat. 35, 1169–1177.

Greenblatt, M., Solomon, M.H., Evans, A.S. & Brooks, G.W. (eds) (1965) Drug and Social Therapy in Chronic Schizophrenia, Springfield, IL, Charles C. Thomas.

Gross, H.S. (1974) Curr. Ther. Res. 16, 696–705.

Gross, M. & Reeves, W.P. (1961) in Mental Patients in Transition (ed. Greenblatt, M.), pp. 313–321, Springfield, IL, Charles C. Thomas.

Hershon, H.I., Kennedy, P.F. & McGuire, R.J. (1972) Br. J. Psychiat. 120, 4150.

Herz, M.I., Glazer, W.M., Mostert, M.A. et al. (1990) Clin. Neuropharmacol. 13 (Suppl. 2), 426–427.

Herz, M.I., Glazer, W.M., Mostert, M.A. et al. (1991) Arch. Gen. Psychiat. 48, 333–339.

Hirsch, S.R., Gaind, R., Rohde, P.D. et al. (1973) Br. Med. J. 1, 633–637.

Hogarty, G.E. & Goldberg, S.C. (1973) Arch. Gen. Psychiat. 28, 54–64.

Hogarty, G.E. & Ulrich, R.F. (1977) Arch. Gen. Psychiat. 34, 297–301.

Hogarty, G.E., Goldberg, S.C., Schooler, N.R., Ulrich, R.F., Collaborative Study Group (1974) Arch. Gen. Psychiat. 31, 603–608.

Hogarty, G.E., Ulrich, R.F., Mussare, F. & Aristigueta, H. (1976) Dis. Nerv. Syst. 37, 494–500.

Hogarty, G.E., Schooler, N.R., Ulrich, R. et al. (1979) Arch. Gen. Psychiat. 1283–1294.

Hogarty, G.E., Anderson, C.M., Reiss, D.J. et al. (1986) Arch. Gen. Psychiat. 43, 633–642.

Hogarty, G.E., McEvoy, J.P., Munetz, M. et al. (1988) Arch. Gen. Psychiat. 45, 797–805.

Hogarty, G.E., Anderson, C.M., Reiss, D.J. et al. (1991) Arch. Gen. Psychiat. 48, 340–347.

Hunt, J.I., Singh, H. & Simpson, G.M. (1988) J. Clin. Psychiat. 49, 258–261.

Johnson, D.A.W. (1976a) Br. J. Psychiat. 128, 246–250.

Johnson, D.A.W. (1976b) Acta Psychiat. Scand. 53, 298–301.

Johnson, D.A.W. (1979) Br. J. Psychiat. 135, 524–530.

Johnson, D.A.W. (1981) J. Psychiat. 139, 89–101.

Johnson, D.A.W. & Wright, N.F. (1990) Br. J. Psychiat. 156, 827–834.

Johnson, D.A.W., Pasterski, J.M., Ludlow, J.M. et al. (1983) Acta Psychiat. Scand. 67, 339–352.

Johnson, D.A.W., Ludlow, J.M., Street, K. & Taylor, R.D.W. (1987) Br. J. Psychiat. 151, 634–638.

Jolley, A.G., Hirsch, S.R., McRink, A. & Manchanda, R. (1989) Br. Med. J. 298, 985–990.

Jolley, A.G., Hirsch, S.R., Morrison, E. et al. (1990) Br. Med. J. 301, 837–846.

Kane, J.M. (ed.) (1984) Drug Maintenance Strategies in Schizophrenia, Washington, DC, American Psychiatric Press.

Kane, J.M., Rifkin, A., Woerner, M. *et al.* (1983) *Arch. Gen. Psychiat.* **40**, 893–896.
Kinross-Wright, J. & Charalampous, K.D. (1965) *Int. J. Neuropsychiat.* **1**, 66–70.
Leff, J.P. & Wing, J.K. (1971) *Br. Med. J.* **2**, 599–604.
Leff, J., Kuipers, L., Berkowitz, R. *et al.* (1982) *Br. J. Psychiat.* **141**, 121–134.
Leff, J., Berkowitz, R., Shavit, N. *et al.* (1990) *Br. J. Psychiat.* **157**, 571–577.
Levine, J., Schooler, N., Serene, F. *et al.* (1980) In *Long-Term Effects of Neuroleptics* (ed. Cattabeni, E.), pp. 483–484, New York, Raven Press.
Mantel, N. & Haenszel, W. (1959) *J. Natl. Cancer Inst.* **22**, 719–748.
Marder, S.R., Van Putten, T., Mintz, J. *et al.* (1987) *Arch. Gen. Psychiat.* **44**, 518–521.
Marriott, P. & Hiep, A. (1976) *Aust. New Zealand J. Psychiat.* **10**, 163–116.
May, P.R.A., Tuma, A.H. & Dixon, W.J. (1976a) *Arch. Gen. Psychiat.* **33**, 474–478.
May, P.R.A., Tuma, A.H., Yale, C. *et al.* (1976b) *Arch. Gen. Psychiat.* **33**, 481–486.
Melnyk, W.T., Worthington, A.G. & Laverty, S.G. (1966) *Can. Psychiat. Assoc. J.* **11**, 410–413.
Morgan, R. & Cheadle, J. (1974) *Acta Psychiat. Scand.* **50**, 78–85.
Morton, M.R. (1968) *Am. J. Psychiat.* **124**, 1585–1588.
Nishikawa, T., Tsuda, A., Tanaka, M. *et al.* (1982) *Psychopharmacology* **77**, 301–304.
Peet, M. (1991) *J. Clin. Psychiat.* (Letter to the Editor) **52**, 90.
Prien, R.F. & Cole, J.O. (1968) *Arch. Gen. Psychiat.* **18**, 482–495.
Prien, R.F., Cole, J.O. & Belkin, N.F. (1969) *Br. J. Psychiat.* **115**, 679–686.
Prien, R.F., Levine, J. & Switalski, R.W. (1971) *Hosp. Community Psychiat.* **22**, 4–7.
Prusoff, B.A., Williams, D.H., Weissman, M.M. *et al.* (1979) *Arch. Gen. Psychiat.* **36**, 569–575.
Rassidakis, N.C., Kondakis, X., Papanastassiou, A. *et al.* (1970) *Bull. Menninger Clin.* **34**, 216–222.
Rifkin, A., Quitkin, F., Rabiner, C.J. *et al.* (1977) *Arch. Gen. Psychiat.* **34**, 43–47.
Ruskin, P.E. & Nyman, G. (1991) *J. Nerv. Mental Dis.* **179**, 212–214.
Schauver, J., Gorham, D.R., Leskin, L.W. *et al.* (1959) *Dis. Nerv. Syst.* **20**, 452–457.
Schiele, B.C. (1975) *Dis. Nerv. Syst.* **36**, 361–364.
Schooler, N.R., Levine, J. & Severe, J.B. (1979) *Psychopharmacol. Bull.* **15**, 44–47.
Singh, H., Hunt, J.L., Vitiello, B. & Simpson, G.M. (1990) *J. Clin. Psychiat.* **51**, 319–321.
Siris, S.G., Morgan, V., Fagerstrom, R. *et al.* (1987) *Arch. Gen. Psychiat.* **44**, 533–539.
Siris, S.G., Mason, S.E., Beranzohn, P.C. *et al.* (1990) *Psychopharmacol. Bull.* **26**, 91–94.
Tarrier, N., Barrowclough, C., Vaughn, C. *et al.* (1988) *Br. J. Psychiat.* **153**, 532–542.
Tegeler, J. & Lehmann, E. (1981) *Prog. Neuro-Psychopharmacol.* **5**, 79–90.
Troshinsky, C.H., Aaronson, H.G. & Stone, R.K. (1962) *Pennsylvania Psychiat. Quart.* **2**, 11–15.
Vaughn, C.E. & Leff, J.P. (1976) *Br. J. Psychiat.* **129**, 125–137.
Vaughn, C.E., Snyder, K.S., Jones, S. *et al.* (1984) *Arch. Gen. Psychiat.* **41**, 1169–1177.
Whitaker, C.B. & Hoy, R.M. (1963) *Br. J. Psychiat.* **109**, 422–427.
Wistedt, B. (1981) *Acta Univ. Upsal.* 391–397.

CHAPTER 13

DEPOT NEUROLEPTICS

D.A.W. Johnson

University Hospital of South Manchester, Manchester, UK

Table of Contents

13.1 Introduction

Neuroleptic drug administration in the form of long-acting depot injection was introduced into clinical practice in June 1966. Initial evaluations of its efficacy were all based on the so-called 'mirror image' methodology in which identical intervals before and after the introduction of depot medication are compared. All these studies were open and uncontrolled, although they had the advantage of measuring treatment under normal clinical conditions. Each study reported a major reduction in the number of relapses experienced on depot injections (30–70% reduction) together with a substantial reduction in the length of time spent in hospital (Denham & Adamson, 1971; Johnson & Freeman, 1972; Gottfries & Green, 1974; Marriott & Hiep, 1976). At first it was not universally accepted that the clinical advantages resulted from regular medication; it was thought by some that they came from increased support and contact with services. However, a double-blind placebo trial by Hirsch *et al.* (1973) demonstrated that the therapeutic benefit did indeed come from the use of regular drug treatment.

Subsequently, a number of carefully executed trials have demonstrated that under research conditions, maintenance therapy with oral medication can be as successful as treatment by depot injections (Del Guidice *et al.*, 1975; Rifkin *et al.*, 1977; Falloon *et al.*, 1978; Schooler *et al.*, 1980). It would be surprising if this were not the case, since whatever the method of drug administration it is the same drug molecule that acts on the brain. However, each of these studies was highly atypical of maintenance treatment under the normal conditions of clinical practice. Patient samples were highly selected in a way that often led to the specific exclusion of unstable, poor prognosis or non-compliant patients. All the studies included a considerable investment of resources with a substantial increase in staff–patient contact, sometimes resulting in more than one contact in a week. Since only one study (Hogarty et al., 1979) compared treatments for more than 1 year, it is doubtful if these studies truly attempted to evaluate long-term maintenance therapy. In the second year, Hogarty et al. (1979) reported an increased relapse rate on oral medication (42% versus 8%), which only failed to reach a level of statistical significance because of the small numbers of patients remaining in the 2-year analysis.

These limitations must leave the advantages of maintenance treatment of schizophrenia by depot injections unchallenged. Hogarty (1984) concluded that the prophylactic efficacy of maintenance medication is probably the strongest clinical effect that has been demonstrated in psychiatry. This enormous potential for therapeutic benefit must not be placed in jeopardy. The longest prospective monitoring of maintenance treatment comparing oral and depot injections is over 3 years. This single-blind study suggests a survival of 60% of patients free from relapse over this period compared to 20–40% of patients on no regular medication or oral medication (Johnson, 1981a).

The main advantage claimed for oral medication is the flexibility of prescriptions provided by its short duration of action. The assumption is that a dose reduction or drug discontinuation will result in a rapid lowering of drug levels with an almost immediate resolution of side-effects – particularly extrapyramidal symptoms. This conclusion overlooks the fact that neuroleptic drugs are highly soluble in the body lipids and consequently can be stored in fatty tissues, creating their own secondary depot sites. Active metabolites may also remain in the body for extended periods. For both these reasons oral medication may cease to be truly short-acting drugs after a few weeks of regular treatment. As a consequence, oral medication then begins to share perhaps the greatest drawback of the depot injections: a delay in the response of extrapyramidal side-effects to dose change. Unfortunately, this extended action of oral medication after a few weeks is all too frequently overlooked in drug trials which allow only a short washout period.

The depot injection method of drug administration has a number of important advantages. It overcomes the problems of absorption and bypasses the metabolic actions of the gut wall and liver cells. As a result the blood levels produced are more constant, not only in single individuals but also between patients (Curry et al., 1973). This is the likely reason why a smaller total dose is required for successful maintenance therapy. A steady blood level may also result in fewer extrapyramidal side-effects in patients with correctly adjusted dose regimens.

13.2 Compliance

Perhaps the most important clinical advantage and the one most clearly demonstrated is the level of improved compliance. It has been demonstrated repeatedly that non-compliance with oral medication is very high in the community (37-65% after only 4-6 weeks). This is true not only with psychiatric patients but with all drug treatments. Even in highly motivated groups such as mothers administering medication to infants, or seriously ill patients with potentially lethal conditions (Ley & Spelman, 1967). In psychiatric inpatients urinalyses have demonstrated both the absence of prescribed drugs in 6-8% of patients and the presence of drugs to which it was believed they had no access in 10% (Ballinger et al., 1974, 1975). These results should be less surprising when we remember that no more than 50% of essential information is retained by a patient after a consultation and that most information about both illness and treatment is claimed by patients to come from non-medical sources. The problems of compliance are complex and depend not only upon the patient, but also their family's attitudes towards mental illness and its treatment by drugs (Johnson, 1986a). It is not a situation where patients either take their drugs appropriately or discontinue medication. The degree of compliance may vary enormously. For doctors to make a sensible decision concerning future management, whether for therapeutic benefits or for the treatment of side-effects, they must have a knowledge of the exact dose and type of drug actually received by the patient. This can be achieved only by the use of depot injections.

It must be accepted that maintenance treatment of schizophrenia with depot injections has its own problems of compliance. A 1973 survey reported that 10-15% of patients refused the prescription of depot injections and the same percentage defaulted over a 2-year period. In a repeat survey (1987-90) only 5% of patients treated in the community refused to start depot therapy but 10-15% still defaulted from treatment over a 2-year interval (Johnson & Freeman, 1973; Johnson & Wright, 1990). Curson et al. (1985) followed up the research sample of Hirsch et al. (1973) and found after 7 years that 73% of the original sample were still successfully on depot injections even after this long interval, with a positive correlation between survival and compliance. This level of non-compliance is an enormous reduction on the expectation for oral medication.

The use of depot medication also reduces the availability of drugs for overdose or abuse. This is a potentially important consideration not only for the patient but also for the whole family. Depression is common in the course of schizophrenia and 10-15% of schizophrenic patients die by suicide (Johnson, 1990a). In the United Kingdom, the most common source of drugs used in overdose is medication prescribed for the patient, the next most common source is medication belonging to another member of the family.

13.3 Delivery service

A further important consideration is the organization required to make regular drug administration by depot injection a success. The selection of depot injections is not an easy alternative to the prescription of oral drugs. It requires careful planning, extra resources and additional staff time. The depot injection service should be much more than a delivery system for drugs alone. It should act as the fulcrum for long-term treatment and ensure the continued supervision of care and redistribution of resources when necessary. However, it is not a substitute for the continued attendance at a normal psychiatric outpatient clinic, but rather a complementary service offering additional support and regular evaluation of mental state, social functioning and drug side-effects. Its advantage is that it promotes regular contact between staff and patients which make it ideal for detecting early changes. It has been suggested that prodromal non-specific changes are present before many major florid symptoms and that a treatment at this time may prevent some psychotic episodes at least (Herz & Melville, 1980; Johnson et al., 1987; Johnson, 1988a,b; Carpenter et al., 1990; Jolley et al., 1990).

There is an ongoing debate whether the depot injection should be given in a hospital (depot injection clinic), at a local community clinic, by the family doctor or on a domiciliary basis by community nurses. It is likely that no single solution will meet the needs of all patients. The nature of the illness within individual patients and the environmental setting of a particular service are two important factors to be considered. Whichever delivery service is selected for individual patients it is essential to have a central master register which is carefully monitored by a single responsible member of staff. If depot clinics are developed then it is important to give careful thought to the hours of access. Usually it should be available on at least two separate days each week, including one early evening to meet the needs of patients who are working or those who need assistance from members of the family who work. The clinic should be staffed by a stable group of psychiatrically trained nurses for whom the service represents a substantial part of their normal work. They should have special training in the early detection of side-effects and change of mental state. Sufficient time should be allocated to the staff to enable them to fulfil the full functions of the clinic. Educational meetings should be held for both patients and relatives since it is essential that they have a clear understanding of both the illness and treatment goals. This not only improves treatment compliance but may also help to modify environmental influences and lead to the early reporting of changes by the family. Drug prescriptions should be valid for a maximum period of 6 months to ensure a regular review by the medical team. A system of flagging the non-attendance of patients is required together with planning for first reminding and, when necessary, visiting defaulters. On each attendance a checklist should be completed to include weight, extrapyramidal side-effects, tardive dyskinesia, change of mental state/physical state/social or work function (Johnson, 1990b).

13.4 Risk of side-effects

It has been suggested that there are special risks of side-effects from the use of depot injections. In particular, it has been suggested that there is an increased risk of extrapyramidal symptoms and an increased frequency of depression. This is quite untrue and a full understanding of this form of drug delivery supports this conclusion. However the drug is delivered to the central nervous system it is the same drug, with the same properties, that produces both the therapeutic and unwanted effects. Nevertheless, it should be acknowledged that there are special considerations.

It is universally accepted that all neuroleptics produce extrapyramidal symptoms although the exact risks may remain controversial. Reported prevalence rates vary between 23 and 88%, although most cluster around 40%. The interpretation of these studies is difficult. Most have been carried out on long-term patients of uncertain diagnosis, possibly with secondary complications. In nearly all studies essential dependent variables have been omitted, including the duration of observation, dosage of drugs, pharmacological classification of the antipsychotic and the presence of any other drugs. The possibility that side-effects may have resulted from an unnecessarily high dosage or polypharmacy has been consistently overlooked. The extent to which polypharmacy and high doses are used was reported, after a series of surveys, by Johnson & Wright (1990). It has been acknowledged already that there is a problem of delay following a dose adjustment before extrapyramidal symptoms resolve, but at the same time it has been explained that oral medication develops an identical problem in the setting of maintenance therapy, so the intervals of delay become increasingly similar. A knowledge of this risk, regular evaluation of early signs and the proper use of anticholinergic medication during the interval before dose reduction results in side-effect resolution should minimize this difficulty. Having prescribed anticholinergic drugs it is essential to review their need since studies conclusively demonstrate that most patients on these drugs do not develop side-effects once stopped (McClelland *et al.*, 1974; Rifkin *et al.*, 1978; Johnson 1978; Jellinek *et al.*, 1981).

The perception of some of the problems arising from the early experiences with depot injections were based upon unrealistic expectations. Depot fluphenazine injections were introduced as a treatment that should be prescribed in a dose range of 25–50 mg every 2 weeks in the enanthate form, and every 3 weeks in the later decanoate preparation. This resulted in too high a dose for many patients, and an inflexible approach to prescribing with regards to the interval between injections. We now know that the correct approach is a flexible, personalized prescription that is regularly monitored, and that for many patients, perhaps 50%, the dose can be halved or substantially reduced over 12 months. It has been clearly demonstrated that in 40–50% of patients the side-effects can be abolished by dose reduction alone without any loss of control (Johnson, 1973, 1975). The first drug introduced as a depot injection, and in many countries the only drug available for over a decade, was fluphenazine. This belongs to the piperazine derivatives which are known to have higher risks of extrapyramidal side-effects than some other phenothiazine derivatives. It must also be remembered that the stability of plasma levels produced by depot injections may be an advantage in actually reducing the risks of extrapyramidal symptoms for some neuroleptics. It is certainly true that some research suggests that a change of blood levels may produce symptoms, and clinically it is recognized that the risks may be increased 2–5 days after an injection and less certainly a few days before an injection is due. For haloperidol there is some evidence that the overall risks for extrapyramidal symptoms are less with the depot decanoate preparation than for oral preparations.

In forming clinical impressions it should not be forgotten that with the depot injection preparations the patient is known to receive the medication. With the oral preparations any apparent reduction of side-effects may be due to some level of non-compliance.

Concern that depot injections may give rise to increased risks of depression probably originate from a well-publicized paper by de Alarcon & Carney (1969). During their initial experience with depot treatment they observed a number of serious depressions and suicides and quite properly called for a close supervision of patients and asked whether there was any association with the drug. Further experience with maintenance depot treatment led Carney to conclude that depression is not a simple pharmacological effect of the drug (Carney & Sheffield, 1973).

Depression and suicide in schizophrenia is a complex topic. In recent years it has been researched in some depth. It has become recognized as one of the most frequent symptoms in schizophrenia irrespective of whether the patients are on neuroleptic medication. There are a wide range of possible aetiologies (Johnson, 1986a, 1988a,b). If true pharmacogenic depression exists it is likely to be responsible for only a small minority of depressive symptoms. However, 'akinetic' depression, which is an extrapyramidal syndrome, may be mistaken for true depression and has been identified as being responsible for 10–15% of patients identified as depressed (Johnson, 1981a,b). Because of any increased delay in response to drug dose reduction it is possible that 'akinetic' depression may be more common in patients on depot injections, but any such increase is marginal. The patients who experience least depression are those patients in a stable mental state living in the community on regular maintenance therapy.

It must not be forgotten that there might be different influences on mood by different drugs. It has been shown that flupenthixol in low dosage has an antidepressant effect in non-psychotic patients when given either orally or by depot injection (Frolund, 1974; Rosenberg et al., 1976; Johnson, 1979; Young et al., 1976). It has also been suggested that flupenthixol decanoate may have a mood-elevating effect in acute schizophrenia (Johnson & Malik, 1975). Caution must be exercised in reaching any final conclusion on the direct influence upon mood by neuroleptic drugs since the issues are complex. Depressive symptoms may emerge as the patient recovers from an acute episode due to a differential response of existing symptoms rather than new symptoms developing (Knights & Hirsch, 1981; McGlashan & Carpenter, 1976). The apparent mood change observed may be more dependent upon the response of the psychosis than a true mood change. The non-specific sedative effect may further complicate the issues.

13.5 Conclusions

The introduction of neuroleptics, in parallel with the social changes in psychiatric practice, was undoubtedly a major step forward in the care and prognosis for chronic psychosis. The introduction of the long-acting depot injection has allowed psychiatrists to develop the full therapeutic potential of maintenance medication. The initial unfettered enthusiasm for the therapeutic advantages of neuroleptic drugs has been tempered by an increasing knowledge of their limitations and unwanted effects. As a consequence, much recent research has focused on the better use of neuroleptics with particular emphasis on dose reduction, low-dose strategies and the effectiveness of monitored intermittent treatment. Properly used, the depot injections present no significant increased risks or handicaps. It is likely that many of the reported difficulties arise from the prescribing practices rather than from inherent difficulties in the depot injection. It cannot be stressed too often that their use requires careful planning and supervision by experienced staff. It must never be allowed to become a routine that is delegated to junior or inexperienced staff.

References

de Alarcon, R. & Carney, M.W.P. (1969) *Br. Med. J.* **3**, 564–567.
Ballinger, B.R., Simpson, E. & Stewart, M.J. (1974) *Br. J. Psychiat.* **125**, 202–207.
Ballinger, B.R., Ramsay, A.C. & Stewart, M.J. (1975) *Br. J. Psychiat.* **127**, 494–498.
Carney, M.W.P. & Sheffield, B.F. (1973) *Curr. Med. Res. Opinion* **1**, 423–426.
Carpenter, W.T., Hanlon, T.E., Heinrichs, D.W. *et al.* (1990) *Am. J. Psychiat.* **149**(9), 1138–1148.
Curry, S.H., Lewis, D.M., Samuel, G. *et al.* (1973) *Intern. Drug Ther. Newslett.* **6**, 53–60.
Curson, D.A., Barnes, T.R.E., Bamber, R.W. *et al.* (1985) *Br. J. Psychiat.* **146**, 464–480.
Del Guidice, J., Clarke, W.G. & Gocks, E.F. (1975) *Psychosoma. Med.* **16**, 32–36.
Denham, J. & Adamson, L. (1971) *Acta Psychiat. Scand.* **47**, 420.
Falloon, I., Watt, D.C. & Shepherd, M. (1978) *Psychol. Med.* **8**, 59–70.
Frolund, F. (1974) *Curr. Med. Res. Opinion* **2**, 78.
Gottfries, C.G. & Green, L. (1974) *Acta Psychiat. Scand. Suppl.* **255**, 15–23.
Herz, M.I. & Melville, C. (1980) *Am. J. Psychiat.* **137**, 801–805.
Hirsch, G.R., Gaind, R., Rhode, P.D. *et al.* (1973) *Br. Med. J.* **i**, 633–637.
Hogarty, G.E. (1984) *J. Clin. Psychiat.* **45**(5), Sec. 2, 36–42.
Hogarty, G.E., Schooler, N.R., Ulrich, R.F. *et al.* (1979) *Arch. Gen. Psychiat.* **36**, 1283–1294.
Jellinek, T., Gardos, G. & Cole, J.O. (1981) *Am. J. Psychiat.* **138**, 1567–1571.

Johnson, D.A.W. (1973) *Br. J. Psychiat.* **123**, 519-522.

Johnson, D.A.W. (1975) *Br. J. Psychiat.* **126**, 457-461.

Johnson, D.A.W. (1978) *Br. J. Psychiat.* **132**, 27-30.

Johnson, D.A.W. (1979) *Acta Psychiat. Scand.* **59**, 1-8.

Johnson, D.A.W. (1981a) In *Epidemiological Impact of Psychotropic Drugs* (eds Tognoni, G., Bellantuono, C. & Lader, M.), Amsterdam, North Holland, Elsevier.

Johnson, D.A.W. (1981b) *Br. J. Psychiat.* **139**, 89-101.

Johnson, D.A.W. (1986a) *Int. Med. Suppl.* **11**, 14-17.

Johnson, D.A.W. (1986b) In *Contemporary Issues in Schizophrenia* (eds Kerr, A. & Snaith, P.), pp. 451-459, London, Gaskell.

Johnson, D.A.W. (1988a) *Br. J. Psychiat.* **152**, 320-323.

Johnson, D.A.W. (1988b) In *Depression in Schizophrenics* (eds Williams, R. & Dalby, J.T.), pp. 193-203, New York, Plenum Press.

Johnson, D.A.W. (1990a) *Int. Rev. Psychiat.* **2**, 341-353.

Johnson, D.A.W. (1990b) *Pract. Rev. Psychiat. Series 2* **10**, 1-4.

Johnson, D.A.W. & Freeman, N.L. (1972) *The Practitioner* **208**, 395-400.

Johnson, D.A.W. & Freeman, H.L. (1973) *Psychol. Med.* **3**, 115-119.

Johnson, D.A.W. & Malik, N.A. (1975) *Acta Psychiat. Scand.* **51**, 257-267.

Johnson, D.A.W. & Wright, N. (1990) *Br. J. Psychiat.* **156**, 827-834.

Johnson, D.A.W., Ludlow, J.M., Street, K. & Taylor, R.D.W. (1987) *Br. J. Psychiat.* **151**, 634-638.

Jolley, A.G., Hirsch, S.R., Morrison, E. *et al.* (1990) *Br. Med. J.* **301**, 837-842.

Knights, A. & Hirsch, S.R. (1981) *Arch. Gen. Psychiat.* **38**, 806-811.

Ley, P. & Spelman, M.S. (1967) *Communicating with the Patient*, London, The Trinity Press.

McClelland, H.A., Blessed, G. & Bater, S. (1974) *Br. J. Psychiat.* **124**, 151-159.

McGlashan, T.H. & Carpenter, W.T. (1976) *Arch. Gen. Psychiat.* **33**, 231-239.

Marriott, P. & Hiep, A. (1976) *Aust. NZ J. Psychiat.* **10**, 163-167.

Rifkin, A., Quitkin, F., Rabiner, C.J. *et al.* (1977) *Arch. Gen. Psychiat.* **34**, 43-47.

Rifkin, A., Quitkin, F., Kane, J. *et al.* (1978) *Arch. Gen. Psychiat.* **35**, 483-489.

Rosenberg, I.U., Ostensen, A.I. & Fonnelop, H. (1976) *T. norsk Laegelforening* **96**, 229.

Schooler, N.R., Levine, J., Severe, J.V. *et al.* (1980) *Arch. Gen. Psychiat.* **37**, 16-24.

Young, J.P.R., Hughes, W.C. & Lader, M.H. (1976) *Br. Med. J.* **i**, 1116-1118.

CHAPTER 14

THE SIDE-EFFECTS OF ANTIPSYCHOTIC DRUGS.
I. CNS AND NEUROMUSCULAR EFFECTS

Thomas R.E. Barnes[1] and J. Guy Edwards[2]

[1]Department of Psychiatry, Charing Cross and Westminster Medical School, University of London, UK and [2]Southampton University Department of Psychiatry, Royal South Hants Hospital, Southampton, UK

Table of Contents

It has not proved possible to show consistently that there is a significant difference between antipsychotic drugs in their effectiveness on specific symptoms, syndromes or types of schizophrenia. Nor has it been possible to identify a pattern of symptoms, signs or demographic variables that could help to predict the response of an individual patient to a particular drug. Thus, for the antipsychotic drugs currently available, it is their side-effect profiles that tend to determine clinical choice. This chapter reviews the neuropsychiatric adverse effects associated with these drugs, principally the consequences of their actions on the autonomic system, effects on cognition and behaviour, epileptogenic effects, the acute extrapyramidal phenomena and the late-onset movement disorders such as tardive dyskinesia.

14.1 Neuropsychiatric effects

14.1.1 Cognitive and behavioural effects

The effects of psychotropic drugs on cognition and psychomotor performance are extremely complex. They are influenced by numerous interrelated variables that affect different people in different ways. These variables relate to both the subject and the task undertaken. The personality and affective state of the subject, motivation and practice, as well as age and sex, all have to be taken into account. Behaviour is influenced by the type of activity, and performance on boring and repetitive tasks is likely to be different to that on interesting, challenging tests. Similarly, there may be differences in performance on laboratory or simulation tasks compared with that in real life situations. In the real world, subjects use their past experience of interacting with the environment to compensate for drug-induced decrements in functioning.

Our knowledge of cognitive and behavioural effects on patients is limited also by the fact that most research has been carried out in relatively small samples of normal subjects, often after single doses of drugs. A wide variety of tests with different sensitivities has been used and different methodologies have been adopted by different researchers. The tests do not allow for accurate predictions of behaviour outside the test situation. Cognition and behaviour are also affected by the illness being treated, but the effects of this (and other variables in the subject) on test results can be assessed by adequate within-group and between-group controls, and serial measures following the administration of the drug.

More cognitive and psychomotor research has been carried out on anxiolytic/ sedative drugs and antidepressants than on antipsychotic agents. The studies of neuroleptics that have been undertaken have yielded inconsistent results. In a comprehensive review of the literature published during the last 25 years, King (1990) found that treatment with antipsychotic drugs was mostly associated with an improvement in cognitive function that occurred in parallel with clinical recovery.

The effects of the more sedating neuroleptics, such as chlorpromazine and thioridazine, on psychomotor performance are greater at high doses and in susceptible individuals, while schizophrenic patients are less susceptible to the sedative effects than normal subjects (Okuma et al., 1976). The reasons for this are not known, but differences in rates of absorption and in levels of arousal have been considered as possible explanations. Non-smokers are more prone to chlorpromazine-induced drowsiness than are smokers, possibly due to stimulation in smokers of enzymes involved in the metabolism of chlorpromazine (Swett, 1974).

Little is known about the effects of antipsychotic drugs on driving and other potentially dangerous activities or on precision and productivity in industry, but it is advisable to err on the side of safety and, especially when prescribing more sedating neuroleptics, warning patients of the possible risks. These are more likely to occur when treatment is started, doses are increased and drugs are used in combination with alcohol or other sedating substances.

Concern over the possibility that neuroleptics could cause depression was highlighted by a report by de Alarcon & Carney (1969) on the occurrence of severe depression, but Carney & Sheffield (1975) found that patients receiving fluphenthixol and decanoate. It was suspected that fluphenazine might be especially likely to cause depression, but Carney & Sheffield (1975) found that patients receiving fluphenthioxol decanoate also had depression that sometimes led to suicide. By 1980, more than 30 published papers had drawn attention to the relationship between antipsychotic drugs and depression (Ananth & Ghadirian, 1980).

But as with other drugs, there are several reasons why it is difficult to establish a cause and effect relationship (Edwards, 1981, 1989). First, the differential diagnosis of depression in schizophrenia includes a syndrome of demoralization as might accompany any chronic, disabling disorder; dysphoria as part of a prodromal syndrome heralding a psychotic relapse; emotional and social withdrawal representing a patient's attempt to cope with and minimize interpersonal and other social stresses; and negative symptoms such as flattened affect. Second, depression is a well-established symptom of schizophrenia (Hirsch *et al.*, 1990). The risk of suicide in schizophrenic patients is much higher than in the general population, but a direct causal relationship between successful or attempted suicide and treatment with antipsychotic drugs has not been demonstrated (Johnson, 1986; Roy, 1986a,b; Edwards, 1992). Third, some cases of neuroleptic-induced parkinsonism have features similar to those of a depressive illness, and in individual cases distressing extrapyramidal symptoms may contribute to a patient's low mood (see below). Fourth, claims have been made that some antipsychotic drugs have mood-elevating effects in schizophrenic patients and even antidepressant effects when used in low doses for depressive illness (Robertson & Trimble, 1982). Most studies confirm that depressive symptoms are a regular feature of schizophrenia, being most common during the acute florid phase of the illness, when they may be seen in up to half of the patients, and gradually becoming less prevalent during remission (Johnson, 1981; Knights & Hirsch, 1981; House *et al.*, 1987). Leff and co-workers (1988) reviewed the studies in which depressive and psychotic symptoms had been monitored over time in samples of schizophrenic patients treated with antipsychotic drugs but not antidepressant drugs. He concluded that the depressive and negative symptoms tended to run a parallel course in response to treatment, and that this constituted strong evidence for regarding depressive symptoms as an integral part of schizophrenia.

The use of relatively high doses of neuroleptics may be associated with violent, disturbed behaviour and a deterioration in mental state (Barnes & Bridges, 1980; Baldessarini *et al.*, 1988; Herrera *et al.*, 1988; Van Putten *et al.*, 1990). The violent behaviour may be a response to the stressful, subjective experience of akathisia or a less specific 'behavioural toxicity' (Van Putten & Marder, 1987; Herrera *et al.*, 1988; Van Putten *et al.*, 1990). Such episodes may respond to decreasing the dose of drug (Van Putten, 1974).

14.1.2 Epileptogenic effects

Antipsychotic drugs can precipitate convulsive seizures (Logothetis, 1967; Toone & Fenton, 1977). There is usually no preceding aura, focal disturbance or residual neurological deficit. Convulsions are more likely to occur when neuroleptics are given in high doses or in combination with other potentially epileptogenic drugs, or when there is a rapid change in dose. Other risk factors include pre-existing brain damage or epilepsy. The differential effects of neuroleptics on dopaminergic and cholinergic transmission have been said to be important in determining the relative epileptogenic potential of antipsychotic drugs, as is the case with extrapyramidal effects (Cools et al., 1975; Remick & Fine, 1979). In therapeutic doses, low potency neuroleptics may be more likely to cause seizures, possibly due to their higher anticholinergic activity. Patients receiving antipsychotic drugs may have a slowing of the electro-encephalogram with a decrease in alpha and beta activity and an increase in theta and, to a lesser extent, delta waves. These drugs may also induce spikes or sharp waves and paroxysmal features (Fink, 1969; Itil, 1978).

14.1.3 Other neuropsychiatric effects

Neuroleptics can cause non-specific neuropsychiatric symptoms, such as headache, but these often occur in normal subjects and as side-effects of placebo treatment. The symptoms are seen in such a wide variety of disorders that it is usually difficult to relate them directly to drug treatment. In large doses, antipsychotic drugs cause cerebellar signs, including nystagmus, dysarthria and ataxia of the extremities. Muscle pain, spasms, twitches and weakness may also be encountered. Chlorpromazine may aggravate myasthenia gravis presumably because of its neuromuscular blocking action (McQuillen et al., 1963).

The central nervous effects discussed above are reversible. However, a study by Lyon et al. (1981) suggested that permanent drug-induced effects might occur. These investigators carried out brain density measurements using computerized tomography printout matrices of chronic schizophrenic patients who had received prolonged treatment with various neuroleptics. Despite the methodological limitations of the study, the investigators found a significant correlation between density measurements in the posterior quadrants of both hemispheres and lifelong drug consumption.

14.2 Neuromuscular effects

The motor disorders associated with antipsychotic drugs are major disadvantages. They are common, often distressing and disabling, and a major cause of poor compliance with treatment, which has implications for relapse, hospitalization and morbidity. Furthermore, the overlap in symptoms between some of the drug-induced movement disorders and psychiatric symptoms can confound the clinical assessment of patients. The acute extrapyramidal symptoms, usually occurring soon after starting antipsychotic treatment or after a dose increase, are acute akathisia, acute dystonia and parkinsonism. The later-onset conditions, which tend to develop in patients on maintenance treatment, are tardive dystonia, chronic akathisia and tardive dyskinesia.

217

14.2.1 Parkinsonism

14.2.1.1 Clinical features

The main clinical features of neuroleptic-induced parkinsonism are muscle rigidity, tremor and bradykinesia. Other characteristic signs are impaired postural reflexes, seborrhoea of the face, excessive salivation and failure to habituate to the glabellar tap. Drug-induced parkinsonism resembles idiopathic Parkinson's disease in most respects and the two conditions are often considered indistinguishable. However, some authors suggest that the typical festinant gait and pill-rolling (3–5 Hz) tremor of the idiopathic disease are not characteristic of drug-induced parkinsonism (Schwab & England, 1968; Hershey *et al.*, 1982).

With passive movement of the limbs, two types of stiffness can be detected. The first is 'lead pipe' rigidity, where the resistance is steady and even. This rigidity can usually be enhanced by reinforcement, where the patient is asked to move the contralateral limb. This may be helpful where there is uncertainty about the presence of the phenomenon in an uncooperative, tense or apprehensive patient (Barnes, 1992a). The second is 'cogwheel' rigidity, where resistance is overcome in a ratchet-like fashion. Cogwheel rigidity is the result of tremor being superimposed upon the stretch reflex (Findley *et al.*, 1981).

Bradykinesia (or akinesia) is another motor side-effect that is usually considered as a feature of parkinsonism. It manifests itself as lack of spontaneity, diminished facial expression, paucity of gesture, mask-like facies and slow monotonous speech (Rifkin *et al.*, 1975). Bradykinesia may be misdiagnosed as retarded depression, referred to by Van Putten & May (1978) as 'akinetic depression'. The condition is also a major confounding factor in the assessment of the negative symptoms of schizophrenia such as affective flattening (Barnes & Liddle, 1990).

Signs of parkinsonism may develop within days of starting antipsychotic medication. The reported incidence of the disorder severe enough to warrant treatment varies widely, with figures up to 40% being cited. However, as McClelland (1976) points out, high prevalence figures do not necessarily reflect morbidity: 'When a patient might be said to be suffering from drug-induced parkinsonism is quite a different matter'. Although the natural history of the condition is poorly documented, it is said to improve spontaneously within 3 months in many cases, due to the development of tolerance in the nigrostriatal system to the dopamine receptor antagonism of these drugs.

14.2.1.2 Pathophysiology

It is thought that drug-induced parkinsonism is due to antagonism of postsynaptic dopamine receptors in the basal ganglia, leading to a functional deficiency of dopamine in the nigrostriatal system (Marsden & Jenner, 1980). The emergence of the disorder may be related to dopaminergic function falling below a critical threshold. This may be the consequence of a combination of the dopamine receptor blockade and an age-related, but subclinical, decline in dopaminergic function (Waddington, 1992). This notion fits with the observation that older patients require lower doses of antipsychotic drugs to induce parkinsonism.

14.2.2 Acute dystonia

14.2.2.1 Clinical features

Acute dystonia presents as sustained muscle contraction causing contorting, twisting, repetitive movements or abnormal postures (Ayd, 1961; Rupniak et al., 1986; Burke, 1992). It may present as sustained contraction of the masticatory muscles (trismus), forceful, sustained eye closure (blepharospasm), facial grimacing, oculogyric spasm (characterized by a brief, fixed stare, followed by upward and lateral rotation of the eyes so that only the sclera are visible), dysarthria and dysphagia (due to glossopharyngeal contractions) and torticollis. The extremities may be involved with dystonic limb and trunk movements and bizarre postures and gait.

Subtle forms of dystonia, such as tightness of the neck and shoulder muscles or mild lingual or laryngeal dystonia causing difficulties in speaking or chewing, may go unnoticed. However, in contrast to the other extrapyramidal effects, patients usually complain of the reaction, as the spasms are often painful and distressing and sometimes frightening. The consequences of neuroleptic-induced dystonia may be severe. For example, dislocation of the jaw has been reported (Abelson, 1968; Ryan & LaDow, 1968; Smith, 1973). Flaherty & Lahmeyer (1978) and Brown & Kocsis (1984) suggested that dystonia could be a possible cause of sudden death in patients receiving antipsychotic drugs. Laryngeal dystonia can lead to respiratory distress and asphyxia, and acute dystonia of respiratory muscles can cause life-threatening dyspnoea. Modestin et al. (1981) reported a case of unexpected, sudden death in a woman administered high doses of haloperidol. They postulated that drug-induced laryngeal spasms had precipitated vagal reflexes which led to cardiac arrest.

Dystonic reactions may be misinterpreted as dissociative phenomena, malingering, seizures or posturing associated with psychosis. They may even be regarded on occasion as an attempt by the patient to persuade the doctor to prescribe anticholinergic agents.

14.2.2.2 Incidence

Acute dystonic reactions in patients receiving antipsychotic drugs have generally been considered as relatively rare, with a reported incidence of around 2-5% (Rupniak et al., 1986). However, a study by Addonzio & Alexopoulos (1988) suggested the much higher overall figure of 25%. Children and young adults are the most commonly affected. The reactions usually occur within a day or two of starting treatment, with the majority of cases occurring within 4–5 days (Ayd, 1961). Acute dystonia can also occur 24 h or more after drug withdrawal – even after a single dose.

14.2.2.3 Pathophysiology

Marsden & Jenner (1980) proposed that dystonia was due to a compensatory increase in dopamine synthesis and presynaptic release, provoked by the acute administration of antipsychotic drugs, in association with an acute supersensitivity of postsynaptic dopamine receptors. As the antipsychotic drug concentration decreases, either following a single dose or between doses, the acutely supersensitive receptor becomes exposed to an enhanced presynaptic release of the neurotransmitter. This leads to an exaggerated dopaminergic response which is manifested as the dystonic reaction. This explanation could account for the early onset of dystonic reactions as well as their transient nature and emergence as withdrawal phenomena.

The response of dystonia to anticholinergic agents suggests an alternative mechanism related to a dopaminergic–cholinergic imbalance, with relative dopaminergic hypofunction, as may underlie drug-induced parkinsonism (Stahl *et al.* (1982). A recent critical review by Waddington (1992) concluded that it was not yet possible to provide a systematic pathophysiological explanation for dystonia.

14.2.3 Tardive dystonia

14.2.3.1 Clinical features

Acute dystonia, an early-onset side-effect of antipsychotic drugs, has long been recognized as a distinct clinical entity. The term 'dystonia tarda' was first used in a case report by Keegan & Rajput (1973) to refer to dystonic phenomena occurring as a discrete side-effect of chronic antipsychotic drug treatment. However, the occurrence of persistent dystonia in association with neuroleptic treatment has only been widely recognized for a decade or so (Burke *et al.*, 1982). These researchers described the dystonic movements as particularly disabling, likely to be persistent and difficult to treat. Clinically, tardive dystonia is not clearly distinguishable from acute dystonia except by duration; it is persistent rather than transient. Like acute dystonia, the face and neck muscles are involved in the vast majority of cases, with blepharospasm, torticollis and retrocollis being the most common presentations. Blepharospasm is a characteristic, early sign of the disorder (Wojcik *et al.*, 1991). Oculogyric spasm may also be a relatively common, recurrent problem that Sachdev (1993) found to be largely ignored by clinicians. The trunk and limbs are less commonly involved (Kang *et al.*, 1986), but Burke (1992) described the arms being forcibly extended at the elbow and the trunk involved in arching of the back, with excessive lordosis or flexion. Axial dystonia, if unilateral, may cause the trunk to lean laterally, a presentation of tardive dystonia called the Pisa syndrome for obvious reasons (Yassa, 1985). Davis *et al.* (1988) have reported rarer phenomena such as laryngospasm and spasmodic dysphonia which present with difficulty in talking, for example hypophonia, a 'strained, strangled hoarse whisper' and speech limited to 'gutteral inflections'.

One typical feature of tardive dystonia is the patients' use of tactile manoeuvres to control partially the muscle spasms. Examples of these characteristic 'sensory tricks' are a light touch to the chin with the hand to overcome torticollis or touching the brow to control blepharospasm (Burke, 1992). One female patient who exhibited lingual dystonia when she tried to talk found that sucking a sweet provided some relief. Patients with arching of the back or hyperextension of the neck may choose to sit in a chair against a wall, or stand against a wall to prevent the movements.

14.2.3.2 Diagnosis

Tardive dystonia is diagnosed by Burke *et al.* (1982) on the basis of the following criteria: the presence of chronic dystonia; exposure to antipsychotic drugs prior to the onset; exclusion of other known causes of dystonia; and a negative family history for dystonia.

In addition to the disorders that have to be considered in the differential diagnosis of acute dystonia, discussed above, tardive dystonia should be distinguished from idiopathic torsion dystonia or dystonia secondary to conditions such as Huntington's disease, Wilson's disease, Hallevorden–Spatz disease and Meige's syndrome (Marsden & Quinn, 1990; Burke, 1992). The condition also needs to be distinguished from tardive dyskinesia, with which it may coexist. The involuntary movements of tardive dystonia are distinct from those of tardive dyskinesia in terms of their nature and site, and the two conditions differ in prevalence, course, outcome and clinical pharmacology (Kang *et al.*, 1988; Barnes, 1990; Wojcik *et al.*, 1991). For example, while tardive dystonia sometimes partially responds to anticholinergic medication, such medication almost invariably worsens tardive dyskinesia. There are also epidemiological differences, with tardive dyskinesia occurring more often in older patients while tardive dystonia occurs at all ages.

14.2.3.3 Prevalence

The reported prevalence is around 1.5-2% (Yassa *et al.*, 1986; Anon., 1988). However, these figures probably relate to more obvious or disabling cases. Within populations of psychiatric patients receiving long-term antipsychotic medication, subtle dystonic movements and postural abnormalities coexist with a variety of other abnormal involuntary movements and may therefore be overlooked or misdiagnosed (Barnes *et al.*, 1983).

14.2.3.4   Risk factors

While the clear relationship between acute dystonia and antipsychotic drug treatment suggests that the medication may contribute to the appearance of tardive dystonia, the rigorous, prospective, epidemiological studies necessary to establish a causal connection have not been carried out (Kang *et al.*, 1988; Burke & Kang, 1988). Nevertheless, a frequent association has been found between persistent dystonia and treatment with neuroleptics. Burke (1992) identified 42 reports that described 250 patients who had developed persistent dystonia while receiving antipsychotic drugs, and Burke adduced further evidence for a causal relationship. First, a 12% remission rate has been found following drug withdrawal (Kang *et al.*, 1986) while spontaneous improvement is unusual for idiopathic, non-focal dystonia. Second, there is a strong tendency for tardive dystonia to coexist with orofacial dyskinesia and chronic akathisia. Third, persistent dystonia is suppressed by dopamine antagonists, and in this regard it is like tardive dyskinesia but unlike other forms of dystonia.

A review of 32 cases of tardive dystonia by Wojcik *et al.* (1991) supported previous opinions regarding general risk factors, that is, the majority of cases are under 50 years of age and most are male. However, there are no reliable predictors of tardive dystonia. Even the appearance of acute dystonia does not appear to predict the later development of the disorder (Anon., 1988). Furthermore, there are no reliable treatment guidelines that can be followed to minimize the risk of the condition, as no relationship has been demonstrated between tardive dystonia and any particular antipsychotic drug, maximum dose administered or total dosage received. Exposure to neuroleptics need not necessarily be prolonged for tardive dystonia to emerge (Giron, 1987). Cases of persistent dystonia have been reported in which symptoms began within 3 days of starting drug therapy (Burke *et al.*, 1982; Miller & Jankovic, 1992). In a retrospective view of 67 cases by Kang and colleagues (1988), 21, that is nearly a third, had developed the condition within the first year of drug treatment.

14.2.4   Acute akathisia

Drug-induced akathisia was first reported by Sigwald *et al.* (1947) during a clinical trial of promethazine. Soon after the introduction of antipsychotic drugs into clinical practice in the 1950s, Steck (1954) noted that patients administered these drugs exhibited jittery, restless or rhythmic movements, often of the feet, which he called 'neuroleptic-induced akathisia'. This condition is now recognized as perhaps the most common and most distressing motor disturbance associated with antipsychotic drug administration (Barnes, 1992b).

The term 'akathisia' is derived from the Greek and literally means 'not to sit'. It was coined by Haskovec (1901, 1902) early this century to describe a few psychoneurotic patients who were unable to remain seated. He considered the condition to be compulsive, and other authors later suggested a psychogenic origin (Oppenheim,

1911; Bing, 1939). Subsequently, the term was also employed to describe a similar and relatively rare condition of restlessness occurring in patients with idiopathic and postencephalitic parkinsonism (Bing, 1923; Sicard, 1923; Wilson, 1928).

During later years, the condition seemed to engender limited research interest. Clinically, akathisia often went unrecognized or was misdiagnosed as agitation or psychotic excitement (Kruse, 1960; Van Putten, 1975; Weiden et al., 1987). There may be several reasons for this. First, the clinical diagnosis tended to rest, somewhat unreliably, upon a subjective report of 'inner restlessness' (Barnes & Braude, 1985; Van Putten & Marder, 1987). Secondly, a clear description of the typical experience of restlessness and distress associated with akathisia may be particularly difficult to elicit in psychotic patients. Lastly, the lack of delineation of the motor phenomena associated with akathisia may have led to difficulty in distinguishing the condition from other movement disorders associated with antipsychotic drugs, particularly tardive dyskinesia affecting the limbs and agitation and restlessness related to the psychiatric illness being treated.

14.2.4.1   Clinical features

Characteristically, patients with akathisia describe a subjective sense of inner restlessness, mental unease, irritability or dysphoria which can be intense (Braude et al., 1983; Marder et al., 1991). Typically, they also report that they are unable to keep their legs still and feel a compulsion to move. Many patients complain that the condition is least tolerable when they are required to stand still. Also, patients with akathisia are sometimes aware of tension and discomfort in their limbs, with paraesthesiae and unpleasant 'pulling' or 'drawing' sensations in their legs (Braude et al., 1983). These complaints are akin to symptoms found in the 'restless legs', or Ekbom's, syndrome (Blom & Ekbom, 1961).

The subjective experience of akathisia can be intense and distressing, and this can hinder therapeutic endeavours in a number of ways. It can adversely affect compliance (Van Putten, 1974). Patients may abandon their drug treatment because the intense sense of restlessness and discomfort is intolerable. Also, the condition may contribute to aggressive behaviour or impulsive suicidal or homicidal behaviour (Van Putten & Marder, 1987), although this remains a controversial area. Furthermore, it has been suggested that akathisia may be responsible for aggravating the psychotic illness being treated (Duncan et al., 1989). Van Putten and Marder (1987) noted that the clinical picture seen with worsening of the psychotic illness related to akathisia tended to be similar to that of the original illness rather than a toxic psychosis.

Clinical diagnosis involves specific enquiry to elicit the subjective experience of akathisia. Patients should be questioned about the experience of inner restlessness, and whether they can locate restless, fidgety feelings in any part of their body. Symptoms referrable to the lower limbs seem to be the most characteristic. In addition, patients should be asked if they have any awareness of difficulty sitting comfortably for long periods, an increasing restlessness and tension when required to stand still, or feel compelled to move.

The diagnosis also rests on the observation of characteristic movements that are not dyskinetic in nature but more akin to normal, restless movement. Perhaps the commonest movements associated with the subjective experience of akathisia are rocking from foot to foot and walking on the spot when standing. When seated, patients who have akathisia tend to shuffle or tramp their feet and swing one leg on the other. In severe cases, patients are unable to stand without walking or pacing (Braude et al., 1983; Gibb & Lees, 1986). In addition to restless movements in the lower limbs, rocking of the trunk and fidgety movements of the upper limbs may be seen, although such movements are less typical (Walters et al., 1989).

14.2.4.2 Acute akathisia as a risk factor for tardive dyskinesia

Based on clinical observation, Chouinard et al. (1979) concluded that patients with 'hyperkinetic' symptoms of parkinsonism, such as tremor or akathisia, might be more likely to develop tardive dyskinesia than patients with 'hypokinetic' symptoms such as bradykinesia and rigidity. A series of case reports suggested an association between acute akathisia and the later appearance of tardive dyskinesia (De Veaugh-Geiss, 1982; Goswami & Channabasavanna, 1984; Barnes & Braude, 1984). Subsequently, prospective studies of tardive dyskinesia in relatively young psychiatric patients in the early phase of drug treatment (Kane et al., 1982) and in elderly patients starting antipsychotic medication (Saltz et al., 1991) provided more substantial evidence that the early occurrence of akathisia can be associated with a significantly increased risk of developing tardive dyskinesia (see below).

14.2.4.3 Pathophysiology

The most plausible explanation of the pathophysiological basis of akathisia remains the hypothesis put forward by Marsden & Jenner (1980) over a decade ago, which was based on evidence from animal work that has been substantially replicated (Murray & Kerwin, 1988; Weinberger, 1988). These investigators proposed that the condition resulted from dopamine receptor blockade in the mesocortical dopamine system. Animal experiments had indicated that the prefrontal systems regulate subcortical dopamine activity. Specifically, they may exert an inhibitory effect on spontaneous locomotor behaviour (Iversen, 1971; Tassin et al., 1978). Lesions of the prefrontal cortex can lead to increased activity in the subcortical dopamine systems, with an associated increase in locomotor activity (Pycock et al., 1980). Marsden & Jenner (1980) suggested that the equivalent result in man, following mesocortical dopamine receptor blockade by antipsychotic drugs, was the psychological and motor manifestations of akathisia.

Data from PET studies of both healthy controls and schizophrenic subjects given neuroleptics persuasively link D_2 receptor occupancy with the development of extrapyramidal side-effects, including akathisia (Farde, 1992; Farde et al., 1992). While akathisia correlated well with the time-course of the occupancy of the D_2 striatal receptors by neuroleptics, similar results were obtained with the administration of a highly selective D_1 antagonist. This suggests that akathisia may result from blockade of either D_1 or D_2 receptors. This may provide a possible explanation for the finding that, while clozapine has a low liability for parkinsonism, two study reports (Claghorn et al., 1987; Cohen et al., 1991) claim that the prevalence and severity of akathisia are similar to those in patients treated with standard neuroleptic drugs.

The response of akathisia to β-adrenergic receptor blockers such as propranolol has led to tentative theories regarding the role of noradrenergic pathways. De Keyser et al. (1987) suggested that akathisia may be an expression of an overactive β-adrenergic state, possibly generated by the blockade of presynaptic dopamine terminals on noradrenergic pathways by antipsychotic drugs. Other investigators have hypothesized that an imbalance between central dopaminergic and noradrenergic systems may be involved (Yassa et al., 1988). Lipinski et al. (1988) postulated that β-blockers alleviate akathisia by antagonizing the inhibitory effect of noradrenergic input to the ventral tegmental area, the origin of the mesocortical and mesolimbic dopamine systems, leading to enhanced dopamine neurotransmission.

The development of akathisia during treatment with antidepressant drugs also has implications for understanding the pathophysiology of this condition. Tricyclic antidepressants might induce akathisia by enhancing noradrenergic neurotransmission which causes a degree of inhibition of dopamine neurotransmission, particularly in neurons in the ventral tegmental area (Zubenko et al., 1987; Lipinski et al., 1989). Similarly, akathisia associated with fluoxetine could be explained by enhanced 5-HT-mediated inhibition of dopamine neurons in the ventral tegmental area (Lipinski et al., 1989).

14.2.4.4 Association with serum iron

The relationship noted between iron deficiency and Ekbom's syndrome (Ekbom, 1960) prompted speculation that there might be a similar association with akathisia. This proved to be the case in a study by Brown et al. (1987). Both serum iron and its percentage saturation were significantly decreased in 13 patients with akathisia compared with the same number of control patients without akathisia, while total iron binding capacity (TIBC) was correspondingly increased. The researchers also found a significant, negative correlation between the serum iron levels and ratings of severity of akathisia. A similar finding was reported by Horiguchi (1991) who noted that patients with akathisia or dystonia had significantly lower serum concentrations of iron than patients without those movement disorders.

Several neuropharmacological explanations have been put forward for the alleged association between akathisia and low serum iron levels. Ben-Schachar et al. (1985)

225

suggest that, as the D_2 dopamine receptor is an iron-containing protein, low serum iron may cause hypofunction of the receptor, rendering patients on antipsychotic drugs vulnerable to akathisia. Similarly, it has been suggested that the capacity of antipsychotic drugs to ligate with iron is related to their ability to induce akathisia (Blake et al., 1986). There is also evidence that antipsychotic medication may lead to an accumulation of iron in certain brain structures (Campbell et al., 1985; Hunter et al., 1968) although this may be compatible with, and even the result of, functional depletion of iron due to ligation and the subsequent deposition of iron complexes in the central nervous system.

While serum iron is a measure of physiologically active iron and plasma ferritin is a reflection of total body iron, the relevance of CSF iron concentration to the pathogenesis of akathisia has not yet been explored. The role of ferritin was investigated by Barton et al. (1990) in a replication of the study of Brown et al. (1987). They reported that, in akathisic patients, plasma ferritin was significantly decreased and that it correlated with measurements of severity of akathisia. The investigators considered that their findings gave broad support to the proposed relationship between akathisia and depletion of iron stores. However, while plasma iron, transferrin and percentage saturation of transferrin were low in patients with akathisia, they were not below the normal range.

In contrast to these reports, no significant associations between low serum iron levels and akathisia were found in subsequent studies of patients with acute akathisia (O'Loughlin et al., 1991; Sachdev & Loneragan, 1991) or chronic akathisia (Barton et al., 1990; Nemes et al., 1991; Barnes et al., 1992). In a sample of 105 long-stay schizophrenic inpatients, Barnes et al. (1992) failed to find a significant correlation between serum iron concentration and severity of akathisia, while serum iron, TIBC and percentage saturation did not differ significantly between patients with chronic akathisia and those without akathisia. O'Loughlin et al. (1991) studied six patients who developed acute akathisia but did not have low levels of serum iron or transferrin. In their follow-up assessments 2–3 weeks later, the investigators found that severity scores for akathisia were highly correlated with serum transferrin levels, and that iron and transferrin levels had decreased significantly only in those patients with akathisia. The results of further studies are awaited to resolve this issue.

14.2.5 Chronic (tardive) akathisia

Akathisia is thought of as an early-onset, relatively transient phenomenon but it can be a persistent problem in approximately a quarter of patients receiving long-term antipsychotic drug treatment (Braude & Barnes, 1983; Barnes & Braude, 1985; Barnes et al., 1992). Chronic akathisia often follows a fluctuating course over many years (Kruse, 1960) and can even continue after drug withdrawal (Weiner & Luby, 1983). Burke et al. (1989) reported 27 patients withdrawn from dopamine antagonists in whom the condition persisted for a mean of 2.7 years (range 0.3–7 years).

Barnes & Braude (1985) studied 89 chronic schizophrenic outpatients receiving maintenance antipsychotic treatment and a control group of 55 surgical outpatients. Twenty-nine (35%) of the former had both the subjective experience and motor manifestations of akathisia. None of the control subjects were diagnosed as having akathisia, although eight reported symptoms consistent with Ekbom's syndrome (Ekbom, 1960; Gibb & Lees, 1986). In a study of a similar population of 196 schizophrenic outpatients receiving long-term antipsychotic medication, Kahn *et al.* (1992) found virtually the same prevalence, 36%.

14.2.5.1 Chronic akathisia subtypes

Pseudoakathisia   Some patients may exhibit the complex, repetitive movements characteristic of acute akathisia but not report a sense of restlessness, compulsion to move or dysphoria. This syndrome was identified by Munetz & Cornes (1982), who called it pseudoakathisia. A typical feature is rocking from foot to foot while standing. The condition is more likely to be seen in older patients and in those with negative schizophrenic symptoms, and commonly coexists with orofacial dyskinesia (Barnes & Braude 1985; Brown & White, 1991). Barnes & Braude (1985) diagnosed pseudo-akathisia in 12% of their outpatient population (mean age 44 years) and in a later study (Barnes *et al.*, 1992) found the condition in 18% of a sample of 120 drug-treated, long-stay inpatients (mean age 53 years).

One view of pseudoakathisia is that it represents an end-stage akathisia, where the subjective sense of restlessness has faded. An alternative view is that the condition is a variant of tardive dyskinesia (Munetz, 1986). However, according to this hypothesis, non-dyskinetic limb movements are being included within the tardive dyskinesia syndrome which traditionally comprises dyskinetic, choreiform movements.

Acute persistent akathisia   In some cases, chronic akathisia appears to represent the persistence of acute akathisia. Although the symptoms have been present for several years, review of the case notes may reveal that at the onset there was the typical picture of acute akathisia, usually associated with an increase in drug dosage (Barnes & Braude, 1985).

Tardive akathisia   In patients receiving long-term antipsychotic drug treatment, akathisia may appear when the drug is withdrawn or the dose reduced. This phenomenon has been reported by several investigators (Jeste & Wyatt, 1982; Fahn, 1983; Braude & Barnes, 1983; Barnes & Braude, 1985), being termed 'tardive' akathisia on the basis that it shared the pharmacological characteristics of tardive dyskinesia, that is, it seemed to be exacerbated or provoked by antipsychotic drug reduction or withdrawal and improved at least temporarily when medication was restarted or the dose increased. The findings of a study by Dufresne & Wagner (1988) provided supportive evidence for the existence of the tardive akathisia subtype. Of 33 chronic schizophrenic patients withdrawn from antipsychotic drug treatment for at least 2 weeks, 13 experienced akathisia.

The prevalence figures for the subtypes of chronic akathisia in the surveys of outpatient and inpatient populations described above are relatively consistent. But the clinical information necessary to distinguish tardive and acute persistent akathisia is not always available, and it is not clear whether the peripheral movements of akathisia and those of tardive dyskinesia can always be reliably differentiated. The two conditions commonly occur together (Barnes *et al.*, 1983; Dufresne & Wagner, 1988; Burke *et al.*, 1989).

Whether these akathisia subtypes represent stages in the progression of the condition is unclear. While it is plausible that chronic akathisia could represent a transitional stage in the natural history of the disorder, and pseudoakathisia could be the final stage of the evolution, there are no follow-up data to support this notion. Whether the akathisia subtypes represent separate clinical entities will only be established by prospective studies, perhaps using drug withdrawal and pharmaco-logical challenges.

14.2.6 Tardive dyskinesia

14.2.6.1 Clinical features

Tardive dyskinesia comprises orofacial dyskinesia and trunk and limb dyskinesia of a choreiform nature. The orofacial movements include protrusion or twisting of the tongue, smacking, pursing and sucking movements of the lips, puffing of the cheeks and chewing and lateral motion of the jaw. These movements are more obvious in endentulous patients, although the constant movement and dry mouth associated with the dyskinesia may be partly responsible for the failure to persist with dentures. In addition to these orofacial phenomena, most descriptions of tardive dyskinesia include a range of trunk and limb movements. The involuntary limb movements are purposeless, jerky and often stereotypic in nature; they are usually described as choreiform or choreoathetoid. Athetosis of the extremities, and axial and limb dystonia are sometimes included as part of the syndrome, as are grunting and respiratory arrhythmias and abnormalities of gait and trunk posture, such as lordosis, rocking and swaying, shoulder shrugging and rotary movements of the pelvis.

There is evidence from several sources that orofacial and trunk and limb dyskinesia should be considered as distinct subsyndromes of tardive dyskinesia. These subsyndromes originally emerged from multivariate statistical analyses, and have subsequently been shown to differ in their pharmacological responses and their correlation with clinical and demographic variables. Thus, the two regional subsyndromes of tardive dyskinesia may have distinct pathophysiologies, and in research studies it is probably appropriate to analyse ratings from the two regions separately (Waddington *et al.*, 1987; Barnes, 1990, Kane *et al.*, 1992, p. 22).

Disability   Patients are usually unaware of tardive dyskinesia (Macpherson & Collis, 1992) and complaints are often prompted by relatives or friends. Nevertheless, the condition can be both socially and physically disabling. Disability may be directly related to the movements, causing impairment of mobility, and interference with eating, speech and respiration sometimes leading to dysphagia or choking (Yassa & Lal, 1986; Gregory *et al.*, 1992). Patients with this condition may carry an excess burden of morbidity and mortality due to respiratory tract infections and cardiovascular disorders (Youssef & Waddington, 1987). The condition can also be a serious social handicap, especially if the movements are severe. Odd, sometimes grotesque, movements of the face, lips, tongue and jaw can stigmatize patients and sabotage rehabilitation programmes to improve the patients' functioning in the community.

14.2.6.2   Diagnosis

Diagnostic criteria suggested by Jeste & Wyatt (1982) and Schooler & Kane (1982) refer to choreiform, athetoid or rhythmic abnormal, involuntary movements that are reduced by voluntary movement of the affected areas and exacerbated by the voluntary movement of unaffected body sites. These abnormal movements should have been present for at least 4 weeks in patients exposed to neuroleptics for a minimum of 3 months.

Individual patients may show a wide variation in the site and severity of dyskinesia, related to alteration of medication, such as change in dosage of antipsychotic or anticholinergic drugs, or changes in posture, mobility or level of physiological arousal. Also, apparently spontaneous fluctuations in the severity of the movements may occur from day to day or even within hours or minutes. This intra-patient variability is great enough to contribute to the likelihood of false negative assessments of tardive dyskinesia, particularly if patients are observed for only brief periods.

14.2.6.3   Prevalence and incidence

Tardive dyskinesia is perceived as a common problem in individuals receiving long-term antipsychotic drug treatment. The reported prevalence figures vary widely, from 0.5% to 56% (Tepper & Haas, 1979; Kane & Smith, 1982), reflecting variables such as the age of the study sample and the diagnostic criteria used. Overall, the literature suggests that only 20% or so of such patients will develop the problem, and of these, the dyskinesia will be severe in 10% or less (Kane & Smith, 1982; Yassa & Jeste, 1992).

A major prospective study by Kane *et al.* (1985) found that in the first 8 years or so of treatment with antipsychotic drugs, the incidence was 3–4% each year. The findings of this study suggest that the cumulative incidence of tardive dyskinesia in the early years of drug treatment steadily increases with the duration of drug exposure.

14.2.6.4   Natural history

Follow-up studies of tardive dyskinesia generally show little change in prevalence over a few years. Thus, it appears that the proportion of patients with tardive dyskinesia remains relatively stable. However, closer scrutiny of the data often reveals that underlying this apparent stability there is substantial change within individual patients, with spontaneous remissions being relatively common, particularly in younger patients (Barnes et al., 1983; Chouinard et al., 1986; Gardos et al., 1988). The results from two 10-year follow-up studies (Yagi & Itoh, 1987; Casey & Guardos, 1990) provide further support for this view.

Overall, the data from follow-up studies suggest that tardive dyskinesia is not usually progressive, and tends to follow a fluctuating course with spontaneous remissions (Gardos et al., 1988), although there are occasional reports of tardive dyskinesia worsening during continued drug therapy (Jus et al., 1979; Mehta et al., 1977; Levine et al., 1980; Gardos & Cole, 1983; Casey & Gerlach, 1986).

If drug treatment is stopped, tardive dyskinesia may have a more favourable outcome than is often assumed (Casey, 1985a; Casey & Gerlach, 1986). If the condition does not rapidly improve after drug discontinuation, it will generally follow a course of gradual improvement or stabilization over many years. In a proportion of patients whose abnormal involuntary movements appear to be irreversible, in that they persist for years after the withdrawal of antipsychotic drugs, the movements probably represent manifestations of the psychotic illness or spontaneous dyskinesia of the elderly (Marsden, 1985).

14.2.6.5   Risk factors

The identification of variables that contribute to individual susceptibility to tardive dyskinesia could be of value in the prediction of the condition and the development of preventive strategies. However, the predictive value of potentially relevant patient and treatment variables has not been systematically investigated in long-term, prospective studies and reviews have had to derive evidence from cross-sectional and retrospective studies, case reports and short-term follow-up studies (Barnes, 1988; Waddington, 1989).

Antipsychotic drugs   Some debate still lingers over the extent to which antipsychotic drug treatment is either necessary or sufficient to produce abnormal involuntary movements in various psychiatric populations. Kane et al. (1992) concluded that antipsychotic drugs do play a major role in producing or evoking abnormal involuntary movements, but recognized that abnormal involuntary movements occurring in schizophrenic patients were observed in the pre-antipsychotic drug era (Kraepelin, 1919; Bleuler, 1950) and more recently among chronic schizophrenic patients never treated with antipsychotic drugs (Owens et al., 1982; Waddington et al., 1987).

In a sample of 441 schizophrenic inpatients, Owens *et al.* (1982) identified 47 who had never been exposed to antipsychotic drugs. Comparison of the drug-treated and non-drug-treated groups failed to reveal many significant differences with regard to the prevalence, severity and distribution of abnormal, involuntary movements. Owens (1985) later analysed the data further, taking the age difference between the two patient samples into account. There was a significant linear relationship between the prevalence of abnormal involuntary movements and exposure to antipsychotic medication, and a particular susceptibility to orofacial dyskinesia in drug-treated patients. Nevertheless, such movements were seen in 30% of those cases never treated with drugs, which suggests that spontaneous, involuntary, orofacial movements can be a feature of chronic schizophrenia that has not been influenced by the administration of neuroleptic drugs.

Antipsychotic drug treatment variables Although some relationship between the emergence of tardive dyskinesia and drug variables is usually assumed, this has not been clearly established in clinical studies. Those studies which have reported a significant relationship between tardive dyskinesia and antipsychotic drug dosage or duration of treatment have involved samples of patients in the early years of treatment (Kane & Smith, 1982). But the vast majority of cross-sectional studies and follow-up studies that have addressed this issue have failed to find a significant association between the development of tardive dyskinesia and variables such as the length of time on medication, the total amount administered, the type or class of drug, current dosage, or plasma drug concentrations (Kane & Smith, 1982; Jeste & Wyatt, 1981; Dahl, 1986; Gardos *et al.*, 1988). Several possible reasons for this have been put forward. First, any dose–response relationship would only exist in the minority of patients who are vulnerable to the disorder and this subgroup is difficult to identify and study separately (Kane & Leiberman, 1992). Second, the high doses of drug administered to most patients might obscure any relationship between dose and risk of tardive dyskinesia (Baldessarini *et al.*, 1988). Third, older patients are not only more likely to exhibit tardive dyskinesia but they are also invariably administered lower doses of antipsychotic medication. Thus, it is a common finding that patients with tardive dyskinesia are receiving significantly lower doses of drug than their non-dyskinetic fellows, although this could be due to dyskinetic patients being significantly older (Barnes *et al.*, 1989).

Age It has been repeatedly demonstrated in clinical studies that advancing age is a major predisposing factor for tardive dyskinesia (Smith & Baldessarini, 1980; Kane & Smith, 1982). Increasing age remains the most consistently implicated factor for the risk of development of tardive dyskinesia, and elderly patients exposed to antipsychotic drugs for the first time seem to have an incidence of tardive dyskinesia over 1 year that is 5–10 times that of younger patients (Saltz *et al.*, 1991; Harris *et al.*, 1992). Patients in their sixth decade may be at the highest risk of developing orofacial dyskinesia (Kidger *et al.*, 1980; Barnes *et al.*, 1983). Although age and duration of drug exposure to antipsychotic drugs are likely to be confounded in clinical investigations, it has been shown that the effect of age cannot be explained in terms of a longer duration of antipsychotic drug treatment (Kane & Smith, 1982; Barnes et al., 1983).

Advancing age is not only associated with an increased occurrence of tardive dyskinesia but also greater severity and a reduced likelihood of spontaneous remission. Smith & Baldessarini (1980) found that tardive dyskinesia in those less than 60 years of age was over three times more likely to remit spontaneously. Furthermore, the older a patient is when he first receives antipsychotic medication, the more likely he is to develop the condition early in treatment. A prospective study of tardive dyskinesia in 160 elderly patients (mean age 77 years) found an incidence of 31% after only 43 weeks of cumulative administration of neuroleptics (Saltz et al., 1991). Yassa et al. (1992) carried out a 5-year, follow-up study of the condition in 162 first-admission, elderly, psychiatric patients who had not previously received neuroleptics. Of the 99 patients in the sample who received these drugs, 35% were found to have tardive dyskinesia. These two studies confirm the high vulnerability of elderly psychiatric patients to the development of tardive dyskinesia.

Gender There is some evidence that women have a greater prevalence of severe dyskinesia, although this may only be true within the geriatric age range, that is, over 70 years of age (Kane & Smith, 1982). Smith & Dunn (1979) identified 13 studies reporting statistically significant differences supporting female vulnerability, with the average unweighted female to male prevalence ratio in the patient samples being 1.7. In a more recent review of the relevant literature, Yassa & Jeste (1992) concluded that, overall, the prevalence in women (26.6%) was significantly higher than that in men (21.6%). In men, prevalence reaches a peak in the 50–70 years age-band, while for women the prevalence continued to rise after the age of 70 years. However, the prospective study of tardive dyskinesia in the elderly conducted by Saltz et al. (1991) failed to find a significant relationship between sex and incidence. Indeed, the incidence was slightly higher in males, although they were significantly younger than the females.

As a vulnerability factor, gender has far less influence than age, although there seems to be an interaction between the two variables. There is no clear explanation for the preponderance of women, although it has been suggested that neuroendocrine factors may be relevant (Hruska & Silbergeld, 1980; Davila et al., 1991).

Acute extrapyramidal side-effects Susceptibility to acute drug-induced extrapyramidal side-effects as a predictor of tardive dyskinesia was first suggested by Crane (1972). He considered that tardive dyskinesia was more likely to develop in patients who had exhibited parkinsonian side-effects than in those who had not. Subsequently, the findings of several studies and case reports supported the notion that patients presenting with symptoms of either parkinsonism or acute akathisia are more likely to manifest tardive dyskinesia (Chouinard et al., 1979; De Veaugh-Geiss, 1982; Barnes & Braude, 1984).

More convincing evidence has been provided by prospective studies of risk factors for tardive dyskinesia. Analysis of data from the first 5 years of a follow-up study by Kane *et al.* (1985) showed that a history of early, clinically significant parkinsonism indicated susceptibility to the subsequent development of tardive dyskinesia, particularly for those patients developing the disorder within the first 2 years of exposure to antipsychotic drugs. The patients in this study were relatively young, the mean age at recruitment into the study being 27 years. Saltz *et al.* (1991) carried out a prospective study of elderly patients starting antipsychotic medication for the first time. The 160 patients (mean age 77 years) were followed up for up to 18 months. Those individuals showing parkinsonism and akathisia early in treatment with antipsychotic drugs were significantly more likely to have developed tardive dyskinesia by the end of the follow-up period.

Psychiatric diagnosis
Affective disorder   There is accumulating evidence that patients with primary affective disorder may be at particular risk of tardive dyskinesia if administered antipsychotic drugs for long periods (Davis *et al.*, 1976; Rush *et al.*, 1982; Yassa *et al.*, 1992). In the prospective study of tardive dyskinesia mentioned above, Kane *et al.* (1985) found that after 6 years of treatment with antipsychotic drugs, the cumulative incidence of tardive dyskinesia in patients with affective or schizoaffective disorder (26%) was significantly greater than that of patients with a diagnosis of schizophrenia (18%). In addition, Mukherjee *et. al* (1986) found persistent tardive dyskinesia in 35% of a sample of bipolar patients who had received maintenance antipsychotic drugs (the condition was not present in any patient who had not received neuroleptics).

Schizophrenia   The schizophrenic illness itself may be a risk factor (Barnes & Liddle, 1985; Waddington, 1989). The condition has long been known to be characterized by abnormal involuntary movements, which were well described in psychiatric patients, particularly those with catatonic features, before the advent of neuroleptics. The movements described include stereotypies and mannerisms, perseverative movements, tics, grimaces and lack of coordination. The terminology used to refer to the motor phenomena tends to reflect the observer's conceptual notion of the aetiology (Marsden, 1985; Rogers, 1985). Some observers noted spasmodic movements of the orofacial muscles, which were considered choreiform in nature (Kraepelin, 1919; Farran-Ridge, 1926), although Marsden *et al.* (1975) concluded that true chorea and athetosis were only rarely found in chronic psychiatric patients before drug treatment, much of the motor disorder being attributable to organic neurological disorder such as encephalitis and syphilis.

Barnes & Liddle (1985) put forward three explanations for the association between schizophrenia and movement disorder. First, both the motor disturbance and schizophrenia are the product of organic brain disease: the two conditions occur together when the brain disease is also responsible for symptomatic schizophrenia, as, for example, when schizophrenia appears in patients with conditions such as

233

encephalitis, Wilson's disease or Huntington's disease (Davison & Bagley, 1969). Second, the movements may be secondary to the disturbance of will, thought and emotion that occurs in psychotic illness (Kraepelin, 1919; Bleuler, 1950). Third, the schizophrenic illness and motor disturbance may both be a consequence of the same underlying neuropathological process. According to this last notion, the schizophrenic illness can be seen as a psychomotor disorder with an inherent, increased risk of motor disorder. Antipsychotic drug treatment may interact with disease-related and/or age-related cerebral dysfunction to hasten or provoke the appearance of such movement disorder (Barnes & Liddle, 1985; Owens, 1985). However, specific aspects of the schizophrenic illness may be related to the risk of developing abnormal involuntary movements. For example, the follow-up study of young psychotic patients by Yarden & DiScipio (1971) suggested that abnormal involuntary movements can be a manifestation of a disease process which predisposes to a severe, progressive course. Such a notion is inherent in the classifications of schizophrenia by Crow (1980) and Murray & O'Callaghan (1991) which identify a subgroup of schizophrenic patients who are more likely to manifest abnormal involuntary movements, and are characterized by poor outcome and negative symptoms. The consistent finding of an association between negative symptoms and tardive dyskinesia (Waddington, 1987; Barnes, 1988) raises the possibility that the pathological processes underlying the former involve neuronal systems relevant to the manifestation of tardive dyskinesia, or at least the orofacial subsyndrome (Pantelis *et al.*, 1992; Brown & White, 1992). If this were so, then patients with negative symptoms might be expected to be more vulnerable to the development of tardive dyskinesia. In accordance with this hypothesis, Barnes *et al.* (1989) found that schizophrenic patients with negative symptoms were more likely to exhibit orofacial dyskinesia at an earlier age than those without negative symptoms.

Alcohol abuse   Recent studies hint that alcohol abuse may be a risk factor for tardive dyskinesia. For example, in an epidemiologically based prevalence study of schizophrenia, Duke *et al.* (1992) found no difference between patients with and without a history of problem drinking in their ratings for tardive dyskinesia, although the former group had a significantly shorter duration of illness. However, peak alcohol consumption showed a significant, positive correlation with orofacial dyskinesia. Dixon *et al.* (1992) studied 75 consecutive admissions with schizophrenia, assessing tardive dyskinesia and lifetime diagnosis of alcohol and drug use. Patients with a lifetime diagnosis of drug or alcohol abuse had significantly higher scores for tardive dyskinesia compared with non-abusers, and this association seemed to be independent of other known risk factors for tardive dyskinesia.

14.2.6.6   Cognitive impairment

The literature suggests that cognitive impairment is more common in schizophrenic patients who develop tardive dyskinesia than in those who do not. Waddington (1989) reviewed 21 studies in schizophrenic patients and 17 reported that patients exhibiting abnormal involuntary movements showed significantly greater cognitive dysfunction. The association between cognitive dysfunction and involuntary movements has been considered to be particularly robust in relation to orofacial dyskinesia rather than trunk and limb dyskinesia (Waddington *et al.*, 1987, 1990; DeWolfe *et al.*, 1988) and in relation to persistent rather than transient dyskinesia (Struve & Wilner, 1983). In contrast, Brown & White (1991, 1992) found cognitive impairment associated with trunk and limb dyskinesia but not orofacial dyskinesia.

There are three ways of conceptualizing the relationship between tardive dyskinesia and cognitive impairment. The cognitive deficit may reflect a pre-existing dysfunction that makes the patients vulnerable to tardive dyskinesia (Waddington, 1987; King, 1990), or both conditions may be manifestations of neuroleptic toxicity (Famuyiwa *et al.*, 1979; Wade *et al.*, 1987). Alternatively, tardive dyskinesia and cognitive impairment may occur together in a particular schizophrenic subgroup, such as premorbid asocials, Type II or neurodevelopmental schizophrenia, which are also characterized by negative symptoms. These possible explanations are not mutually exclusive, and probably overlap to some extent.

14.2.6.7 Pathophysiology

The dopamine supersensitivity theory   Pathophysiological theories for tardive dyskinesia were initially based on analogy with conditions characterized by choreiform movements, such as Huntington's disease and L-dopa-induced dyskinesia, that are thought to be related to hyperactivity in central dopamine systems. The predominant hypothesis was that tardive dyskinesia had its basis in striatal dopaminergic hyperfunction, specifically an increase in number (supersensitivity) of postsynaptic D_2 dopamine receptors in the striatum (caudate/putamen) (Klawans, 1973). The explanation was that this supersensitivity represented a response to chronic blockade of these receptors by neuroleptics (so-called disuse or denervation supersensitivity). This notion has its origins in animal studies, and the limitations of the present animal models of tardive dyskinesia have been discussed by Waddington (1992).

The validity of this hypothesis has been challenged further by the findings of post-mortem investigations and work in clinical psychopharmacology (Jeste & Wyatt, 1981; Barnes, 1988). Perhaps the most obvious inconsistency is that only a proportion of patients receiving long-term antipsychotic medication will manifest dyskinesia even though the development of dopamine receptor supersensitivity appears to be an inevitable consequence of such treatment (Reynolds & Cutts, 1992).

D_1 receptor agonists have been shown to cause tongue protrusion and chewing movements in animals. This prompted Gerlach (1991) to postulate a refinement of the supersensitivity theory. Neuroleptics block postsynaptic D_2 receptors, inducing parkinsonism. But the simultaneous blockade of presynaptic D_2 autoreceptors leads to increased synthesis and release of dopamine which stimulates the unblocked postsynaptic D_1 receptor, causing dyskinesia in predisposed individuals.

One prediction from the supersensitivity theory would be an association between the presence and severity of dyskinesia and the number of postsynaptic dopamine receptors in the critical brain areas. However, post-mortem studies in schizophrenia, using radiolabelled ligand-binding techniques have failed to reveal any clear relationship between the presence of dyskinesia in life and dopamine D_1 and D_2 receptor numbers in the basal ganglia (Cross *et al.*, 1985; Seeman, 1985). Furthermore, Kornhuber *et al.* (1989) found no differences in D_2 receptor binding in the putamen between patients with and without tardive dyskinesia in life. Reynolds *et al.* (1989) reported a decrease in caudate D_2 receptors in the brains of some patients with tardive dyskinesia compared with controls, although further studies from these investigators have suggested that D_2 receptor changes in the pallidum, rather than the striatum alone, may be more relevant to the production of dyskinesia (Reynolds & Cutts, 1992; Reynolds *et al.*, 1992).

Despite the evidence against the supersensitivity hypothesis, it remains a plausible explanation for a number of clinical observations. First, dyskinesia may worsen or disappear for the first time following drug dose reduction or withdrawal. This would be explained as increased exposure of the supersensitive receptors to the neurotransmitter. Second, reinstitution of antipsychotic drugs or an increase in dose will temporarily relieve the symptoms. The eventual reappearance of dyskinesia may be seen as a consequence of the development of further supersensitivity (Kazamatsuri *et al.*, 1972). Third, the administration of anticholinergic agents may uncover or aggravate the condition, a result of tipping the postulated balance between cholinergic and dopaminergic activity in the striatum further in the direction of relative dopamine dominance.

The GABAergic theory   Elaborations of the dopamine supersensitivity hypothesis have addressed the changes occurring in the basal ganglia with antipsychotic treatment, starting with dopamine blockade and extending to secondary biochemical and functional changes in striatal projection areas. One theory has been that while changes in dopamine receptors in the basal ganglia nuclei have not differentiated between drug-treated individuals who develop tardive dyskinesia and those who do not, perhaps changes in GABA content or metabolism might (Thaker *et al.*, 1987). GABA-mediated striatal and nucleus accumbens efferent projections may become involved with chronic antipsychotic administration. The best known of these is the GABAergic pathway from striatum to substantia nigra which is thought to be inhibitory on dopamine cell firing. However, the interaction between GABA and nigrostriatal dopamine systems is now known to be considerably more complex, with dopamine inhibiting some GABA pathways (for example, the pathway from the anterior striatum to the lateral segment of the globus pallidus) and stimulating others (for example, from the posterior striatum to the pars reticulata of the substantia nigra and to the median segment of the globus pallidus).

Scheel-Kruger & Arnt (1985) concluded that GABA, because of its influence on both dopaminergic and non-dopaminergic neurons, is an important mediator and moderator of dopamine-related functions in the striatal and limbic systems. These authors also concluded that in addition to a dopamine hypothesis for basal ganglia disorder, such as tardive dyskinesia, a 'dopamine–GABA' hypothesis should be considered. In summary, the present formulation of such a hypothesis seems to be that the pathophysiology of tardive dyskinesia stems from chronic blockade of dopamine receptors in the striatum (Tamminga & Thaker, 1989). It is then mediated via activity in the striatonigral GABAergic pathway and finally manifests itself as disturbance of GABA transmission in the pars reticulata of the substantia nigra, a key area for processing motor information within the basal ganglia.

14.2.7 Neuroleptic malignant syndrome

The neuroleptic malignant syndrome (NMS) is an idiosyncratic response following treatment with antipsychotic drugs that was first reported by Delay et al. (1960). The term 'neuroleptic malignant syndrome' was coined by Delay & Deniker (1968).

14.2.7.1 Clinical features

The clinical features include muscle rigidity, with cogwheeling as occurs in parkinsonism, or sometimes the waxy flexibility of catatonia, diffuse and coarse tremor, fluctuating levels of consciousness and the akinetic mutism of stupor. Altered thermoregulation results in pyrexia, sometimes with profuse sweating. Autonomic dysregulation may manifest itself as pallor, tachycardia, tachypnoea, labile blood pressure and incontinence. There is often an elevated white blood cell count and a rise in the serum level of skeletal muscle creatinine phosphokinase, reflecting myonecrosis from intense, sustained muscle contractions (Rampertaap, 1986).

The clinical course is typically rapid. Potentially fatal complications may ensue, including dehydration, pneumonia, pulmonary embolism and renal failure. The mortality rate is 20–30% (Caroff, 1980; Shalev et al., 1989) which may, in part, be due to a delay in diagnosing and treating the disorder.

14.2.7.2 Incidence

Fortunately the condition is relatively rare, although the precise incidence is uncertain, with 100-fold variation in published reports, from 0.02% to 2.4% (Keck et al., 1991). There is a suspicion that the disorder was under-reported in the past, as NMS was confused with other conditions such as extrapyramidal side-effects of antipsychotic medication or catatonia (Renwick et al., 1992). Hermesh et al. (1992)

used the diagnostic criteria for full-blown NMS suggested by previous investigators (Levenson, 1985; Pope *et al.*, 1986; Lazarus *et al.*, 1989) in a prospective study of two samples of acute psychiatric patients. The first group of 120 schizophrenic patients were treated with haloperidol while the second group of 103 psychotic patients received diverse antipsychotics. Five patients developed NMS, giving an incidence of 2.2%.

14.2.7.3   Risk factors

There are few clear risk factors, although the condition is most common in young men, 20–40 years of age. There is no consistent evidence to implicate any particular class or type of antipsychotic drug as more or less likely to produce NMS. Lazarus *et al.* (1989) noted that high-potency drugs were involved in approximately half of the reported cases of NMS but did not consider that patients on such treatment necessarily had an increased risk of developing the condition. It has been suggested that the use of intramuscular and intravenous routes of administration may increase the risk of NMS, possibly related to the rapid achievement of high peak plasma drug concentrations. There is some evidence that patients are at a greater risk of developing the condition at the start of drug treatment or following a dose increase (Shalev & Munitz, 1986), and most reviews of the literature suggest that the use of low to medium doses reduces the incidence (Gratz *et al.*, 1992).

The differential diagnosis includes extrapyramidal side-effects, heat stroke, malignant hyperthermia and the disputed syndrome of lithium–haloperidol toxicity (Gratz *et al.*, 1992). In patients presenting with a clouding of consciousness and a stiff neck, meningitis or a subarachnoid haemorrhage will need to be excluded, while septicaemia will need to be considered in those with pyrexia and hypotension related to the autonomic instability of NMS (Sagar, 1991). There is overlap between the symptoms of NMS and the syndrome of hyperpyrexia and motor disturbance occurring in psychotic patients in the last century, that was described as lethal catatonia (Kellam, 1987). Catatonia in this context referred to extreme behavioural agitation rather than rigidity, and the lethal catatonia was characterized by exhaustion and sometimes death. Whether the patients with this presentation suffered from some unidentified medical disorder remains unknown.

Mann *et al.* (1986) reported 292 cases of lethal catatonia diagnosed since 1960, 60% of whom had died, and suggested that NMS is a iatrogenic form of the condition. However, the motor manifestations of the two disorders differ markedly, in that lethal catatonia begins with psychotic excitement while the early signs of NMS are muscle rigidity and hyperthermia. A more difficult diagnostic distinction is between NMS and severe parkinsonian rigidity or dystonia. Indeed, several authors have suggested that NMS is the extreme end of the spectrum of extrapyramidal side-effects (Fogel & Goldberg, 1985).

Patients who develop NMS are not necessarily predisposed to develop it again if antipsychotic drugs are reintroduced, but a neuroleptic re-challenge within 2 months is more likely to precipitate a recurrence than a challenge at a later time (Rosebush *et al.*, 1989; Pope *et al.*, 1991). In all cases, an antipsychotic drug should only be reintroduced cautiously, aiming at the lowest effective dose. Atypical neuroleptic drugs such as clozapine may have a role in the management of patients who have had a previous episode of NMS (Addonzio *et al.*, 1987; Weller & Kornhuber, 1992).

14.3 Autonomic effects

Most clinically recognizable autonomic effects of neuroleptics are due to their cholinergic and α-adrenergic blocking actions, but their adrenergic, antihistaminic and antiserotonergic actions could also be involved because of the complexity of the actions on neurotransmission, the effects of these drugs on the autonomic nervous system are difficult to predict. However, they occur more often during treatment with aliphatic and piperazine phenothiazines, with the effects being mild and decreasing in severity as tolerance develops.

14.3.1 Sedation

In addition to the antipsychotic effect, neuroleptics possess a less specific, sedative effect that occurs as soon as adequate blood levels are reached. Patients commonly experience feelings of slowness, lethargy and weakness. While a sedative action may be desirable in agitated, excited psychotic patients, it is generally undesirable in other patients.

The sedation produced by antipsychotic drugs is related to their antihistaminergic action and α_1-adrenergic blockade, which is also responsible for the postural hypotension many patients experience. It has been suggested that the ratio between the capacity of a particular drug to block α_1-adrenoceptors and its potency at dopaminergic, principally D_2, receptors probably determines the extent to which the drug causes sedation in therapeutic doses (Hirsch, 1986). For chlorpromazine and thioridazine this ratio is high and, therefore, these drugs have a greater tendency to produce sedation and orthostatic hypotension. Pimozide and sulpiride are considerably more active at dopamine receptors than α_1-adrenoceptors and are thought less likely to induce sympatholytic effects.

14.3.2 Anti-α-adrenergic effects

The effects of α-adrenergic receptor antagonism include nasal congestion, inhibition of ejaculation and postural hypotension. Hypotension may be caused by depression of medullary vasopressor reflexes leading to decreased peripheral vascular resistance, as well as a α-adrenoceptor blockade (Alexander & Nino, 1969). In those rare patients with phaeochromocytomas, phenothiazines administered parenterally may produce a particularly sudden and severe drop of blood pressure with generalized circulatory failure (Brody, 1959; Lund-Johansen, 1962). Chlorpromazine-induced hypotension, like drowsiness, occurs more often in non-smokers, possibly due to the stimulation in smokers of enzymes concerned with the metabolism of chlorpromazine (Swett *et al.*, 1977). Hypotension is a particular hazard in the elderly. It can result in falls, fractures, cerebrovascular ischaemia (with toxic confusional states, strokes or unconsciousness) and myocardial ischaemia with or without infarction.

Like sedation, the tendency for individual neuroleptics to cause hypotension is partly related to their capacity to block α-adrenoceptor sites (Creese *et al.*, 1978). It is therefore a greater risk with low potency neuroleptics such as chlorpromazine and thioridazine. In most instances, tolerance to the hypotensive effects of antipsychotic drugs occurs, but in some patients orthostatic hypotension can persist for as long as the drug is continued.

Phenothiazines have central (hypothalamic) and peripheral (anti-α-adrenergic) effects on temperature regulatory mechanisms. Interference with temperature regulation may cause hyperthermia and, less frequently, hypothermia. The effects are influenced by the ambient temperature and the rate of heat production that is in turn affected by physical activity and the physiological state of the patient. Hypothermia may be accompanied by vasodilation, an increase in superficial temperature of the extremities and suppression of shivering. Chlorpromazine can precipitate hypothermic coma in myxoedematous patients (Jones & Meade, 1964). In contrast, hyperpyrexia with profuse perspiration may occur (Garmany *et al.*, 1954) and the combination of heat, physical exertion and neuroleptics can be life-threatening or even lethal (Mann & Boger, 1978; Cooper, 1979; Kilbourne *et al.*, 1982; Stadnyk & Glezos, 1983). Heat stroke can be aggravated by antiparkinsonian drugs as these drugs decrease sweating.

14.3.3 Anticholinergic effects

Antipsychotic drugs are dissimilar in their intrinsic anticholinergic activity. Studies in rat brains, suggest that drugs such as thioridazine and chlorpromazine are several hundred times more potent as muscarinic cholinergic receptor blockers than, say, haloperidol or fluphenazine. Nevertheless, clinical studies suggest that the incidence of anticholinergic side-effects during treatment with the different drugs is similar (Borison, 1985). Peripheral cholinergic receptor blockade by antipsychotic drugs produces a number of adverse effects, which are often compounded by the concomitant use of anticholinergic agents, such as procyclidine, orphenadrine or benzhexol, prescribed to combat extrapyramidal side-effects. These anticholinergic drugs cause drowsiness, as well as such non-specific symptoms of dizziness, muzziness or light-headedness (Critchley, 1958).

Patients may complain of dry mouth (xerostomia) due to decreased salivary flow that may promote the development of dental caries and cause polydipsia. Blurred vision may occur in association with dilated pupils (mydriasis) due to paralysis of accommodation. Tachycardia, with or without palpitations, and urinary hesitancy or retention may also be encountered. Decreased oesophageal and gastric sphincter tone may occur while reduced gastrointestinal motility can lead to constipation. The most serious anticholinergic effects are the precipitation of angle-closure glaucoma, urinary retention and paralytic ileus, although fortunately these are uncommon.

14.3.3.1 Withdrawal effects

In a small proportion of cases, discontinuation of anticholinergic drugs can produce a range of unpleasant withdrawal symptoms, including nausea, diarrhoea, abdominal pain, dizziness, headache, restlessness and insomnia (Grove & Crammer, 1972; Gardos et al., 1978; Jellinek et al., 1981). These are principally symptoms of excessive cholinergic activity and are sometimes referred to as cholinergic rebound phenomena. However, restlessness and anxiety may be features of emergent akathisia which had been effectively kept in abeyance by the anticholinergic (Jellinek et al., 1981). Similar symptoms are also seen on withdrawal of low-potency antipsychotic drugs, such as thioridazine and chlorpromazine, that possess relatively potent anticholinergic properties (Chouinard et al., 1984; Eppel & Mishra, 1984).

References

Abelson, C.B. (1968) J. Oral Surg. 26, 649–650.
Addonzio, G. & Alexopoulos, G.S. (1988) Am. J. Psychiat. 145, 869–871.
Addonzio, G., Susman, V.L. & Roth, S.D. (1987) Biol. Psychiat. 22, 1004–1020.
Alexander, C.S. & Nino, A. (1969) Am. Heart J. 78, 757–769.
Ananth, N. & Ghadirian, A.M. (1980) Int. Pharmacopsychiat. 15, 59–73.
Anon. (1988) Drug Ther. Bull. 26, 33–36.
Ayd, J. (1961) J. Am. Med. Assoc. 175, 1054–1060.
Baldessarini, R.J., Cohen, B.M. & Teicher, M.H. (1988) Arch. Gen. Psychiat. 45, 79–91.
Barnes, T.R.E. (1988) In Recent Advances in Psychiatry (ed. Granville-Grossman, K.), Vol. 6, pp. 185–207, London, Churchill-Livingstone.
Barnes, T.R.E. (1990) Int. Rev. Psychiat. 2, 355–366.
Barnes, T.R.E. (1992a) J. Psychopharmacol. 6, 214–221.
Barnes, T.R.E. (1992b) In Adverse Effects of Psychotropic Drugs (eds Kane, J.M. & Lieberman, J.A.), pp. 201–217, New York, Guilford Press.
Barnes, T.R.E. & Braude, W.M. (1984) Postgrad. Med. J. 60, 51–53.
Barnes, T.R.E. & Braude, W.M. (1985) Arch. Gen. Psychiat. 42, 874–878.
Barnes, T.R.E. & Bridges, P.K. (1980) Br. Med. J. 281, 274–275.
Barnes, T.R.E. & Liddle, P.F. (1985) In Schizophrenia: New Pharmacological and Clinical Developments (eds Schiff, A.A., Roth, Sir Martin & Freeman, H.L.), p. 81, London, Royal Society of Medicine Services Ltd., International Congress and Symposium Series, Number 94.

Barnes, T.R.E. & Liddle, P.F. (1990) In *Modern Problems of Pharmacopsychiatry, Schizophrenia: Positive and Negative Symptoms and Syndromes* (ed. Andreasen, N.C.), pp. 43-72, Basel, Karger.

Barnes, T.R.E., Kidger, T. & Gore, S.M. (1983) *Psychol. Med.* **13**, 71-81.

Barnes, T.R.E., Liddle, P.F., Curson, D.A. *et al.* (1989) *Br. J. Psychiat.* **155** (Suppl. 7), 99-103.

Barnes, T.R.E., Halstead, S.M. & Little, P.W.A. (1992) *Br. J. Psychiat.* **161**, 791-796.

Barton, A., Bowie, J. & Ebmeier, K. (1990) *J. Neurol. Neurosurg. Psychiat.* **53**, 671-674.

Ben-Schachar, D., Finberg, J.P.M. & Youdim, M.D.H. (1985) *J. Neurochem.* **145**, 999-1005.

Bing, R. (1923) *Schweiz. Med. Wochenschr.* **53**, 167-171.

Bing, R. (1939) *Textbook of Nervous Diseases* (5th edition), London, Henry Kimpton.

Blake, D.R., Williams, A.C., Pall, H. *et al.* (1986) *Br. Med. J.* **292**, 1393.

Bleuler, E. (1950) *Dementia Praecox or the Group of Schizophrenias* (1911 edition), translated by J. Zinkin, New York, International Universities Press.

Blom, S. & Ekbom, K.A. (1961) *Acta Med. Scand.* **170**, 689-694.

Borison, R.L. (1985) *J. Clin. Psychiat.* **4**, 25-28.

Braude, W.M. & Barnes, T.R.E. (1983) *Am. J. Psychiat.* **140**, 611-612.

Braude, W.M., Barnes, T.R.E. & Gore, S.M. (1983) *Br. J. Psychiat.* **143**, 139-150.

Brody, I.A. (1959) *J. Am. Med. Assoc.* **169**, 1749-1751.

Brown, K.W. & White, T. (1991) *Acta Psychiat. Scand.* **84**, 107-109.

Brown, K.W. & White, T. (1992) *Psychol. Med.* **22**, 923-927.

Brown, K.W., Glen, S.E. & White, T. (1987) *Lancet* **i**, 1234-1236.

Brown, R.P. & Kocsis, J.H. (1984) *Hosp. Community Psychiat.* **35**, 486-491.

Burke, R.E. (1992) In *Adverse Effects of Psychotropic Drugs* (eds Kane, J.M. & Lieberman, J.A.), pp. 198-200, New York, Guilford Press.

Burke, R.E. & Kang, U.J. (1988) In *Advances in Neurology*, Vol. 49, *Facial Dyskinesias* (eds Jankovic, J. & Tolosa, E.), pp. 199-210, New York, Raven Press.

Burke, R.E., Fahn, S., Jankovic, J. *et al.* (1982) *Neurology* **32**, 1335-1346.

Burke, R.E., Kang, U.J., Jankovic, J. *et al.* (1989) *Movement Disorders* **4**, 157-175.

Campbell, W.G., Raskind, M.A., Gordon, T. *et al.* (1985) *Am. J. Psychiat.* **142**, 364-365.

Carney, M.W.P. & Sheffield, B.F. (1975) *Curr. Med. Res. Opinion* **3**, 447-452.

Caroff, S.N. (1980) *J. Clin. Psychiat.* **41**, 79-83.

Casey, D.E. (1985) In *Dyskinesia - Research and Treatment* (eds Casey, D.E., Chase, T.N., Christensen, A.V. & Gerlach, J.), pp. 88-97, Berlin, Springer-Verlag.

Casey, D.E. & Gardos, G. (1990) *Schizophrenia Res.* **3**, 11.

Casey, D.E. & Gerlach, J. (1986) In *Tardive Dyskinesia and Neuroleptics: From Dogma to Reason* (eds Casey, D.E. & Gardos, G.), pp. 75-97, Washington, DC, American Psychiatric Press.

Chouinard, G., Annable, L., Ross-Chouinard, A. *et al.* (1979) *Am. J. Psychiat.* **136**, 79-83.

Chouinard, G., Bradwejn, J., Annable, L. *et al.* (1984) *J. Clin. Psychiat.* **45**, 500-502.

Chouinard, G., Annable, L., Mercier, P. *et al.* (1986) *Psychopharmacol. Bull.* **22**, 259-263.

Claghorn, J., Honigfeld, G., Abuzzahab-FS. Sr, *et al.* (1987) *J. Clin. Psychopharmacol.* **7**, 377-384.

Cohen, B.M., Keck, P.E., Satlin, A. *et al.* (1991) *Biol. Psychiat.* **29**, 1215-1219.

Cools, A.R., Hendriks, G. & Korten, J. (1975) *J. Neural Transm.* **36**, 91-105.

Cooper, R.A. (1979) *Am. J. Psychiat.* **136**, 466-467.

Crane, G.E. (1972) *Arch. Neurol.* **27**, 426-430.

Creese, I., Burt, D.R. & Snyder, S.A. (1978) In *Handbook of Psychopharmacology*, Vol. 10, *Neuroleptics and Schizophrenia* (eds Iversen, L.L., Iversen, S.D. & Snyder, S.H.), New York, Plenum Press.

Critchley, M. (1958) *Br. Med. J.* **ii**, 1214-1215.

Cross, A.J., Crow, T.J., Ferrier, I.N. *et al.* (1985) In *Dyskinesia: Research and Treatment* (eds

Casey, D.E., Chase, T.N. & Christensen, A.V.), pp. 104-110, Berlin, Springer-Verlag.

Crow, T.J. (1980) *Br. Med. J.* **280**, 66-68.

Dahl, S.G. (1986) *Clin. Pharmacokinet.* **11**, 36-61.

Davila, R., Andia, I., Miller, J.C. *et al.* (1991) *Acta Psychiatr. Scand.* **83**, 1-3.

Davis, K., Berger, P. & Hollister, L. (1976) *Psychopharmacol. Commun.* **2**, 125-130.

Davis, R.J., Cummings, J.L. & Hierholzer, R.W. (1988) *Behav. Neurol.* **1**, 41-47.

Davison, K. & Bagley, C. (1969) In *Current Problems in Neuropsychiatry* (ed. Herrington, R.N.), *Br. J. Psychiat.* Special Publication 4, pp. 113-184, Ashford, Kent, Headley Brothers.

de Alarcon, R. & Carney, M.W.P. (1969) *Br. Med. J.* **3**, 564-567.

De Keyser, J., Ebinger, G. & Herregodts, P. (1987) *Lancet* **ii**, 336.

Delay, J. & Deniker, P. (1968) In *Handbook of Clinical Neurology* (eds Vinken, P.J. & Bruyn, G.W.), Amsterdam, North Holland.

Delay, J., Pichot, P., Lemperiere, T. *et al.* (1960) *Ann. Medico-Psychol.* **118**, 145-152.

De Veaugh-Geiss, J. (1982) In *Tardive Dyskinesia and Related Involuntary Movement Disorders* (ed. DeVeaugh-Geiss, J.), pp. 161-178, Boston, John Wright & Sons.

DeWolfe, A.S., Ryan, J.J. & Wolf, M.E. (1988) *J. Nerv. Mental Dis.* **176**, 270-274.

Dixon, L., Weiden, P.J., Haas, G. *et al.* (1992) *Compr. Psychiat.* **33**, 121-122.

Dufresne, R.L. & Wagner, R.L. (1988) *J. Clin. Psychiat.* **49**, 435-438.

Duke, P.J., Pantelis, C. & Barnes, T.R.E. (1992) *Schizophrenia Res.* **6**, 122.

Duncan, E., Angrist, B., Adler, L. *et al.* (1989) *Schizophrenia Res.* **2**, 242.

Edwards, J.G. (1981) In *Handbook of Biological Psychiatry. Part VI. Practical Applications of Psychotropic Drugs and Other Biological Treatments* (eds van Praag, H.M., Lader, M.H. Raphaelsen, O.J. & Sachar, E.J.), pp. 1-38, New York, Marcel Dekker.

Edwards, J.G. (1989) In *Depression, An Integrative Approach* (eds Herbst, K.R. & Paykel, E.S.), pp. 81-108, Oxford, Heinemann.

Edwards, J.G. (1992) In *Suicidal Behaviour in Europe. Recent Research Findings* (eds Crepet, P., Ferrari, G., Platt, S. & Bellini, M.), pp. 131-142, Rome, John Libbey.

Ekbom, K.A. (1960) *Neurology* **10**, 868-873.

Eppel, A.B. & Mishra, R. (1984) *Can. J. Psychiat.* **29**, 508-509.

Fahn, S. (1983) In *Advances in Neurology*, Vol. 37, *Experimental Therapeutics of Movement Disorders* (eds Fahn, S., Calne, D.B. & Shoulson, I.), New York, Raven Press.

Famuyiwa, O.O., Eccleston, D., Donaldson, A.A. *et al.* (1979) *Br. J. Psychiat.* **135**, 500-504.

Fann, W.E., Stafford, J.E., Malone, R.L. *et al.* (1977) *Am. J. Psychiat.* **134**, 759-762.

Farde, L. (1992) *Psychopharmacology* **107**, 23-29.

Farde, L., Norstrom, A.-L., Wiesel, F.-A. *et al.* (1992) *Arch. Gen. Psychiat.* **49**, 538-544.

Farran-Ridge, C. (1926) *J. Mental Sci.* **72**, 513-523.

Findley, L.J., Gresty, M.A. & Halmagyi, G.M. (1981) *J. Neurol. Neurosurg. Psychiat.* **44**, 534-546.

Fink, M. (1969) *Ann. Rev. Pharmacol.* **9**, 241-258.

Flaherty, J.A. & Lahmeyer, H.W. (1978) *Am. J. Psychiat.* **135**, 1414-1415.

Gardos, G. & Cole, J.O. (1983) *J. Clin. Psychiat.* **44**, 177-179.

Gardos, G., Cole, J.O. & Tarsy, D. (1978) *Am. J. Psychiat.* **135**, 1321-1324.

Gardos, G., Cole, J.O., Haskell, D. *et al.* (1988) *J. Clin. Psychopharmacol.* **8** (Suppl.), 31-37.

Garmany, G., May, A.R. & Folkson, A. (1954) *Br. Med. J.* **2**, 439-441.

Gerlach, J. (1991) *Pharmacopsychiatry* **24**, 47-48.

Gibb, W.R.G. & Lees, A.J. (1986) *J. Neurol. Neurosurg. Psychiat.* **49**, 861-866.

Giron, L.T. Jr. (1987) *J. Family Pract.* **24**, 405-406.

Goswami, U. & Channabasavanna, S.M. (1984) *Clin. Neurol. Neurosurg.* **86**, 107-110.

Gratz, S.S., Levinson, D.F. & Simpson, G.M. (1992) In *Adverse Effects of Psychotropic Drugs* (eds Kane J.M. & Lieberman, J.A.), pp. 266-284, New York, Guilford Press.

Gregory, R.P., Smith, P.T. & Rudge, P. (1992) *J. Neurol. Neurosurg. Psychiat.* **55**, 1203-1204.

Grove, L. & Crammer, J.L. (1972) *Br. Med. J.* **i**, 276-279.

Harris, M.J., Panton, D., Caligiuri, M.P. *et al.* (1992) *Psychopharmacol. Bull.* **28**, 87-92.

Haskovec, L. (1901) *Arch. Boheme Med. Clin.* 193-200.

Haskovec, L. (1902) *Rev. Neurol.* **9**, 1107-1109.

Hermesh, H., Aizenberb, D., Weizman, A. *et al.* (1992) *Br. J. Psychiat.* **161**, 254-257.

Herrera, J.N., Sramek, J.J., Costa, J.F. *et al.* (1988) *J. Nerv. Mental Dis.* **176**, 558-561.

Hershey, L.A., Gift, T. & Rivera-Calimlin, L. (1982) *Lancet* **ii**, 49.

Hirsch, S.R. (1986) In *The Psychopharmacology and Treatment of Schizophrenia* (eds Bradley, P.B. & Hirsch, S.R.), pp. 286-339, Oxford, Oxford University Press.

Hirsch, S.R., Jolley, A. & Barnes, T.R.E. (1990) In *Depression in Schizophrenia* (ed. DeLisi, L.E.), pp. 27-37, Washington, DC, American Psychiatric Press.

Horiguchi, J. (1991) *Acta Psychiat. Scand.* **84**, 301-303.

House, A., Bostock, J. & Cooper, J. (1987) *Br. J. Psychiat.* **151**, 773-779.

Hruska, R.E. & Silbergeld, E.K. (1980) *Eur. J. Pharmacol.* **61**, 397-400.

Hunter, R., Blackwood, W. & Smith, M.C. (1968) *J. Neurol. Sci.* **7**, 263-273.

Itil, T.M. (1978) In *Principles of Psychopharmacology* (2nd edition) (eds Clark, W.G. & de Guidice, J.), pp. 261-277, New York, Academic Press.

Iversen, S.D. (1971) *Brain Res.* **31**, 295-311.

Jellinek, T., Gardos, G. & Cole, J.O. (1981) *Am. J. Psychiat.* **138**, 1567-1571.

Jeste, D.V. & Wyatt, R.J. (1981) *Am. J. Psychiat.* **138**, 297-309.

Jeste, D.V. & Wyatt, R.J. (1982) *Understanding and Treating Tardive Dyskinesia*, New York, Guilford Press.

Jeste, D.V., Lohr, J.B., Clark, K. *et al.* (1988) *J. Clin. Psychopharmacol.* **8** (Suppl.), 38-48.

Johnson, D.A.W. (1981) *Br. J. Psychiat.* **139**, 89-101.

Johnson, D.A.W. (1986) In *Contemporary Issues in Schizophrenia* (eds Kerr, A. & Snaith, P.), pp. 451-458, London, Gaskell.

Jones, I.H. & Meade, T.W. (1964) *Geront. Clin.* **6**, 252-256.

Jus, A., Jus, K. & Fontaine, P. (1979) *J. Clin. Psychiat.* **40**, 72-77.

Kahn, E.M., Munetz, M.R., Davies, M.A. *et al.* (1992) *Compr. Psychiat.* **33**, 233-236.

Kane, J.M. & Lieberman, J. (1992) In *Adverse Effects of Psychotropic Drugs* (eds Kane, J.M. & Lieberman, J.A.), pp. 235-245, New York, Guilford Press.

Kane, J.M. & Smith, J.M. (1982) *Arch. Gen. Psychiat.* **39**, 473-481.

Kane, J.M., Woerner, M., Weinhold, P. *et al.* (1982) *J. Clin. Psychopharmacol.* **2** 345-349.

Kane, J.M. Woerner, M. & Lieberman, J. (1985) In *Dyskinesia - Research and Treatment* (eds Casey, D.E., Chase, T.N., Christensen, A.V. & Gerlach, J.), pp. 72-78, Berlin, Springer-Verlag.

Kane, J.M., Woerner, M. & Borenstein, M. (1986) *Psychopharmacol. Bull.* **22**, 254-258.

Kane, J.M., Jeste, D.V., Barnes, T.R.E. *et al.* (1992) *Tardive Dyskinesia: A Task Force Report of the American Psychiatric Association*, Washington, DC, APA.

Kang, U.J., Burke, R.E. & Fahn, S. (1986) *Movement Disorders* **1**, 193-208.

Kang, U.J., Burke, R.E. & Fahn, S. (1988) *Adv. Neurol.* **50**, 415-429.

Kazamatsuri, H., Chien, C.P. & Cole, J.O. (1972) *Arch. Gen. Psychiat.* **27**, 95-99.

Keck, P.E., Pope, H.G. & McElroy, S.L. (1991) *Am. J. Psychiat.* **148**, 880-882.

Keegan, D.L. & Rajput, A.H. (1973) *Dis. Nerv. Syst.* **38**, 167-169.

Kellam, A.M.P. (1987) *Br. J. Psychiat.* **150**, 752-759.

Kidger, T., Barnes, T.R.E., Trauer, T. *et al.* (1980) *Psychol. Med.* **10**, 513-520.

Kilbourne, E.M., Choi, K., Jones, S. *et al.* (1982) *J. Am. Med. Assoc.* **247**, 3332-3336.

King, D.J. (1990) *Br. J. Psychiat.* **157**, 799-811.

Klawans, H.L. (1973) *Am. J. Psychiat.* **130**, 82-86.

Knights, A. & Hirsch, S.R. (1981) *Arch. Gen. Psychiat.* **38**, 806–811.
Kornhuber, J., Riederer, P., Reynolds, G.P. *et al.* (1989) *J. Neural Transm.* **75**, 1–10.
Kraepelin, E.P. (1919) *Dementia Praecox and Paraphrenia*, translated by R.M. Barclay, Edinburgh, E. & S. Livingstone.
Kruse, W. (1960) *Am. J. Psychiat.* **117**, 152–153.
Lazarus, A., Mann, S.C. & Caroff, S.N. (1989) *The Neuroleptic Malignant Syndrome and Related Conditions*, Clinical Practice Series No. 6, Washington, DC, American Psychiatric Press.
Leff, J., Tress, K. & Edwards, B. (1988) *Schizophrenia Res.* **1**, 25–30.
Levenson, J. (1985) *Am. J. Psychiat.* **142**, 1137–1145.
Levine, J., Schooler, N.C., Severe, J. *et al.* (1980) *Psychopharmacology* **24**, 483–493.
Lipinski, J.F., Jr., Keck, P.E., Jr. & McElroy, S.L. (1988) *J. Clin. Psychopharmacol.* **8**, 409–416.
Lipinski, J.F., Jr., Mallya, G., Zimmerman, P. *et al.* (1989) *J. Clin. Psychiat.* **50**, 339–342.
Logothetis, J. (1967) *Neurology* **17**, 869–877.
Lund-Johansen, P. (1962) *Acta Med. Scand.* **172**, 525–529.
Lyon, K., Wilson, J., Golden, C.J. *et al.* (1981) *Psychiat. Res.* **5**, 33–37.
McClelland, H.A. (1976) *Br. J. Clin. Pharmacol.* (Suppl.), 401–403.
Macpherson, R. & Collis, R. (1992) *Br. J. Psychiat.* **160**, 110–112.
McQuillen, M.P., Gross, M. & Jones, R.J. (1963) *Arch. Neurol.* **8**, 286–290.
Mann, S.C. & Boger, W.P. (1978) *Am. J. Psychiat.* **135**, 1097–1100.
Mann, S.C., Caroff, S.N., Bleier, H.R. *et al.* (1986) *Am. J. Psychiat.* **143**, 1374–1381.
Marder, S.R., Van Putten, T., Wirsching, W.C. *et al.* (1991) In *Biological Psychiatry* (eds Racagni, G. *et al.*), Amsterdam, Elsevier Science Publishers.
Marsden, C.D. (1985) In *Dyskinesia – Research and Treatment* (eds Casey, D.E., Chase, T.N., Christensen, A.V. & Gerlach, J.), pp. 64–71, Berlin, Springer-Verlag.
Marsden, C.D. & Jenner, P. (1980) *Psychol. Med.* **10**, 55–72.
Marsden, C.D. & Quinn, N.P. (1990) *Br. Med. J.* **300**, 139–144.
Marsden, C.D., Tarsy, D. & Baldessarini, R.J. (1975) In *Psychiatric Aspects of Neurological Disease* (eds Benson, D.F. & Blumer, D.), pp. 219–265, New York, Grune & Stratton.
Mehta, D., Mehta, S. & Mathew, P. (1977) *J. Am. Geriatr. Soc.* **25**, 545–547.
Miller, L.G. & Jankovic, J. (1992) *Movement Disorders* **7**, 62–63.
Modestin, J., Krapf, R. & Boker, W. (1981) *Am. J. Psychiat.* **138**, 1616–1617.
Mukherjee, S., Rosen, A.M., Caracci, G. *et al.* (1986) *Arch. Gen. Psychiat.* **43**, 342–346.
Munetz, M.R. (1986) *Arch. Gen. Psychiat.* **43**, 1015.
Munetz, M.R. & Cornes, C.L. (1982) *Compr. Psychiat.* **23**, 345–352.
Murray, R.M. & Kerwin, R.W. (1988) *Arch. Gen. Psychiat.* **45**, 1052–1053.
Nemes, Z.C., Rotrosen, J., Angrist, B. *et al.* (1991) *Biol. Psychiat.* **29**, 411–413.
Okuma, T., Koga, I. & Uchida, Y. (1976) *Psychopharmacology* **5**, 101–105.
O'Loughlin, V., Dickie, A.C. & Ebmeier, K.P. (1991) *J. Neurol. Neurosurg. Psychiat.* **54**, 363–364.
Oppenheim, H. (1911) *Textbook of Nervous Diseases for Physicians and Students*, Edinburgh, Otto Schulze.
Owens, D.G.C. (1985) In *Dyskinesia: Research and Treatment* (eds Casey, D.E., Chase, T.N., Christensen, A.V. & Gerlach, J.), pp. 79–87, Berlin, Springer-Verlag.
Owens, G.C., Johnstone, E.C. & Frith, C.D. (1982) *Arch. Gen. Psychiat.* **39**, 452–461.
Pantelis, C., Barnes, T.R.E. & Nelson, H.E. (1992) *Br. J. Psychiat.* **160**, 442–460.
Pope, H.G., Keck, P.E. & McElroy, S.L. (1986) *Am. J. Psychiat.* **143**, 1227–1233.
Pope, H.G., Aizley, H.G., Keck, P.E. *et al.* (1991) *J. Clin. Psychiat.* **52**, 208–212.
Pycock, C.J., Kerwin, R.W. & Carter, C.J. (1980) *Nature* **286**, 74–76.
Remick, R.A. & Fine, S.H. (1979) *J. Clin. Psychiat.* **40**, 78–80.

Renwick, D.S., Chandraker, A. & Bannister, P. (1992) *Br. Med. J.* **304**, 831-832.
Reynolds, G.P. & Cutts, A.J. (1992) *Schizophrenia Res.* **6**, 137.
Reynolds, G.P., McCall, J.C. & Mackay, A.V. (1989) *Schizophrenia Res.* **2**, 106.
Reynolds, G.P., Brown, J.E., McCall, J.C. *et al.* (1992) *J. Neural Transm.* **87**, 225-230.
Rifkin, A., Quitkin, F. & Klein, D.F. (1975) *Arch. Gen. Psychiat.* **32**, 672-674.
Robertson, M.M. & Trimble, M.R. (1982) *J. Affective Dis.* **4**, 173-193.
Rogers, D. (1985) *Br. J. Psychiat.* **147**, 221-232.
Rosebush, P.I., Stewart, T.D. & Gelenberg, A.J. (1989) *J. Clin. Psychiat.* **50**, 295-298.
Roy, A. (1986a) In *Suicide* (ed. Roy, A.), pp. 97-112, Baltimore, Williams & Wilkins.
Roy, A. (1986b) *Psychiat. Clin. North Am.* **9**, 193-206.
Rupniak, N.M.J., Jenner, P. & Marsden, C.D. (1986) *Psychopharmacology* **88**, 403-419.
Rush, M., Diamond, F. & Alpert, M. (1982) *Biol. Psychiat.* **17**, 387-392.
Ryan, M. & LaDow, C. (1968) *J. Oral. Surg.* **26**, 646-648.
Sachdev, P. (1993) *Movement Disorders* **8**, 93-97.
Sachdev, P. & Loneragan, C. (1991) *Psychopharmacology* **103**, 138-139.
Sagar, S.M. (1991) *J. Roy. Soc. Med.* **84**, 500-501.
Saltz, B., Woerner, M., Kane, J.M. *et al.* (1991) *J. Am. Med. Assoc.* **266**, 2402-2406.
Scheel-Kruger, J. & Arnt, J. (1985) In *Dyskinesia – Research and Treatment* (eds Casey, D.E., Chase, T.N., Christensen, A.V. & Gerlach, J.), pp. 46-57, Berlin, Springer-Verlag.
Schooler, N.R. & Kane, J.M. (1982) *Arch. Gen. Psychiat.* **39**, 486-487.
Schwab, R.S. & England, A.C. Jr. (1968) In *Handbook of Clinical Neurology, Diseases of the Basal Ganglia*, Vol. 6 (eds Vinken, P.J. & Bruyn, G.W.), p. 227, Amsterdam, North-Holland.
Shalev, A. & Munitz, H. (1986) *Acta Psychiat. Scand.* **73**, 337-347.
Shalev, A., Hermesh, H., Munitz, H. *et al.* (1989) *J. Clin. Psyciat.* **50**, 18-22.
Sicard, J.A. (1923) *La Presse Medicale* **31**, 265-266.
Sigwald, J., Grossiord, A. & Duriel, P. (1947) *Rev. Neurol. (Paris)* **79**, 638-687.
Smith, A.J. (1973) *Br. J. Oral Surg.* **10**, 349-351.
Smith, J.M. & Baldessarini, R.J. (1980) *Arch. Gen. Psychiat.* **37**, 1368-1373.
Smith, J.M. & Dunn, D.D. (1979) *Am. J. Psychiat.* **136**, 1080-1082.
Stadnyk, A.N. & Glezos, J.D. (1983) *Can. Med. Assoc. J.* **128**, 957-959.
Stahl, S.M., Davis, K.L. & Berger, P.A. (1982) *J. Clin. Psychopharmacol.* **2**, 321-328.
Steck, H. (1954) *Ann. Medico-Psychol.* **112**, 734-743.
Struve, F.A. & Wilner, A.E. (1983) *Br. J. Psychiat.* **143**, 597-600.
Swett, C. (1974) *Arch. Gen. Psychiat.* **31**, 211-213.
Swett, C., Cole, J.O., Hartz, S.C. *et al.* (1977) *Arch. Gen. Psychiat.* **34**, 661-663.
Tamminga, C.A. & Thaker, G.K. (1989) *Curr. Opin. Psychiat.* **2**, 12-16.
Tassin, J.P., Stinus, L., Simon, H. *et al.* (1978) *Brain Res.* **141**, 267-281.
Tepper, S.J. & Haas, J.F. (1979) *J. Clin. Psychiat.* **40**, 508-516.
Thaker, G.K., Tamminga, C.A., Alphs, L.D. *et al.* (1987) *Arch. Gen. Psychiat.* **44**, 522-529.
Toone, B.K. & Fenton, G.W. (1977) *Psychol. Med.* **7**, 265-270.
Van Putten, T. (1974) *Arch. Gen. Psychiat.* **31**, 67-72.
Van Putten, T. (1975) *Compr. Psychiat.* **16**, 43-47.
Van Putten, T. & Marder, S.R. (1986) *Arch. Gen. Psychiat.* **43**, 1015-1016.
Van Putten, T. & Marder, S.R. (1987) *J. Clin. Psychiat.* **48** (Suppl. 9), 13-19.
Van Putten, T. & May, P.R. (1978) *Arch. Gen. Psychiat.* **35**, 1101-1107.
Van Putten, T., Marder, S.R. & Mintz, J. (1990) *Arch. Gen. Psychiat.* **47**, 754-758.
Waddington, J.L. (1987) *Human Psychopharmacol.* **2**, 11-22.
Waddington, J.L. (1989) *Int. Rev. Neurobiol.* **31**, 297-353.
Waddington, J.L. (1992) In *Adverse Effects of Psychotropic Drugs* (eds Kane, J.M. & Lieberman, J.A.), pp. 246-265, New York, Guilford Press.

Waddington, J.L., Youssef, H.A., Dolphin, C. *et al.* (1987) *Arch. Gen. Psychiat.* **44**, 907–912.

Waddington, J.L., Youssef, H.A. & Kinsella, A. (1990) *Psychol. Med.* **20**, 835–842.

Wade, J.B., Taylor, M.A., Kasprisin, A. *et al.* (1987) *Biol. Psychiat.* **22**, 393–395.

Walters, A.S., Hening, W., Chokroverty, S. *et al.* (1989) *J. Neurol.* **236**, 435.

Weiden, P.J., Mann, J.J., Haas, G. *et al.* (1987) *Am. J. Psychiat.* **144**, 1148–1153.

Weinberger, D.R. (1988) *Arch. Gen. Psychiat.* **45**, 1053–1054.

Weiner, W.J. & Luby, E.D. (1983) *Ann. Neurol.* **13**, 466–467.

Weller, M. & Kornhuber, J. (1992) *Br. J. Psychiat.* **161**, 855–856.

Wilson, S.A.K. (1928) *Modern Problems in Neurology*, London, Edward Arnold.

Wojcik, J.D., Falk, W.E., Fink, J.S. *et al.* (1991) *Am. J. Psychiat.* **148**, 1055–1059.

Yagi, G. & Itoh, H. (1987) *Am. J. Psychiat.* **144**, 1496–1498.

Yarden, P.E. & DiScipio, W.J. (1971) *Am. J. Psychiat.* **128**, 317–323.

Yassa, R. (1985) *Br. J. Psychiat.* **146**, 93–95.

Yassa, R. & Jeste, D.V. (1992) *Schizophrenia Bull.* **18**, 701–715.

Yassa, R. & Lal, S. (1986) *Acta Psychiat. Scand.* **73**, 506–510.

Yassa, R., Nair, V. & Dimitry, R. (1986) *Acta Psychiat. Scand.* **73**, 629–633.

Yassa, R., Iskandar, H. & Nastase, C. (1988) *J. Clin. Psychopharmacol.* **8**, 283–285.

Yassa, R., Nastase, C., Dupont, D. *et al.* (1992) *Am. J. Psychiat.* **149**, 1206–1211.

Youssef, H.A. & Waddington, J.L. (1987) *Acta Psychiat. Scand.* **75**, 74–77.

Zubenko, G.S., Cohen, B.M. & Lipinski, J.F. (1987) *J. Clin. Psychopharmacol.* **7**, 254–257.

_____ **CHAPTER 15**_____

THE SIDE-EFFECTS OF ANTIPSYCHOTIC DRUGS.
II. EFFECTS ON OTHER PHYSIOLOGICAL SYSTEMS

J. Guy Edwards[1] and Thomas R.E. Barnes[2]

[1]*Southampton University Department of Psychiatry, Royal South Hants Hospital, Southampton, UK and* [2]*Department of Psychiatry, Charing Cross and Westminster Medical School, University of London, UK*

Table of Contents

It is not surprising when dealing with a category of psychotropic drugs, in this case neuroleptics, that behavioural, psychiatric and neurological effects are the types of adverse reactions most often encountered, and it is for this reason that the whole of the previous chapter was devoted to them. Here we discuss a much wider range of unwanted effects on other physiological systems. Fortunately, many of these are uncommon and some occur in patients who have disorders in which pathological disturbances of tissue sensitivity and pharmacokinetics predispose to exaggerated effects. This means that at least in some cases the untoward effects may be predictable and preventable. The wide range of effects that can occur reminds us as psychiatrists that our earlier acquired knowledge of general medicine should not be locked away in inaccessible recesses of our memory, but needs to be drawn on from time to time for the recognition and treatment of adverse reactions. This is particularly the case in areas where psychiatrists do not have easy access to advice from colleagues in other disciplines.

15.1 Endocrine and metabolic disorders

Antipsychotic drugs may influence hypothalamic–pituitary function through their effects on neurotransmission, as a non-specific action mediated haemodynamically or via their influence on thermoregulation (de Wied, 1967). Neuroleptics stimulate the release of prolactin, melanocyte-stimulating hormone (MSH) and antidiuretic hormone (ADH), while they suppress corticotrophin (ACTH), growth hormone (GH), thyrotrophin (TSH), follicle-stimulating hormone (FSH) and luteinizing hormone (LH).

The release of prolactin is inhibited by dopamine, other less important neurotransmitters and peptides collectively known as prolactin inhibitory factor (PIF). Prolactin controls its own release by enhancing the release of PIF– that is, by 'negative feedback'. Antipsychotic drugs decrease the availability of dopamine at its receptors by receptor blockade; that in turn leads to increased plasma prolactin levels (Beumont *et al.*, 1974a,b; Meltzer & Fang, 1976; Gruen *et al.*, 1978; Rubin & Hays, 1980; Beumont, 1981).

Only some of the known hormonal changes are associated with clinical effects. Neuroleptic-induced hyperprolactinaemia, for instance, may produce galactorrhoea while increased MSH may lead to ocular and cutaneous hyperpigmentation. Amenorrhoea may result from specific inhibitory effects associated with changes in FSH and LH, while its occurrence with drug-induced galactorrhoea suggests that it is mediated via the hypothalamus (Shader & DiMascio, 1970). However, amenorrhoea is difficult to relate to antipsychotic drugs because it often occurs as a symptom of the psychoses being treated. The tendency for drugs to produce hormonal effects may be related to dose, duration of treatment and predisposing factors, such as those thought to exist in the hypothalamic–pituitary–mammary gland axis in the case of galactorrhoea (Shader & DiMascio, 1970).

Inappropriate lactation has been reported with frequencies ranging from 10 to 80%, depending on the degree of awareness of the effect, whether or not the breasts are examined specifically for lactation, and the concomitant use of other drugs such as oral contraceptives. Phenothiazines may produce a false positive pregnancy test (Marks & Shackeloth, 1966; Paoletti *et al.*, 1966). Gynaecomastia in men is unrelated to neuroleptic-induced lactation and is dependent on the ratio of androgen to oestrogens (Beumont, 1981).

High serum prolactin levels increase the incidence of spontaneously occurring mammary tumours in mice and the growth of established carcinogenic-induced breast tumours in rats. Concern was therefore expressed about the possibility of antipsychotic drugs increasing the risk of carcinoma of the breast in humans. Fortunately, epidemiological studies have failed to show such an increase (Burgmans *et al.*, 1973; Ettigi *et al.*, 1973; Overall, 1978; Schyve *et al.*, 1978; Wagner & Mantel, 1978; Mortensen, 1987).

The syndrome of inappropriate secretion of ADH has been described in patients receiving fluphenazine, thioridazine and haloperidol (Matuk & Kalyanaraman, 1977; Vincent & Emory, 1978; Smith & Clark, 1980; Husband *et al.*, 1981) but also in schizophrenic patients not taking neuroleptics; this leads to difficulty in establishing a cause and effect relationship in individual patients.

Phenothiazines, especially high doses of chlorpromazine, can inhibit insulin secretion and thereby cause hyperglycaemia and glycosuria (Thonnard-Neumann, 1968; Erle *et al.*, 1977). Drug-induced changes in glucose tolerance may precipitate overt diabetes in potential diabetics and cause instability in the control of patients receiving antidiabetic treatment. In some studies the effects of antipsychotic drugs on glucose metabolism are difficult to interpret because of a high prevalence of diabetes mellitus in the cohorts studied (or in their families) and because the research was carried out in older and more obese subjects who may have been intolerant to glucose.

15.1.1 Weight gain

Increase in body weight is a relatively common side-effect of antipsychotic drugs. Obesity of a degree that is considered clinically significant occurs in about a third of patients receiving regular depot injections of fluphenazine decanoate and flupenthixol decanoate (Garrow, 1981). This represents a prevalence about four times that in the general population (Silverstone, 1985). Excessive weight is associated with health risks such as hypertension, maturity-onset diabetes mellitus, respiratory dysfunction and locomotor problems. Furthermore, obesity can be socially embarrassing; it may be a source of distress, and patients may attempt to diet in the face of increased hunger. As a result, patients may be reluctant to continue with their medication.

The precise mechanism by which patients taking antipsychotic drugs gain weight remains unknown. It may be related to stimulation of appetite with increased food consumption, altered food preference such as carbohydrate craving, decreased physical activity, a reduction in basal metabolic rate, or, rarely, water retention which may be accompanied by oedema. Thus, in addition to the type of drug and dosage, research should take into consideration a range of variables that might contribute to weight gain, including diet, smoking, alcohol intake, physical illness and the cost and availability of food (Cookson et al., 1986).

The pharmacological effects that might be relevant are still a matter for speculation. Cookson et al. (1986) suggest that the α_1-adrenergic and 5-HT_2 receptor blocking activity that antipsychotic drugs possess may be relevant, since drugs that stimulate these receptors tend to suppress appetite. On this basis, low-potency neuroleptics such as chlorpromazine and thioridazine might be more likely to cause weight gain because of their relatively potent 5-HT receptor antagonism (Bernstein, 1988).

Weight gain has been reported as a problem with clozapine. Lamberti et al. (1992) reviewed the relevant literature and found incidence figures ranging from less than 1% to one small study where 6 out of 7 patients receiving clozapine put on an average of 25 lb (11.3 kg). In their own study, 36 schizophrenic inpatients (with a mean age of 25 years) were switched from their previous antipsychotic medication to clozapine; three-quarters of them gained at least 10 lb (4.5 kg) in 6 months, while almost a half increased their weight by 20 lb (9.1 kg).

Patients receiving maintenance treatment with antipsychotic drugs should be advised about the risk of weight gain. The need for dietary discretion and a regular programme of exercise should be emphasized, and the advice of a dietician should be sought when necessary. The choice of therapeutic agent may also be relevant. While low-potency antipsychotic drugs should be avoided, certain antipsychotic drugs, specifically haloperidol and molindone, are reputed to have a lower liability for increased appetite and weight gain (Bernstein, 1988). Comparative studies of haloperidol decanoate and fluphenazine decanoate have suggested some advantage for the former in terms of weight gain (Wistedt et al., 1984; Cookson et al., 1986).

15.2 Immunological reactions

Immunological reactions occur in a very small minority of patients. The reactions are not dose-related. Their manifestations are those of protein allergy. They require an induction period following primary exposure but not if the drug is readministered. The reactions disappear when the drug is withdrawn but reappear if it is re-introduced or a chemically related substance administered. Drugs with small molecules cannot on their own stimulate an immunological response. To act as an allergen, the drug or a metabolite must act as a hapten; that is, it must combine with endogenous macromolecules, usually proteins, to produce a covalently bonded complex known as an antigen or immunogen. To elicit an allergic response the antigen forms a bridge between antibody molecules, reacts with complement and releases cytoactive peptides (Assem, 1977; McQueen, 1980).

The clinical manifestations of allergy may be widespread or confined to specific tissues. There may be a generalized anaphylactic reaction, with urticaria or angioneurotic oedema, asthma and/or gastrointestinal symptoms, or serum sickness, with fever, rash, lymphadenopathy, arthritis, periarteritis, oedema and/or haematological abnormalities. Alternatively the patient may have localized urticaria or angioneurotic oedema or reactions against specific organs, such as the liver causing cholestatic jaundice. Identical reactions can be produced by different drugs, or the same drug may produce different reactions in different individuals or in the same individuals at different times.

15.3 Cutaneous reactions

Antipsychotic drugs, particularly phenothiazines, have been alleged to cause many different types of dermatological reactions, although the causal connection between drug and effect is often difficult to establish (Beerman & Kirshbaum, 1975; Cluff *et al.*, 1975; Wintroub *et al.*, 1979; Baker, 1986). Skin disorders such as acne vulgaris, neurodermatitis and allergic reactions to other drugs and chemicals have erroneously been attributed to neuroleptics. Most dermatological symptoms and signs can be caused by drugs but the majority of reactions fall into a number of familiar patterns. Each drug tends to cause a limited range of actions but is capable of producing any type. Cross-sensitivity with a chemically related drug sometimes occurs.

15.3.1 Idiosyncratic reactions

The most frequently reported dermatological effect is an erythematous reaction that sometimes resembles an infectious disease. Most reported cases have allegedly been due to phenothiazines. Eczematous reactions may also occur and very rarely progress to exfoliative dermatitis. Vesicular-bullous eruptions are also rarely encountered. Phenothiazines have been said to cause lichenoid eruptions and erythema that may be of the Stevens–Johnson variety with oro-anal, genital, ophthalmic and respiratory involvement. They have also been alleged to precipitate a systemic lupus erythematosus-like illness and purpura due to a toxic effect on capillaries. Haloperidol has been reported as a cause of an acneiform eruption and loss of hair colour.

One of the most common cutaneous reactions is a chlorpromazine-induced photosensitive sunburn reaction (Epstein, 1968). Rashes may be phototoxic or photoallergic. Drugs that have phototoxic effects increase the reactivity of the skin to visible or ultraviolet light. The reaction does not have an immunological basis and may occur on first exposure to the offending agent. Photoallergic reactions, on the other hand, involve immunological mechanisms. They can be induced by fluorescent lighting.

Allergic contact dermatitis may occur in industrial employees who handle chlorpromazine. The drug is absorbed through the skin and may be stored in the stratum corneum for up to 2 weeks. Fluspiriline, administered by depot injection, may cause toxic necrosis of subcutaneous tissue that is thought to be due to the precipitation of crystals following the rapid absorption of the aqueous vehicle (McCreadle et al., 1979).

15.3.2 Pigmentation

Prolonged treatment with high doses of chlorpromazine can lead to blue-grey or purple-brown pigmentation of the skin (Greiner & Berry, 1964; Satanova & McIntosh, 1967; Bond & Yee, 1980). It occurs more often in women than in men and is most noticeable in parts of the skin exposed to sunlight. It is usually associated with corneal and lenticular opacities. Pigmentary deposits also occur throughout the reticulo-endothelial system and in the parenchymal cells of internal organs such as the heart, lungs, gastrointestinal tract, liver, kidneys, endocrine glands and brain (Greiner & Nicholson, 1964).

Melanin is formed in the cytoplasmic organelles of melanocytes by oxidation of the amino acid tyrosine in the presence of the enzyme tyrosinase. Production is under hormonal and neural control. The main darkening factors are α-MSH, oestrogen and thyroid hormones. The lightening factors include adrenaline, noradrenaline, 5-HT and, most importantly, melatonin. Although the mechanism is uncertain, it has been suggested that phenothiazines disturb the balance between darkening and lightening factors by decreasing the release of adrenaline and noradrenaline, as a result of which there is a relative excess of MSH and overproduction of melanin (Greiner & Nicholson, 1964).

Different views have been expressed on the cause of the purple hue. At one stage it was suggested that 7-hydroxychlorpromazine or another metabolite accumulates in cutaneous and other tissues and becomes converted to a purple compound on exposure to ultraviolet light; the violaceous hue was considered to be due to this purple metabolite or to a pseudo-melanin with a different colour from that of normal melanin (Perry *et al.*, 1964). However, subsequent measurements of skin melanin by reflectance spectrophotometry showed that the pigmentation is due entirely to melanin (Robins, 1972, 1975).

15.4 Ophthalmological reactions

Most ophthalmic effects of antipsychotic drugs occur as part of a more generalized reaction. The eyelids and conjuctiva, for example, may be affected in a widespread allergic skin reaction, cycloplegia and mydriasis may occur as antimuscarinic effects and an oculogyric spasm as a manifestation of extrapyramidal dysfunction.

15.4.1 Glaucoma

Acute glaucoma may result from mydriasis, itself resulting from autonomic paralysis. Mydriasis allows the peripheral part of the iris to occlude access of aqueous humour to the drainage canals. The outflow of humour is thereby impeded and causes raised intraocular pressure. Various mechanisms have been described: angle-closure caused by bunching or bowing forward of the iris in the case of those with narrow irido-corneal angles and over-relaxation of the pupillary muscle that can occur in eyes with or without narrow angles (Reid *et al.*, 1976).

Although glaucoma is a rare complication of neuroleptic treatment, cautious prescribing is indicated for patients with widely dilated pupils, a previous or family history of acute glaucoma, or such symptoms as blurred vision, pain in the eye and seeing coloured rings around lights. In cases where there is concern, the oblique illumination test may be helpful. In dimmed light, the beam of a torch is directed from the temporal side of the eye tangentially towards the pupil. In the normal eye, the nasal and temporal parts of the iris are equally well illuminated, but in those with narrow irido-corneal angles, the nasal part of the iris is in shadow (Vargas & Drance, 1973).

15.4.2 Corneo-lenticular opacities and pigmentary lesions

Phenothiazines, notably chlorpromazine and thioridazine, cause pigmentary changes in the eye as well as in the skin (Greiner & Berry, 1964; Siddall, 1965, 1966, 1968; Mathalone, 1966; Cameron, 1967; Edler *et al.*, 1971; Bond & Yee, 1980). Patients with skin pigmentation invariably have ophthalmic lesions, but most of those with eye changes do not have excessive cutaneous pigmentation. The reported incidence of pigmentation in the eye depends on such variables as the criteria for diagnosis, dose of neuroleptic, duration of treatment, sex of patient, amount of exposure to sunlight and climate. The incidence is higher in women and in those with dark complexions.

Brown pigmentation occurs in exposed parts of the bulbar conjunctiva and cornea. Isolated dust-like specks in the lens may become aggregated and form anterior capsular and subcapsular stellate opacities. Although impaired visual acuity can occur, interference with vision is unusual. Rarely white pearl-like polar cararacts occur. Chlorpromazine may also cause epithelial keratopathy that is thought to be related to high, rather than total, dose of drug. The condition does not impair visual acuity and is at least partially reversible (Johnson & Buffaloe, 1966).

Drug-induced pigmentation also occurs in the fundus. Doses of thioridazine exceeding 800 mg per day and chlorpromazine greater than 300 mg a day can result in pigmentary retinopathy with loss of retinal pigment, epithelium and chorio-capillaries (Connell et al., 1964; Davidorf, 1973; Meredith et al., 1978). The clinical picture resembles that of retinitis pigmentosa with night blindness, transient scotomas in the central part of the visual field and decreased visual acuity. Vision usually improves on stopping treatment though progressive deterioration has been reported in severe cases.

The blood–eye barrier resembles the blood–brain barrier. The ability of a drug to enter the eye depends on its chemical structure, water and lipid solubility, polarity, ionic charge and other factors (Leopold, 1968). In experimental animals (though not albino rabbits) phenothiazines reach concentrations in the uveal tissue 50 times the mean distribution value (Potts, 1962). Chlorpromazine decreases the metabolism of lens epithelium and in large doses produces opacities in guinea-pigs similar to those that occur in humans. It has been suggested that the drug or one of its metabolites acts as a photosensitizing agent, interacts with lens protein and causes denaturation and flocculation. The opacities are thought to be unrelated to melanin as they occur in albino, as well as pigmented animals (Howard et al., 1969).

15.4.3   Other reactions

Other reported effects on the eye include decreased production of tears, meiosis, mydriasis, iridoplegia and cycloplegia induced by phenothiazines and toxic amblyopia caused by perphenazine (Crews, 1962, 1974; Walsh & Hoyt, 1969; Garner et al., 1974; Grant, 1974).

15.5   Haematological reactions

15.5.1   Agranulocytosis

Neuroleptics can cause a variety of haematological abnormalities but the most serious is agranulocytosis. This presents with fever, fatigue and prostration, followed by ulceration at sites where bacteria are normally present in greatest numbers, usually the mouth and throat but also the nose, rectum and vagina. Death is caused by bacteraemia and the mortality rate is about 30%. Fever due to infection may be the only symptom, or a patient may be clinically asymptomatic, and the condition only detected by regular haematological monitoring (Grohmann *et al.*, 1989).

Most cases of agranulocytosis in the past have been associated with phenothiazines (Pisciotta, 1968, 1974; Ayd, 1969; Swett, 1975), with reported prevalance rates ranging from 1 in 700 to 1 in 200 000 (Shepherd *et al.*, 1968; Pisciotta, 1974; Anderson & Griffith, 1977; Krupp & Barnes, 1989). The complication was reported more often during treatment with high doses; it usually occurred during the first three months of drug therapy and often within the first 10 days (Pisciotta, 1971). Some cases have been seen after more prolonged treatment. Agranulocytosis has been reported more often in older subjects and more often in women than men, possibly because phenothiazines have been prescribed more often for females.

The aetiology is not fully understood, but allergic mechanisms were suspected because of the time relationship between introduction of the drug and onset of the dyscrasia and the occurrence in some cases of other hypersensitivity manifestations. It is now thought, however, that agranulocytosis is more likely to result from a toxic effect on white blood cells with limited proliferative potential and reduced DNA synthesis (Pisciotta, 1968, 1974, 1982) and it has been suggested that in those with such a predisposition bone marrow suppression occurs anew each time an antipsychotic agent is introduced (Ducomb & Baldessarini, 1977). There is debate as to whether the aetiological mechanism of clozapine-induced agranulocytosis is mediated via immunological mechanisms or due to toxic depression of the bone marrow (Lieberman *et al.*, 1988).

Reports of agranulocytosis declined after the late 1960s, possibly because of the increased use of non-phenothiazine antipsychotic drugs (Ducomb & Baldessarini, 1977). However, more cases are now being encountered, as a result of treatment with clozapine. This atypical neuroleptic drug is associated with an incidence of agranulocytosis as high as 2% during an exposure period of 1 year (Kane *et al.*, 1988). Granulocytopenia and agranulocytosis associated with this drug were first reported in 1975 when eight Finnish patients died from the complications of secondary infection (Amsler *et al.*, 1977). In view of the high incidence of blood dyscrasias, only patients with normal white blood cell counts and differential counts should be treated with clozapine. Monitoring of the white blood cell count (WBC) should be carried out weekly during the first 3 months, and subsequently every 2 weeks for as long as the patient receives the drug. Clozapine should be withdrawn immediately if the WBC falls below 3000 mm^3 or the absolute neutrophil count falls below 1500 mm^3.

15.5.2 Other reactions

Other haematological reactions allegedly caused by neuroleptics, particularly chlorpromazine, are leucopenia, thrombocytopenia, pancytopenia, leucocytosis, eosinophilia, iron deficiency, haemolytic and aplastic anaemia and a prolonged bleeding time (de Gruchy, 1975; Girdwood, 1976; Wintrobe *et al.*, 1981). In many reported cases the evidence is purely circumstantial.

15.6 Cardiac effects

Antipsychotic drugs, especially thioridazine which has a quinidine-like action on the heart, can cause electrocardiographic (ECG) abnormalities, cardiac conduction defects and arrhythmias (Alexander & Nino, 1969; Lapierre *et al.*, 1969; Ayd, 1970; Crane, 1970; *British Medical Journal*, 1971; Raj & Benson, 1975; Fowler et al., 1976; Deglin *et al.*, 1977; Wheatley, 1981). Prolonged PR and QT intervals, widening of QRS complexes, depression of ST segments and most commonly blunting, flattening or notching of T-waves and the appearance of U-waves may occur. They are observed more often in patients with pre-existing heart disease (Swett & Shader, 1977). In healthy individuals the minor changes are probably harmless and reversible; some resemble those seen in hypokalaemia and may disappear after administering potassium. It has been suggested that phenothiazines affect the T-waves and U-waves by shifting potassium into the intracellular compartment (Alvarez-Mena & Frank, 1973).

Antipsychotic drugs, especially phenothiazines administered in large doses, may cause atrio-ventricular block, bundle branch block, atrial and ventricular extra-systoles, atrial flutter, ventricular tachycardia and ventricular fibrillation. The elderly, notably those who have pre-existing heart disease, are particularly vulnerable to cardiac effects and neuroleptics are capable of precipitating congestive cardiac failure in predisposed subjects. The mechanism of production of cardiac effects if not known, but anticholinergic, anti-adrenergic and other actions have been incriminated.

Lesions in myocardial arterioles and the arteriolar-capillary bed, deposition of mucopolysaccharides and degeneration of myocardial muscle have been demonstrated histologically in patients who have received prolonged treatment with phenothiazines (Richardson *et al.*, 1966). It has been hypothesized that the subendothelial lesions are responsible for the ECG changes and conduction defects, and at one time it was suggested that the temporary increases in plasma aminotransferase activity found in some patients could be due to microinfarcts resulting from the vascular changes (Crane, 1970).

15.6.1 Sudden, unexpected death

There have been many reports published in the literature and sent to drug regulatory authorities of psychiatric patients receiving antipsychotic medication who died suddenly and unexpectedly, and cardiac side-effects have commonly been suspected as the cause (Kelly *et al.*, 1963; Hollister & Kosek, 1965; Leestma & Koenig, 1968; Crane,

1970; Peele & von Loetzen, 1973; Swett & Shader, 1977; Wendkos, 1979; Katal *et al.*, 1979; Modestin *et al.*, 1981; Wagasugi *et al.*, 1986; Huyse & Van Schijndel, 1988). The possible association between antipsychotic drugs and sudden death was investigated by an American Psychiatric Association Task Force (Simpson *et al.*, 1987). The report noted the indirect role of stress in sudden, unexpected death in the healthy population. The authors concluded that there was no clear evidence for an increase of sudden death in patients receiving psychotropic drugs, and even considered that these drugs might prevent sudden death in some patients by virtue of their anti-arrhythmic activity and reduction in vulnerability to stressful reactions. In other patients, however, the drugs could contribute to the cause of sudden death by interacting with the effects of stress and physical activity and increasing the vulnerability to cardiac arrhythmias and other autonomic complications. In the latter cases, the authors suggested that the amount of medication administered could be relevant, although there were no data available to support this view.

Brown & Kocsis (1984) reviewed the evidence for various potential causes of sudden death in patients receiving neuroleptics, including arrhythymias, vascular collapse and asphyxia related to factors such as an impaired gag reflex and laryngeal-pharyngeal dystonia. Death is more likely to be associated with the administration of high doses and to occur when there is pre-existing cardiac disease or general physical disability. Hyperpyrexia, aspiration and asphyxia, vasodilation and hypotension, and inhibition of regulatory centres in the brain have all been suspected as possible mechanisms leading to death, although cardiotoxicity is the most widely accepted explanation. In Finland, a study of sudden death in patients on normal doses of psychotropic drugs found that in most cases the patients were receiving low-potency phenothiazines, and there was a disproportionately large number on thioridazine (Mehtonen *et al.*, 1991). This is consistent with the known dose-related, cardiovascular side-effects of thioridazine and chlorpromazine (Lipscomb, 1980).

One particular cardiac problem related to antipsychotic medication that has been implicated as a possible cause of sudden death is Torsades de pointes. This arrhythmia is a variant of paroxysmal ventricular tachycardia associated with a prolonged QT interval or prominent U-waves (Liberatore & Robinson, 1984; Cleland & Krikler, 1992). Although Torsade de pointes (the term is derived from the ballet) may remit spontaneously, it is potentially lethal in that it can deteriorate into ventricular fibrillation (Krikler & Curry, 1976). This arrhythmia has been reported in association with antipsychotic drugs, specifically thioridazine (Liberatore & Robinson, 1984; Kiriike *et al.*, 1987) and haloperidol (Zee Cheng *et al.*, 1985; Fayer, 1986; Kriwisky *et al.*, 1990; Henderson *et al.* (1991). Henderson *et al.* (1991) recommended caution when using haloperidol in patients with a prolonged QT interval due to other causes, and suggested that any patient who has taken an overdose of the drug or is receiving a high therapeutic dose must be considered at risk of life-threatening arrhythmias and requires careful monitoring. Similarly, Liberatore & Robinson (1984) recommended routine ECG monitoring for patients receiving high doses of thioridazine. Fulop *et al.* (1987) noted that ECG abnormalities had been found in 10% of patients treated with pimozide, leading to recommendations in the USA and UK for periodic ECGs in patients receiving this drug (Committee on Safety of Medicines, 1990). They emphasized that the abnormalities included prolongation of the corrected QT interval (QTc) which increases the risk of potentially fatal arrhythmias.

It has also been suggested that antipsychotic drugs may be responsible for a toxic cardiomyopathy, leading to death by ventricular fibrillation or cardiac arrest. Ultrastructural damage to the heart associated with circulating auto-antibodies, especially those to skeletal muscle, heart, DNA, mitochondria and smooth muscle, has been found in patients who have died from drug-related, fatal arrhythmias (Guillan et al., 1977).

15.7 Respiratory reactions

Antipsychotic drugs given in therapeutic doses have little or no effect on the respiratory system, although respiratory depression may occur if they are taken in overdose or in combination with other drugs that depress respiration, especially in patients with obstructive airways disease. Neuroleptic-induced dystonia and dyskinesia can affect respiratory as well as other muscles. Flaherty & Lahmeyer (1978), for example, reported two patients who were cyanotic and gasping for breath after being treated with haloperidol, probably as a result of laryngeal–pharyngeal dystonia. Asthma can occur as an anaphylactic reaction to phenothiazines, while chlorpromazine has been alleged to cause pulmonary infiltration, together with eosinophilia and other hypersensitivity phenomena (Shear, 1978). There have also been isolated case reports of pulmonary involvement and pleural effusions in patients with systemic lupus erythematosus-like disorders induced by neuroleptics (Dubois et al., 1972; Goldman et al., 1980).

15.8 Gastrointestinal reactions

Antipsychotic drugs can cause oral and gastrointestinal symptoms in isolation or as manifestations of a generalized disturbance. Dryness of the mouth, for example, may occur in isolation or be a manifestation of generalized autonomic dysfunction. It may contribute to the developmental of dental caries, oral candidiasis and bacterial parotitis.

Gastrointestinal reactions may be mediated through central or peripheral anticholinergic or anti-adrenergic mechanisms. They tend to be dose-related and are dependent on individual susceptibility. Pre-existing disorders, such as gastric atrophy, peptic ulceration, coeliac disease and ulcerative colitis, predispose to their occurrence.

Paralytic ileus is a rare but serious unwanted effect of antipsychotic drugs that has a high mortality rate. In one series of cases many of the patients were receiving concomitant treatment with antiparkinsonian drugs (Evans *et al.*, 1979). Death results from the retention of gas and fluids, causing mucosal damage and ischaemia that in turn leads to septicaemia and peritonitis due to invasion by enteric organisms. Constipation and faecal impaction (with or without colonic dilation) induced by antipsychotic drugs occurs much more frequently than adynamic ileus (Goulston, 1976; Sriram *et al.*, 1979).

15.9 Hepatic reactions

The liver is particularly prone to adverse drug effects as it is the principal organ involved in detoxification. However, it is often difficult to relate abnormalities of hepatic function to the administration of drugs, especially in patients with nutritional deficiencies or infectious diseases, in those with a previous history of alcoholism or other disorders that affect liver function and in those who have received other potentially hepatotoxic drugs. Adverse effects are mostly mild, subclinical and only identifiable by liver function tests because of the large functional reserve of the liver. Their severity depends on hepatic blood flow, oxygenation and enzyme activity, and these may be affected by liver disease and the concurrent use of other drugs metabolized in the liver.

Hepatic reactions may be predictable or unpredictable, occurring in susceptible individuals with an immunological defect or an inherent abnormality of hepatic enzymes. The resulting damage may be hepatocellular, cholestatic or mixed. Antipsychotic drugs tend to produce cholestatic jaundice but variations can occur.

15.9.1 Cholestatic jaundice

Cholestatic jaundice may be caused by phenothiazines and rarely other neuroleptics (Fuller *et al.*, 1977; Jones *et al.*, 1983). The clinical picture is similar to that seen in other cases of acute-onset obstructive jaundice with malaise, weakness, fatigue, anorexia, nausea, abnormal discomfort, fever, pale stools, dark urine and hepatosplenomegaly. Laboratory investigations reveal hyperbilirubinaemia; bile in the urine; and increased serum alkaline phosphatase, aspartate aminotransferase, and alanine aminotransferase. Liver biopsy shows centrilobular cholestasis with little or no parenchymal damage and only a mild inflammatory response. Inspissated bile in the hepatic canaliculi may be caused by the intrahepatic precipitation of protein and glycoprotein (Clarke *et al.*, 1972).

Hypersensitivity mechanisms have been incriminated in the aetiology of cholestatic jaundice because it is not dose-related and has even occurred after a single dose of drug.

The reaction mostly appears after a latent period of 2–4 weeks and may be accompanied by other allergic manifestations such as eosinophilia. Jaundice may recur if the offending drug is re-introduced and cross-sensitivity between pheno-thiazines has been said to occur. Antimitochondrial antibodies have been reported in some patients (Rodriguez *et al.*, 1969).

Chlorpromazine-induced jaundice, once relatively common, now occurs much less frequently, possibly because there were impurities in earlier products. Abnormalities of liver function tests (Dickes *et al.*, 1957) and abnormalities found on liver biopsy (Hollister & Hall, 1966) occur more often than overt clinically recognizable reactions. Spontaneous recovery usually occurs, although in some cases there is biochemical and histological evidence of liver cell dysfunction and necrosis. Rarely jaundice is prolonged and the patient develops a clinical picture resembling primary biliary cirrhosis (Kohn & Nyerson, 1961; Read *et al.*, 1961).

15.9.2 Liver cell disease

Liver cell disease occurs during treatment with neuroleptics much less often than does cholestatic jaundice but hypersensitivity mechanisms have been suspected with this reaction also. It has been suggested that damage occurs as a result of covalent-bonding to hepatocyte fractions or an immunological attack directed towards a metabolite-liver cell complex (Read, 1992). The hepatitis is mostly indistinguishable from viral hepatitis and could be due to a coincidental infection. Despite the similarities to a viral disease, spread from one person to another does not occur and the mortality from drug-induced hepatitis (due to necrosis) is higher.

15.10 Sexual dysfunction

Sexual dysfunction associated with antipsychotic drugs has attracted relatively little systematic investigation, although sexual side-effects probably occur more often than is realized (*British Medical Journal*, 1979; Barnes, 1984; Barnes & Harvey, 1993). The data available on prevalence and severity mainly refer to problems in men, and the effects on female sexuality have been studied far less (Smith & Talbert, 1986; Segraves, 1988). Drug-related sexual problems are usually reversible if the medication is withdrawn. However, as most patients receive long-term treatment, sexual dysfunction tends to be persistent and can cause serious problems in relationships.

15.10.1 Loss of sexual drive

The most common problem in both men and women is loss of sexual interest and drive. This has been reported wth phenothiazines (Pomme *et al.*, 1965; Mitchell &

Popkin, 1982) and butyrophenones (Brambilla *et al.*, 1974). There is evidence from animal studies, observations on patients with Parkinson's disease receiving L-dopa and trials of L-dopa on human sexual functioning that the dopamine antagonism of antipsychotic drugs may be responsible (Barnes & Harvey, 1993). Another possible mechanism is interference with the hypothalmo-hypohysial–gonadal axis through increased prolactin secretion (Ghadirian *et al.*, 1982). Gonadal hormones may be suppressed, with low testosterone levels being responsible for the loss of sexual desire. Hyperprolactinaemia due to other causes, such as prolactin-secreting tumours, may cause hypogonadism, with symptoms such as impotence, gynaecomastia and galactorrhoea (Carter *et al.*, 1978). Aside from these neurotransmitter and neuroendocrine mechanisms, other drug-related factors, such as weight gain, sedation and parkinsonism might be relevant in individual cases.

15.10.2   Male sexual dysfunction

15.10.2.1   Erectile and ejaculatory dysfunction

Difficulties achieving and maintaining an erection have been reported with a variety of antipsychotic drugs (Barnes, 1984; Mitchell & Popkin, 1982), especially thioridazine. Kotin *et al.* (1976), for example, found that 25 (44%) of a sample of 57 patients who had been taking thioridazine for a minimum of 2 weeks reported 'difficulties in achieving erection', compared with 12 (19%) out of 64 patients who had received other antipsychotic drugs.

The physiological mechanisms involved in penile erection are not clearly understood (Segraves, 1989), although stimulation of sacral parasympathetic vasodilator fibres, with the possible involvement of sympathetic fibres from the thoraco-lumbar outflow, is thought to be involved. Blood is shunted to the erectile tissue, the two corpora cavernosa and the corpus spongiosum, and the sympathetic system may also contribute further by mediating the constriction of veins in erectile tissue to reduce venous outflow. Erectile dysfunction is thought to occur when these neurophysiological mechanisms are disturbed by the anticholinergic and α-adrenergic receptor blocking action of antipsychotic drugs.

Ejaculatory dysfunction is another common adverse effect (Smith & Talbert, 1986). Ejaculatory problems, typically retrograde ejaculation, have been reported with many antipsychotic drugs, including thioridazine, chlorpromazine, perphenazine, trifluoperazine and haloperidol (Barnes, 1984; Segraves, 1988). Published reports implicate thioridazine more often than any other neuroleptic. Kotin *et al.* (1976) found that a third of their patients treated with thioridazine had this problem.

The neurophysiology of ejaculation is complex, and even less clearly understood than that of erection (Segraves, 1989). The process of ejaculation has been divided into three phases: emission, bladder neck closure and true (anterograde) ejaculation. Emission involves the contraction of the smooth muscle of the vas deferens, seminal vesicles and prostate to release semen into the posterior urethra. There is closure of the bladder neck and the internal urethral sphincter, probably mediated via α-adrenergic stimulation. Anterograde ejaculation is then produced by clonic contractions of the striated bulbocavernosus, ischiocavernosus and urethral muscles. It is possibly mediated via the parasympathetic sacral outflow and somatic efferents. Dopaminergic systems are not clearly implicated in the ejaculatory response.

One plausible explanation for ejaculatory dysfunction is that antipsychotics inhibit the emission phase via α-adrenergic blockade and possibly also their anticholinergic action. Thioridazine is particularly prone to cause retrograde ejaculation, which is probably related to its relatively potent anti-adrenergic effects (Nininger, 1979). Antipsychotic drugs can also cause partial ejaculatory incompetence where emission is unimpaired but there is malfunction of the true ejaculatory phase.

Little is known about the effects of antipsychotic drugs on spermatogenesis but aspermia, without impairment of sexual excitation or the ability to obtain an erection and orgasm, has been reported in patients receiving thioridazine (Shader & DiMascio, 1970).

15.10.2.2 Priapism

Priapism is a persistent and painful erection of the penis which may occur without sexual stimulation and becomes self-perpetuating (Becker & Mitchell, 1965). The condition can constitute a medical emergency and urgent urological consultation may be required if permanent physiological impotence is to be avoided (Mitchell & Popkin, 1982). There is a low reported incidence of priapism in psychiatric patients treated with antipsychotics. The condition seems to be more frequently seen in association with phenothiazines (particularly chlorpromazine and thioridazine) than with butyrophenones (Mitchell & Popkin, 1982; Banos et al., 1989). Priapism has also been reported with a host of other antipsychotic drugs, including fluphenazine, pericyazine, mesoridazine, molindone, chlorprothixene and perphenazine (Griffith & Zil, 1984; Kogeorgos & de Alwis, 1986).

Fishbain (1985) suggested that the α-adrenergic blockade caused by antipsychotic drugs inhibits the sympathetically innervated detumescence, so that cholinergic dominance continues and leads to persistent erection. This hypothesis is supported by case reports of priapism occurring during treatment with the antidepressant, trazodone, which is a potent α-adrenergic antagonist with minimal anticholinergic activity. Priapism has been produced by intracorporeal injections of drugs with α-blocking properties such as phenoxybenzamine, trazodone and chlorpromazine (Brindley, 1983, 1984; Abber et al., 1987). Two reports suggest that anticholinergic agents can be used to treat drug-induced priapism (Osborne, 1974; Fishbain, 1985); it is thought that they work by reversing the cholinergic dominance, thus facilitating detumescence.

15.10.3 Female sexual dysfunction

There is limited information in the literature on neuroleptic-induced sexual problems in women (Barnes, 1984). Orgasmic disturbances have been reported during treatment with thioridazine (Shen & Park, 1982), trifluoperazine (Degen, 1982) and fluphenazine (Ghadirian *et al.*, 1982), but no double-blind studies have assessed the extent to which these drugs are responsible.

One of the few systematic studies (Ghadirian *et al.*, 1982) examined a sample of 29 female schizophrenic outpatients receiving maintenance treatment with either oral or depot fluphenazine. From the time of starting the drug, a third (33%) had noticed a change in the quality of orgasm, and 22% complained of a decreased ability to achieve orgasm. Over 90% of the women in the sample reported disturbance of menstruation after being administered the drugs. Increased irregularity and change in quantity of menstruation were reported by 78% of the sample. However, menstrual irregularities in women with schizophrenia may not be attributable to drug treatment alone; they may also be a consequence of organic brain changes associated with the psychotic illness (Prentice & Deakin, 1992).

Decreased sexual interest and orgasmic difficulties in women have been attributed to the anticholinergic effects of antipsychotic drugs. Degen (1982) reported two women who had delayed orgasm while receiving treatment with the phenothiazines, thioridazine, chlorpromazine and trifluoperazine. When the women were switched to loxapine and fluphenazine, drugs with less anticholinergic and anti-adrenergic activity, their sexual functioning returned to normal.

15.11 Effects on the embryo and newborn

Antipsychotic drugs are prescribed during pregnancy both for the treatment of psychoses and also for complications of pregnancy such as hyperemesis gravidarum. Most antipsychotic drugs cross the placenta and affect the foetus. The rates of transfer from mother to foetus depend on the concentration gradient, surface area and thickness of the placental membrane, rate of blood flow in the intervillous space, placental enzyme activity and molecular weight, configuration, polarity, protein-binding capacity and lipid solubility of the drug (Moya & Thorndike, 1962; Barnes, 1974). The effects of a drug on the embryo and foetus are not the same as those on the mother because of immaturity of detoxification mechanisms and metabolic degradation processes in the foetus. The effects vary depending on the drug, its concentration and the genetic constitution and stage of development of the embryo and foetus. Some drugs have a predilection for specific organs. Prolonged exposure at a low dose is generally more harmful than transient high concentrations at vulnerable stages of development.

15.11.1   Teratogenic effects

Teratogenesis may occur as a direct or indirect effect of the drug; alternatively the drug may act as a co-factor or may sensitize the embryo to the harmful effects of some other substance. Harmful drugs given before the blastocyst is embedded leads to its destruction and resorption. The embryo is most vulnerable during the period of rapid growth between implantation and complete organogenesis; that is from the first to the ninth week. Individual organs are most susceptible at the time of maximum differentiation. Drugs given after the fourth month do not cause teratogenesis but enter the foetal circulation in concentrations similar to those in the mother and produce exaggerated effects because of immaturity of the foetus's metabolic and enzyme systems.

Little is known about the effects of neuroleptics *in utero*. Few conclusions can be drawn from animal experiments because of species differences. Large-scale epidemiological studies have either not been carried out, or, in those that have, methodological limitations do not allow firm conclusions to be reached. Because significant numbers of apparently normal human pregnancies end in spontaneous abortion or the birth of babies with congenital abnormalities, vast numbers of subjects would have to be studied to decide if a small increase in incidence of a common abnormality could be attributed to a drug. Research in this field is complicated further by the facts that mothers often cannot remember the drugs they took during pregnancy, including over-the-counter medication, medical records leave much to be desired, and there is no record at all of other chemicals to which the mother has been exposed.

There have been isolated reports of congenital abnormalities in the offspring of mothers who have taken antipsychotic drugs during pregnancy, but these could be coincidental occurrences. The bulk of the evidence suggests that antipsychotic drugs are not teratogenic (Ananth, 1975) and do not increase the incidence of death *in utero* (Rieder *et al.*, 1975), but some studies have reported a greater than expected incidence of congenital abnormalities, especially cardiovascular malformations, in the offspring of mothers exposed to phenothiazines during pregnancy (Heinonen *et al.*, 1977; Rumeau-Rouquette *et al.*, 1977; Slone *et al.*, 1977).

Animal experiments have suggested that drugs that are teratogens to the CNS may also be behavioural teratogens. Behavioural effects depend on dose and the stage of development of the foetus. The period of susceptibility is longer than that for malformations, although maximum susceptibility occurs at a similar time (Coyle *et al.*, 1976; Vorhees *et al.*, 1979). The implications of these observations for humans is unclear.

15.11.2   Effects on the newborn

Newborn infants, especially if premature, are particularly vulnerable to the effects of drugs received via the placenta, because of deficiencies in the immature liver and kidney of drug-metabolizing enzymes, especially glucuronyl transferase, limited renal clearance, low protein-binding and greater permeability of the blood–brain barrier.

Phenothiazines given to pregnant women can cause hypertonia, tremor, restlessness and athetoid movements (presumably due to extrapyramidal dysfunction), respiratory depression, hypothermia and hypotension in their newborn babies (Hill *et al.*, 1966; Levy & Wisniewski, 1974). Phenothiazines can potentiate analgesics and anaesthetics given during labour to produce neonatal depression with respiratory difficulties (Hodges & Bennett, 1959; Cohen & Olson, 1970).

Most drugs are excreted in breast milk. The concentration in milk depends on the dose, duration of treatment, the mother's hepatic and renal function, the drug's lipid solubility, protein-binding properties, degree of ionization and pharmacokinetics, the volume and constituents of the milk and other factors (Knowles, 1965; Ayd, 1973; *British Medical Journal*, 1979). Little research into the effects of antipsychotic drugs on the newborn due to excretion in breast milk has been carried out, but in general they do not appear to produce serious adverse reactions.

15.12 Drug interactions

Many interactions between neuroleptics and other drugs have been reported, although relatively few are important clinically (Edwards, 1986; Stockley, 1991). The interactions may be mediated through interference with absorption; competition at receptor sites; potentiation or antagonism at the same site or affecting the same process; interference with amine uptake by sympathetic neurons; and stimulation or inhibition of metabolism. As a result, they may interfere with the therapeutic effect of a drug or cause predictable or unpredictable adverse reactions.

The most common effects are due to summation. The anticholinergic effects of antipsychotic drugs summate, for example, with those of antidepressants and antiparkinson agents, causing the problems described in the preceding chapter. Similarly, the anti-α-adrenergic effects of neuroleptics may be added to those of antidepressants or antihypertensive drugs, resulting in an excessive reduction in blood pressure and postural hypotension – an effect that can be particularly troublesome in the elderly. The antidopaminergic effects summate with those of drugs like metoclopramide and can seriously interfere with the treatment of Parkinson's disease with drugs such as L-dopa.

A possible interaction that has caused concern in everyday clinical practice is that between haloperidol and lithium. Fortunately, critical review of the evidence has shown that the alleged risk may have been exaggerated. The two drugs can be safely administered together as long as sensible precautions are taken – for the benefit of the patient and for medico–legal reasons. Serum lithium concentrations should be kept below 1 mmol/litre and the treatment should be suspended if pyrexia occurs alongside severe extrapyramidal symptoms (Johnson *et al.*, 1990).

Interactions of clinical relevance are listed in Table 1.

Table 1 Interactions with neuroleptics.

Neuroleptics interact with:	To cause	Mechanism
Alcohol	Enhanced sedation	Summation
Anaesthetics	Increased hypotension	Summation
Antacids	Decreased absorption of phenothiazines	Formation of adsorption complexes
Anxiolytics/hypnotics	Enhanced sedation	Summation
Anti-arrhythmics	Increased risk of ventricular arrhythmias with drugs that increase QT interval	Summation
Anticonvulsants	Lowered convulsive threshold	Accelerated metabolism
Carbamazepine	Decreased plasma concentration of haloperidol	
Phenytoin	Decreased plasma concentration of clozapine	
Antidepressants		
Tricyclics	Enhanced sedation	Summation
	Enhanced antimuscarinic effects	Summation
MAOIs + oxypertine	CNS excitation Hypertension	
Fluoxetine	Increased plasma concentration of haloperidol	Decreased metabolism
Antihistamines	Increased antimuscarinic effects	Summation
Antihypertensives	Enhanced hypotensive effect	Summation
Adrenergic neuron blockers + high doses of chlorpromazine	Antagonism of hypotensive effect	

Continued

Table 1 (*continued*)

Neuroleptics interact with:	To cause	Mechanism
ACE inhibitors + chlorpromazine and ? other antipsychotics	Severe postural hypotension	
Calcium channel blockers		
Methyldopa Metirosine Rauwolfia alkaloids	Increased risk of extrapyramidal effects	
Antiparkinson drugs		Antagonism
Antimuscarinics (+ phenothiazines)	Increased antimuscarinic effects	Summation
Dopaminergics		Antagonism
Bromocriptine	Decreased hypoprolactinaemic & antiparkinson effects	
L-dopa Lisuride Pergolide	Decreased dopaminergic effect	
Cimetidine	Decreased effects of chlorpromazine, clozapine & ? others	Decreased absorption
Diuretics + pimozide	Increased risk of ventricular arrhythmia	Hypokalaemia
Lithium	Increased risk of extrapyramidal effects Neurotoxicity[a]	Not known
Metoclopramide	Increased risk of extrapyramidal effects	Summation
Propranolol	Increased plasma concentration of chlorpromazine	Inhibition of metabolism
Rifampicin	Decreased plasma concentration of haloperidol	Accelerated metabolism
Tetrabenazine	Increased risk of extrapyramidal effects	Summation

[a]Neurotoxicity = excitation, restlessness, sweating, flushing, pyrexia, tremor, rigidity, coma, death (in extreme cases).
ACE, angiotensin-converting enzyme

15.13 Conclusions

Although this and the previous chapter have highlighted negative aspects of treatment with antipsychotic drugs, that is, their unwanted effects, it should be emphasized that the overall therapeutic advantages of neuroleptics greatly outweigh the disadvantages. Most side-effects are mild and they often disappear with continued treatment. Others can be minimized or prevented by more thoughtful prescribing, such as using the minimum dose required, avoiding unnecessary drug combinations and careful monitoring, especially in the very young, the elderly and those with serious physical illnesses that could predispose to exaggerated reactions.

Clinicians should remain alert for hitherto unrecognized unwanted effects. If delays in the recognition of such effects (as have occurred in the past) are to be avoided, prescribers need to be more cooperative in reporting suspected adverse reactions to regulatory authorities, such as the Committee on Safety of Medicines. The hackneyed ending to a review, 'more research is required', can be added, without apology, especially to less intensively investigated areas such as long-term effects, subtle behavioural effects and effects on the unborn. With regard to the last of these, despite the advice given about avoiding drug treatment during pregnancy, many women take drugs after becoming pregnant (or become pregnant while taking them) and their unborn children thereby become the subjects of uncontrolled and inadequately monitored trials. Research into the short-term and long-term outcome of these cases is of paramount importance.

Finally, a word about the medico–legal aspects of adverse reactions. Doctors practise in an increasingly litiginous world and it is therefore crucial to be fully aware of clinical duties and responsibilities, seen not only from the medical perspective but also from the legal viewpoint. These duties of care have been discussed in great detail by Dukes & Schwartz (1988). A patient can sue for injuries allegedly caused by drugs under the laws of tort– a delict or harm the law will address. If an injury occurs during treatment it does not mean, of course, that the doctor is responsible, as side-effects are an acceptable risk of treatment with any drug. Nevertheless, patients seeking redress may be successful in their litigation if it can be established that the practitioner had a duty of care and was in breach of that duty by, for instance, failing to choose carefully an appropriate drug, failing to assess competently the benefit-risk ratio or failing to administer treatment with the standard of skill reasonably expected. The level of proof required is based on the balance of probabilities and the professional standards against which the doctor will be judged are whether or not his or her treatment reflected a responsible application of existing knowledge, and whether or not the treatment was administered with the due care expected from a doctor with comparable training and experience practising in similar circumstances. A doctor's actions may be defensible even though they deviate widely from recommended and accepted practice, but such deviation places a heavy burden of responsibility on the doctor– and the more cavalier the actions, the greater the risk.

References

Abber, J.C., Lue, T.F., Luo, J. et al. (1987) J. Urol. 137, 1039–1042.

Alexander, C.S. & Nino, A. (1969) Am. Heart J. 78, 757–769.

Alvarez-Mena, S.C. & Frank, M.J. (1973) J. Am. Med. Assoc. 224, 1730–1733.

Amsler, H.A., Teerenhovi, L., Barth, E. et al. (1977) Acta Psychiat. Scand 56, 241.

Ananth, J. (1975) Compr. Psychiat. 16, 437–445.

Anderson, R. & Griffith, R.W. (1977) Eur. J. Clin. Pharmacol 11, 199.

Assem, E.-S. K. (1977) In Textbook of Adverse Reactions (ed. Davies, D.M.), pp. 380–396, Oxford, Oxford University Press.

Ayd, F.J. (1969) Intern. Drug. Ther. Newslett. 4, 13–20.

Ayd, F.J. (1970) Intern. Drug. Ther. Newslett. 5, 1–8.

Ayd, F.J. (1973) Intern. Drug. Ther. Newslett. 8, 33–40.

Baker, H. (1986) In Textbook of Dermatology (4th edition), Vol. 2 (eds Rook, A., Wilkinson, D.S., Ebling, F.J.B., Champion, R.H., Burton, J.L.), pp. 1239–1279, Oxford, Blackwell.

Banos, J.E., Bosch, F. & Farre, M. (1989) Med. Toxicol. 4, 46–58.

Barnes, C.G. (1974) Medical Disorders in Obstetric Practice, London, Blackwell.

Barnes, T.R.E. (1984) In Current Themes in Psychiatry (eds Gaind, R.N., Fawzy, F.I., Hudson, B.L. & Pasnau, R.O.), pp. 51–92, New York, Spectrum Publications.

Barnes, T.R.E. & Harvey, C. (1993) In Sexual Pharmacology (eds Riley, A., Wilson, C. & Peet, M.), Oxford University Press (in press).

Becker, L.E. & Mitchell, A.D. (1965) Surg. Clin. North Am. 45, 1523–1534.

Beerman, H. & Kirshbaum, B.A. (1975) In Dermatology, Vol. 1 (eds Mioschella, S.L., Pillsbury, D.M. & Hurley, H.J.), pp. 350–384, Philadelphia, W.B. Saunders.

Bernstein, J.G. (1988) Clin. Neuropharmacol. 11 (Suppl. 1), 194–206.

Beumont, P. (1981) In Handbook of Biological Psychiatry. Part VI. Practical Applications of Psychotropic Drugs and Other Biological Treatments (eds Van Praag, H.M., Lader, M.H., Raphaelson, O.J. & Sachar, E.J.), pp. 39–56, New York, Marcel Dekker.

Beumont, P., Gelder, M.G., Friesen, H.G. et al. (1974a) Br. J. Psychiat. 124, 413–419.

Beumont, P., Corker, C.S., Friesen, H.G. et al. (1974b) Br. J. Psychiat. 124, 420–430.

Bond, W.S. & Yee, G.C. (1980) Am. J. Hosp. Pharm. 37, 74–78.

Brambilla, F., Guerrini, A., Guastalla, A. et al. (1974) Psychopharmacol. 44, 17–22.

Brindley, G.S. (1983) Br. J. Psychiat. 143, 332–337.

Brindley, G.S. (1984) Lancet i, 220–221.

British Medical Journal (1971) Br. Med. J. 1, 3.

British Medical Journal (1979) Br. Med. J. 1, 642.

Brown, R.P. & Kocsis, J.H. (1984) Hosp. Community Psychiat. 35, 486–491.

Burgmans, J., Verbruggen, F., Dom, J. et al. (1973) Lancet ii, 502–503.

Cameron, M.E. (1967) Br. J. Ophthalmol. 51, 295–305.

Carter, J.N., Tyson, J.E., Tolis, G. et al. (1978) New Engl. J. Med. 299, 847–852.

Clarke, A.E., Maritz, V.M. & Denborough, M.A. (1972) Aust. NZ J. Med. 4, 376–382.

Cleland, J.G.F. & Krickler, D.M. (1992) Br. Heart J. 67, 1–3.

Cluff, L.E., Caranosos, G.J. & Stewart, R.B. (1975) Clinical Problems with Drugs, London, W.B. Saunders.

Cohen, S.N. & Olson, W.A. (1970) Pediat. Clin. North Am. 17, 835–850.

Committee on Safety of Medicines (1990) Current Problems, 29, 1–2..

Connell, M.M., Poley, B.J. & McFarlane, J.R. (1964) Arch. Ophthalmol. 71, 816–821.

Cookson, J.C., Kennedy, J.C. & Gribbon, D. (1986) Int. Clin. Psychopharmacol. 1 (Suppl. 1), 41–48.

Coyle, I., Wagner, M.J. & Singer, A.G. (1976) Pharmacology, Biochemistry and Behavior

4, 191-200.

Crane, G.E. (1970) *Dis. Nerv. Syst.* **31**, 534-539.

Crews, S.J. (1962) *Trans. Ophthal. Soc. UK* **82**, 387-404.

Crews, S.J. (1974) In *Aspects of Neuro-Ophthalmology* (ed. Davidson, S.I.), pp. 148-163, London, Butterworths.

Davidorf, F.H. (1973) *Arch. Ophthalmol.* **980**, 251-255.

Degen, K. (1982) *Psychosomatics* **23**, 959-961.

Deglin, S.M., Deglin, J.M. & Chung, E.K. (1977) *Drugs* **14**, 29-40.

de Gruchy, G.C. (1975) *Drug-Induced Blood Disorders*, London, Blackwell.

de Wied, D. (1967) *Pharmacol. Rev.* **19**, 251-288.

Dickes, R., Schenker, V. & Deutsch, L. (1957) *New Engl. J. Med.* **256**, 1-7.

Dubois, E.L., Tallman, E. & Wonka, R.A. (1972) *J. Am. Med. Assoc.* **221**, 595-596.

Ducomb, L. & Baldessarini, R.J. (1977) *Am. J. Psychiat.* **134**, 1294-1295.

Dukes, M.N.G. & Schwartz, B. (1988) *Responsibility for Drug-induced Injury* Amsterdam, Elsevier.

Edler, K., Gottfies, C.G., Haslund, J. *et al.* (1971) *Acta Psychiat. Scand.* **47**, 377-385.

Edwards, J.G. (1986) In *The Psychopharmacology and Treatment of Schizophrenia* (eds Bradley, P.B. & Hirsch, S.R.), pp. 403-441, Oxford University Press, Oxford.

Epstein, S. (1968) *Arch. Dermatol.* **98**, 354-363.

Erle, G., Basso, M., Federspil, G. *et al.* (1977) *Eur. J. Clin. Pharmacol.* **II**, 15-18.

Ettigi, P., Lal, S. & Friesen, H.G. (1973) *Lancet* **ii**, 266-267.

Evans, D.L., Rogers, J.F. & Peiper, S.C. (1979) *Am. J. Psychiat.* **136**, 970-972.

Fayer, S.A. (1986) *J. Clin. Psychopharmacol.* **6**, 375-376.

Fishbain, D.A. (1985) *Ann. Emergency Med.* **14**, 600-602.

Flaherty, J.A. & Lahmeyer, H.W. (1978) *Am. J. Psychiat.* **135**, 1414-1415.

Fogel, B.S. & Goldberg, R.J. (1985) *New Engl. J. Med.* **313**, 1292.

Fowler, N.O., McCall, D., Chou, T.C. *et al.* (1976) *Am. J. Cardiol.* **37**, 223-230.

Fuller, C.M., Yassinger, S., Donlon, P. *et al.* (1977) *West. J. Med.* **127**, 515-518.

Fulop, G., Phillips, R.A., Shapiro, A.K. *et al.* (1987) *Am. J. Psychiat.* **144**, 673-675.

Garner, L.L., Wang, R.I.H. & Hieb, E. (1974) *Drug Ther.* **4**, 30-37.

Garrow, J.S. (1981) *Treat Obesity Seriously*, Edinburgh, Churchill Livingstone.

Ghadirian, A.M., Chouinard, G. & Annable, L. (1982) *J. Nerv. Mental Dis.* **170**, 463-467.

Girdwood, R.H. (1976) In *Haematological Aspects of Systemic Disease* (eds Israels, M.C.G. & Delaware, I.W.), pp. 495-528, London, W.B. Saunders.

Goldman, L.S., Hudson, J.I. & Weddington, W.W. (1980) *Am. J. Psychiat.* **137**, 1613-1614.

Goulston, E. (1976) *Med. J. Aust.* **2**, 836-844.

Grant, W.M. (1974) *Toxicology of the Eye*, Springfield, IL, Charles C. Thomas.

Greiner, A.C. & Berry, K. (1964) *Can. Med. Assoc. J.* **90**, 663-665.

Greiner, A.C. & Nicholson, G.A. (1964) *Can. Med. Assoc. J.* **91**, 627-635.

Griffith, S.R. & Zil, J.S. (1984) *Psychosomatics* **25**, 629-631.

Grohmann, R., Schmidt, L.G., Spiess-Kiefer, C. *et al.* (1989) *Psychopharmacology* **99** (Suppl.), 109-112.

Gruen, P.H., Sachar, E.J., Langer, G. *et al.* (1978) *Arch. Gen. Psychiat.* **35**, 108-116.

Guillan, R.A., Yang, C.-P. & Hocker, E.V. (1977) *J. Kansas Med. Soc.* **78**, 221-227.

Heinonen, O.P., Sloane, D. & Shapiro, S. (1977) *Birth Defects and Drugs in Pregnancy*, Littledon, MA, Publishing Sciences Group.

Henderson, R.A., Lane, S. & Henry, J.A. (1991) *Human Exp. Toxicol.* **10**, 59-62.

Hill, R.M., Desmond, M.M. & Kay, J.L. (1966) *J. Pediat.* **69**, 589-595.

Hodges, R.J.H. & Bennett, J.R. (1959) *J. Obstet. Gynaecol. Br. Emp.* **66**, 91-98.

Hollister, L.E. & Hall, R.A. (1966) *Am. J. Psychiat.* **123**, 211-212.

Hollister, L.E. & Kosek, J.C (1965) *J. Am. Med. Assoc.* **192**, 1035-1038.

Howard, R.O., McDonald, C.J., Dunn, B. *et al.* (1969) *Invest Opthalmol.* **8**, 413-421.

Husband, C., Mai, F.M. & Carruthers, G. (1981) *Can J. Psychiat.* **26**, 196-197.

Huyse, F. & Van Schijndel, R.S. (1988) *Lancet* ii, 568-569.

Johnson, A.W. & Buffaloe, W.J. (1966) *Arch. Ophthalmol.* **76**, 664-667.

Johnson, D.A.W., Lowe, M.R. & Bachelor, D.H. (1990) *Human Psychopharmacol.* **5** (Suppl.), 262-297.

Jones, I.H. & Meade, T.W. (1964) *Geront. Clin.* **6**, 252-256.

Jones, J.K., Van de Carr, S.W., Zimmerman, H. *et al.* (1983) *Psychopharmacol. Bull.* **19**, 24-27.

Kane, J.M., Honigfeld, G., Singer, J. *et al.* (1988) *Arch. Gen. Psychiat.* **45**, 789-796.

Kelly, H.G., Fay, J.E. & Laverty, S.G. (1963) *Can. Med. Assoc. J.* **89**, 546-554.

Ketal, R., Matthews, J. & Mozdzen, J.J. (1979) *Am. J. Psychiat.* **136**, 112-113.

Kiriike, N., Maeda, Y., Nishiwaki, S. *et al.* (1987) *Biol. Psychiat.* **22**, 99-103.

Knowles, J.A. (1965) *Pediat. Pharmacol. Ther.* **66**, 1068-1082.

Kogeorgos, J. & de Alwis, C. (1986) *Br. J. Psychiat.* **149**, 241-243.

Kohn, N.N. & Myerson, R.M. (1961) *Am. J. Med.* **31**, 665-670.

Kotin, J., Wilbert, D.E., Verburg, D. *et al.* (1976) *Am. J. Psychiat.* **133**, 82-85.

Krickler, D.M. & Curry, P.V.L. (1976) *Br. Heart J.* **38**, 117-120.

Kriwisky, M. and Perry, G.Y., Tarchitsky, D. *et al.* (1990) *Chest* **98**, 482-484.

Krupp, P. & Barnes, P. (1989) *Psychopharmacology* **99** (Suppl.), 118-121.

Lamberti, J.S., Bellnier, T. & Schwarzkopf, S.B. (1992) *Am. J. Psychiat.* **149**, 689-690.

Lapierre, Y.D., Lapointe, L., Bordeleau, J.M. *et al.* (1969) *Can. Psychiat. Assoc. J.* **14**, 517-523.

Leestma, J.E. & Koenig, K.L. (1968) *Arch. Gen. Psychiat.* **18**, 137-148.

Leopold, I.V. (1968) *J. Am. Med. Assoc.* **205**, 631-633.

Levy, W. & Wisniewski, K. (1974) *NY St. J. Med.* **74**, 684-685.

Liberatore, M.A. & Robinson, D.S. (1984) *J. Clin. Psychopharmacol.* **4**, 143-146.

Lieberman, J.A., Johns, C.A., Kane, J.M. *et al.* (1988) *J. Clin. Psychiat.* **49**, 271-277.

Lipscomb, P.A. (1980) *Postgraduate Medicine* **67**, 189-196.

Marks, V. & Shackeloth, P. (1966) *Br. Med. J.* **1**, 617-619.

Mathalone, M.B.R. (1966) *Trans. Ophthal. Soc. UK* **86**, 77-88.

Matuk, F. & Kalyanaraman, K. (1977) *Arch. Neurol.* **34**, 373-375.

McCreadie, R.G., Kiernan, W.E.S., Venner, R.M. *et al.* (1979) *Br. Med. J.* **1**, 522-523.

McQueen, E.G. (1980) In *Drug Treatment: Principles and Practice of Clinical Pharmacology* (ed. Avery, G.S.), pp. 202-235, Edinburgh, Churchill Livingstone.

Mehtonen, O.-P., Aranko, K., Mälkonen, L. *et al.* (1991) *Acta Psychiat. Scand.* **84**, 58-64.

Meltzer, J.Y. & Fang, U.S. (1976) In *Hormones, Behavior and Psychopathology* (ed. Sachar, E.J.), New York, Raven Press.

Meredith, T.A., Aaberg, T.M. & Willerson, D. (1978) *Arch. Ophthalmol.* **96**, 1172-1176.

Mitchell, J.E. & Popkin, M.K. (1982) *Am. J. Psychiat.* **139**, 633-637.

Modestin, J., Krapf, R. & Boker, W. (1981) *Am. J. Psychiat.* **138**, 1616-1617.

Mortensen, P.B. (1987) *Acta Psychiat. Scand.* **75**, 585-590.

Moya, F. & Thorndike, V. (1962) *Am. J. Obstet. Gynecol.* **84**, 1778-1798.

Mortensen, P.B. (1987) *Acta Psychiat. Scand.* **75**, 585-590.

Nininger, J.E. (1979) *Am. J. Psychiat.* **135**, 750-751.

Osborne, M.P. (1974) *Postgrad. Med. J.* **50**, 523-524.

Overall, J.E. (1978) *Arch. Gen. Psychiat.* **35**, 898-899.

Paoletti, F., Juan, A., Vazquez, J. *et al.* (1966) *Am. J. Med. Sci.* **252**, 570-572.

Peele, R. & von Loetzen, I.S. (1973) *Am. J. Psychiat.* **130**, 306-309.

Perry, T.L., Culling, C.F.A., Berry, K. *et al.* (1964) *Science* **146**, 81-83.

Pisciotta, A.V. (1968) In *Psychopharmacology: a Review of Progress 1957-1967* (ed. Efron,

D.F.), Washington, DC, US Government Printing Office.

Pisciotta, A.V. (1971) *Clin. Pharmacol. Ther.* **12**, 13-43.

Pisciotta, A.V. (1974) In *Drugs and Hematologic Reactions, The Twenty-Ninth Hahnemann Symposium* (eds Dimitrov, N.V. & Nodine, J.H.), pp. 233-247, New York, Grune & Stratton.

Pisciotta, A.V. (1982) *Haematologica* **67**, 292-318.

Pomme, B., Girard, J. & Debost, M. (1965) *Ann. Medico-Psychol.* **125**, 551-562.

Potts, A.M. (1962) *Invest. Opthalmol.* **1**, 522-530.

Prentice, D.S. & Deakin, J.F.W. (1992) *Schizophrenia Res.* **6**, 114.

Raj, M.V.J. & Benson, R. (1975) *Postgrad. Med. J.* **51**, 65-68.

Rampertaap, M.P. (1986) *Southern Med. J.* **79**, 331-336.

Read, A.E. (1992) In *Wright's Liver and Biliary Disease* (eds Milward-Sadler, H., Wright, D. & Arthur, M.J.P.), pp. 1233-1261, London, W.B. Saunders.

Read, A.E., Harrison, C.V. & Sherlock, S. (1961) *Am. J. Med.* **31**, 249-257.

Reid, W.W., Blouin, P. & Schermer, M. (1976) *Int. Pharmacopsychiat.* **11**, 163-174.

Richardson, H.L., Graupner, K.I. & Richardson, M.E. (1966) *J. Am. Med. Assoc.* **195**, 114-120.

Rieder, R.O., Rosenthal, D., Wender, P. *et al.* (1975) *Arch. Gen. Psychiat.* **32**, 200-211.

Robins, A.H. (1972) *Br. J. Psychiat.* **121**, 615-617.

Robins, A.H. (1975) *S. Afr. Med. J.* **49**, 1521-1524.

Rodriguez, M., Paronetto, F., Scaffner, F. *et al.* (1969) *J. Am. Med. Assoc.* **208**, 148-150.

Rubin, R.T. & Hays, S.E. (1980) *Psychoneuroendocrinology* **5**, 121-137.

Rumeau-Rouquette, C., Goujard, J. & Huel, G. (1977) *Teratology* **15**, 57-64.

Satanova, A. & McIntosh, J. (1967) *J. Am. Med. Assoc.* **200**, 121-124.

Schyve, P.M., Smithline, F. & Meltzer, H.Y. (1978) *Arch. Gen. Psychiat.* **35**, 1291-1301.

Seeman, P. (1985) In *Dyskinesia-Research and Treatment (Psychopharmacology, Suppl. 2)* (eds Casey, D.E., Chase, T.N., Christensen, A.V., & Gerlach, J.), pp. 2-8. Berlin, Springer-Verlag.

Segraves, R.T. (1988) *Sex Marital Ther.* **14**, 202-207.

Segraves, R.T. (1989) *Arch. Gen. Psychiat.* **46**, 275-284.

Shader, R.I. & DiMascio, A.J. (1970) *Psychotropic Drug Side Effects: Clinical and Theoretical Perspectives*, Baltimore, Williams & Wilkins.

Shear, M.K. (1978) *Am. J. Psychiat.* **135**, 492-493.

Shen, W.W. & Park, S. (1982) *Psychiat. J. Univ. Ottawa* **7**, 249-251.

Shepherd, M., Lader, M.H. & Lader, S.R. (1968) In *Side Effects of Drugs*, Vol. VI, *A Survey of Unwanted Effects of Drugs Reported in 1965-1967* (eds Meyler, L. & Herxheimer, A.), pp. 51-93, Amsterdam, Excerpta Medica.

Siddall, J.R. (1965) *Arch. Ophthalmol.* **74**, 460-464.

Siddall, J.R. (1966) *Can. J. Ophthalmol.* **1**, 190-198.

Siddall, J.R. (1968) *Dis. Nerv. Syst.* **29** (Suppl.), 10-13.

Silverstone, T. (1985) In *Psychopharmacology and Food* (eds Sandler, M. & Silverstone, T.), pp. 139-145, Oxford, Oxford University Press.

Simpson, G.M., Davis, J., Jefferson, J.W. *et al.* (1987) *Sudden Death in Psychiatric Patients: The Role of Neuroleptic Drugs.* An American Psychiatric Association Task Force Report, no. 27.

Slone, D., Siskind, V., Heinonen, O.P. *et al.* (1977) *Am. J. Obstet. Gynecol.* **128**, 486-488.

Smith, P.J. & Talbert, R.L. (1986) *Clin. Pharm.* **5**, 373-383.

Smith, W.O. & Clark, M.L. (1980) *Am. J. Psychiat.* **137**, 1055-1059.

Sriram, K., Schumer, W., Ehrenpreis, S. *et al.* (1979) *Am. J. Surg.* **137**, 87-91.

Stockley, I.H. (1991) *Drug Interactions. A Source Book of Drug Interactions, Their Mechanisms, Clinical Importance and Management*, Second Edition, London,

Blackwell.

Swett, C. (1975) *Arch. Gen. Psychiat.* **32**, 1416–1418.

Swett, C.P. & Shader, R.I. (1977) *Dis. Nerv. Syst.* **38**, 69–72.

Thonnard-Neumann, E. (1968) *Am. J. Psychiat.* **124**, 978–982.

Vargas, E. & Drance, S.M. (1973) *Arch. Ophthalmol.* **90**, 438–439.

Vincent, F.M. & Emory, S. (1978) *Ann. Intern. Med.* **89**, 147–148.

Vorhees, C.V., Brunner, R.L. & Butcher, R.E. (1979) *Science* **205**, 1220–1225.

Wagasugi, C., Nishi, K. & Yamada, M. (1986) *Am. J. Forensic Med. Pathol.* **7**, 165–166.

Wagner, S. & Mantel, N. (1978) *Cancer Res.* **38**, 2703–2708.

Walsh, F.B. & Hoyt, W.F. (1969) *Clinical Neuro-Ophthalmology*, Vol. 3, Baltimore, MD, Williams & Wilkins.

Wendkos, M.H. (1979) *Sudden Death and Psychiatric Illness*, New York, S.P. Medical and Scientific Books.

Wheatley, D. (ed.) (1981) *Stress and the Heart*, New York, Raven Press.

Wintrobe, M.M., Lee, G.R., Boggs, D.R. *et al.* (1981) *Clinical Hematology*, Philadelphia, Lea & Febiger.

Wintroub, B.V., Shiffman, N.J. & Arndt, K.A. (1979) In *Dermatology in General Medicine* (eds Fitzpatrick, T.B., Eisen, A.Z., Wolff, K., Freedberg, I.M. & Austen, K.F.), pp. 555–567, New York, McGraw-Hill.

Wistedt, B., Persson, T. & Hellbom, E. (1984) *Curr. Ther. Res.* **35**, 804–814.

Zee-Cheng, C.S., Mueller, C.E., Seifert, C.F. *et al.* (1985) *Ann. Intern. Med.* **102**, 418.

Index